# Doctor Franklin's Medicine

# DOCTOR FRANKLIN'S MEDICINE

Stanley Finger

UNIVERSITY OF PENNSYLVANIA PRESS

*Philadelphia*

10  9  8  7  6  5  4  3  2  1

Published by
University of Pennsylvania Press
Philadelphia, Pennsylvania 19104-4122

ISBN-13: 978-0-8122-3913-3
ISBN-10: 0-8122-3913-X

A U. S. Library of Congress Cataloging-in-Publication record is available
from the Library of Congress

*To my loving wife Wendy and in memory of our son Robert, who,*
*like Francis Folger Franklin, was taken from us much too soon.*
*This book is also dedicated to our son Brad, his wife Gabrielle, and*
*our first grandchild, Sophia, who at age three months smiled with*
*delight every time I told her about Benjamin Franklin's*
*forays into medicine.*

*He's the best physician that knows*
*the worthlessness of the most medicines.*
—Poor Richard's Almanack, *1732*

# Contents

# Preface

Benjamin Franklin—the only Founding Father of the New Republic to sign the Declaration of Independence, the alliance with France, the peace treaty with Britain, and the Constitution—has long been a favorite of readers and writers of American history. If we count the number of new books, articles, and media presentations involving Franklin, it seems that his popularity is growing with each passing year.

Historians have so admirably covered Franklin's politics, personal life, printing career, economics, science, philosophy, and ethics that one might be tempted to conclude that there is little more that can be discovered or written about this remarkable man. On the pages that follow, however, I shall present a side of Franklin that has not been examined sufficiently and put under one cover in the past—his numerous forays into medicine.

In a sense, this book has three purposes. One is to examine Franklin's major medical contributions in some detail. Another is to show how Franklin was shaped by, and helped to change, the eighteenth-century medical landscape. A third is to look at what he knew about and how he treated his own chronic medical disorders. My efforts here are an initial attempt to survey a wealth of material. Although it is by no means an exhaustive account, it is my hope that it will lead to a greater appreciation of Franklin as a significant figure in the world of medicine. Ideally, it will also shed more light on the status of the healing arts and preventive medicine in America and in Europe during the eighteenth century.

After years of collecting, reading, and taking notes on everything that I could find on Franklin and medicine, I concluded that it would be best to tie Franklin's medical interests and contributions to specific periods in his life. It is clear that he was involved with some problems, such as telling people how to acquire immunity against smallpox, for more than fifty years. But for most subjects, a chronological approach seemed reasonable, and it allowed me to meld his insights and projects with the well-documented narrative of his life and the medical ideas that were being discussed by the physicians and laypeople around him.

Hence, after a general introduction on the nature of eighteenth-century American medicine and Franklin's multifaceted approach to medicine, Part

I will examine his most significant contributions to medicine from the colonies. Part II will turn to what he did as an experimental natural philosopher in the field of medicine while in England, and Part III will do the same for his years in France. Although Franklin was sent to Europe as a diplomat, his mind was never far from medicine, and he interacted with and was respected by some of the most famous physicians of the day, including John Pringle, Thomas Sydenham, and Benjamin Rush. He also corresponded extensively with the leading natural philosophers of the time, and these exchanges aided the development and dissemination of medical advances in Europe and America. Part IV will be devoted to the final years of his life and his death in Philadelphia. Even at an advanced age he invented remarkable devices to compensate for his disabilities, and he experimented and worked with his physicians to manage an annoying skin condition, his recurrent attacks of painful gout, and his large bladder stone.

It has been said that everybody can find their own Franklin and their own unique way of approaching him, even when working with the same resources. My Franklin will differ from the Franklin presented by a social historian, who might draw attention to the changing marketplace for medicine; from the Franklin portrayed by a general biographer, who would be more inclined to concentrate on his politics and social relationships; and from the Franklin constructed by someone intent on knocking him off the high pedestal on which he is often placed.

The Franklin to be presented in this book is constructed by a person who spent more than twenty-five years running a laboratory in the brain and behavioral sciences before turning to the history of science and medicine. As such, I shall concentrate on the medical history and eighteenth-century milieu and let Franklin speak for himself.

I could not have written this book without the editorial help, encouragement, and moral support of my wife Wendy. She deserves a medal or at least a dream vacation for dealing with my ups and downs and hopes and fears, as I read until my eyelids closed and occasionally awoke in a sweat, pondering how best to reach a broad audience.

Robert Lockhart, my editor at the University of Pennsylvania Press, also deserves my special thanks for his insights about how to present this material in a stimulating but factual way, as does my copyeditor, Noreen O'Connor-Abel. In addition, I also must thank Lilla Vekerdy of the Washington University Medical School Rare Books Library for her help, and the Packard Humanties Institute for providing me with a computer disk containing more than 30,000 letters and other pieces from Franklin or sent to him. Without this valuable resource, this book would have taken much longer to complete. Of course, I am also grateful to the many people (too many to name) who looked over one or more of my chapters, and to the American Philosophical Society, Yale University, and the College of Physicians of Philadelphia for allowing me to use their resources.

I hope that everyone involved with this arduous project on Benjamin Franklin and eighteenth-century medicine, even those who might have approached this very challenging topic very differently, will appreciate this first step. My hope is that this volume will stimulate additional research in this area, as there is much more yet to be gleaned about Franklin as a man of medicine.

# Benjamin Franklin's Enlightened Medicine

If you wou'd not be forgotten
As soon as you are dead and rotten,
Either write things worth reading,
Or do things worth the writing.

*—Poor Richard's Almanack*, 1738

In 1784 an experiment was conducted in a sunbathed garden in Passy, a beautiful village along the Seine River, then just a few miles outside Paris. It involved a suggestible twelve-year-old boy with an unspecified medical disorder, his well-connected physician, a select group of observers, and some well-cared-for apricot trees.

While the unnamed boy remained inside a nearby house, his distinguished physician, Charles Deslon (or d'Eslon), proceeded to "magnetize" a single apricot tree in the garden. He then walked behind the other observers, where he would be hidden from the boy's sight. He was allowed, however, to "direct his cane and his countenance toward the tree, in order to augment the action of the magnetism."[1]

After these things had been done, his young patient was brought out of the house with his eyes covered. The "blind" protocol was used to ensure that any overt movements or more subtle cues from the experimenters would not influence him. The boy was then instructed to embrace a number of trees for about two minutes each, knowing only that the physician he greatly trusted had magnetized one of them. He was expected to experience strange feelings throughout his body when he touched the treated tree, but not the "neutral" trees. And this, his physician believed, would allow him to identify the single magnetized tree.

The experiment, as strange as it may seem to us today, was a clever test of a medical theory that had the backing of many practitioners, aristocrats, writers, and ordinary people late in the eighteenth century. But it was also a theory that had thunderous opposition, particularly among the members of France's leading scientific and medical societies.

Franz Anton Mesmer, who held a medical degree, had developed the theory before he had been forced out of conservative Vienna. He maintained that an invisible fluid, which he called animal magnetism, pervades the cosmos, much like Isaac Newton's well-accepted but invisible gravitational force. Mesmer further claimed that this magnetic force could affect all sorts of objects, from animals to trees, and even the human body.

The part of Mesmer's theory that was of greatest concern to the medical community stemmed from his contention that he could manipulate this newly discovered, invisible, magnetic force. Not only could he "magnetize" nonmetallic objects, he could employ the force and even these magnetized objects to cure sick bodies. During the eighteenth century, it was widely believed that blockages caused disorders, a theory that was applied to headaches, palsies, and weak vision, as well as urinary or circulatory problems. In Mesmer's mind, because all diseases shared a common etiology, all could be treated with a single cure, namely the skilled manipulation of the force he called animal magnetism.

Mesmer maintained that the cure he sought was preceded by a "crisis," meaning a noticeable turning point. A common example of a crisis was a fever that peaked before suddenly breaking. But for Mesmer and his disciples, including practitioner Charles Deslon who magnetized the apricot tree in Passy, the crisis was often more dramatic. Many of the patients they treated tended to go into convulsions and even pass out, which brings us back to the boy in the garden. Deslon had chosen him for the experiment because he had been so sensitive to animal magnetism when treated in his clinic.

After a minute at the first tree, which was twenty-seven feet from the treated one, the boy began to perspire, cough up phlegm, and complain of head pain. The second tree was nine feet farther away from the magnetized tree, and here he felt dazed and stupefied, while his headache worsened. At the third tree, his signs and symptoms increased, and he stated that he believed he had to be approaching the magnetized tree, even though it was now almost forty feet away. Finally, at "the fourth tree, one which had not been rendered the object of the procedure, and at a distance of about twenty-four feet from the tree which had, the boy fell into a crisis, he fainted, his limbs stiffened, and he was carried on to a plot of grass, where Deslon hurried to his side and revived him."[2]

Benjamin Franklin was among the eyewitnesses to this well thought out test of Mesmer's theory. In fact, the quotations describing the experiment and boy's crisis were taken from a detailed report that Franklin helped write. Moreover, the experiment took place on the estate on which he was living in 1784, while serving the newly independent United States as minister to France.

The choice of location for this test in a series that included many other tests like it was by no means coincidental. Franklin had been asked to serve as head of a royal commission hastily called for by Louis XVI to evaluate Mesmer's claims. But because gout and a large bladder stone limited Franklin's mobility, the commissioners agreed to do some of the experiments where the distinguished foreigner was in residence.

Franklin and his fellow commissioners ultimately concluded that Mesmer and Deslon were partly right. Mesmerism did cure some people, but their improvements had nothing to do with Mesmer's proposed physical force. The occasional cures documented by Mesmer and Deslon were largely the result of suggestion, and the subjects were very gullible people.

Historians believe that a fair number of the men and women cured by the mesmerists suffered from mental disorders, particularly hysteria (professionals now use the term "conversion disorder"). Today, hysteria is thought of as a psychological problem. But to Franklin and his contemporaries, it was a disorder that actually affected the physical machinery of the body.

In just about every way, Benjamin Franklin, although seventy-eight years old at the time, was the ideal person to lead the royal commission and to sign his name above the others on the *Rapport des Commissaires Chargés par le Roi de l'Examen du Magnétisme Animal.* Having dined with Mesmer and apparently watched him treat some patients, and having read some of his most important writings, Franklin was probably more knowledgeable about Mesmer's theory and claims than any of the other commissioners.

Franklin was also highly respected by all parties for his great intellect and his honesty, and he was the only commissioner who was a foreigner, and therefore not dependent on French governmental support for his position or professional survival. Further, Franklin was a skilled natural philosopher (the old term for a person who studies the laws of nature) and the world's leading authority on another pervasive force that had become faddish in eighteenth-century medicine, namely electricity.

But beyond these credentials and others that he possessed, Franklin had been deeply involved with health and the healing arts since his youth. This was not an intermittent interest. He had helped to shape medicine prior to this time, and he had earned the respect of academic physicians, bedside practitioners, and others involved in the healing arts throughout the world.

The French government officials who asked him to be on the Mesmer commission knew this, as did Lavoisier, Guillotin, and the other commissioners that served with him. This book will explore this important but often overlooked legacy—Benjamin Franklin's many medical contributions, as well as how he fit into the turbulent world of eighteenth-century medicine.[3]

## COLONIAL MEDICAL PRACTITIONERS

Benjamin Franklin did not have any formal medical training—in fact, he had very little schooling. But this was not a barrier to entering and practicing medicine, or conducting medical experiments, in North America in the eighteenth century. In Franklin's America, the mindset about "physicians," college degrees, and regulations was not at all what it is today. In fact, only about 5 to 10 percent of the 3,500 Americans who practiced medicine for a living had college diplomas when the War of Independence started.[4]

One reason for the paucity of degree-bearing physicians during the colonial period was that North Americans did not even have a medical school prior to 1765. Another was that the three major medical schools in Great Britain (Edinburgh, Oxford, and Cambridge) graduated only a few dozen students each year. Moreover, most physicians that graduated abroad aspired to enter "polite society." The smallish cities in the New World could not rival London when it came to establishing elite medical practices befitting proper, well-attired gentlemen, who left surgeries and drug dispensing to the lower sort. Indeed, most colonial physicians had such a hard time supporting themselves in medicine that they also performed occasional surgeries and derived additional income by selling pharmaceuticals as tradesmen.[5]

The observations of some degree-bearing physicians who ventured across the Atlantic did not help. William Douglass, a Scotsman with a degree from Utrecht, viewed colonial medical care as so "perniciously bad" when he arrived in Boston in 1718 that he advised people "to let nature . . . take her course. Frequently there is more danger from the practitioner than the distemper," he warned, "but sometimes nature gets the better of the doctor and the patient recovers."[6]

Douglass was clearly an elitist; he firmly believed that he could offer his patients better treatment than could a practitioner without a college diploma. Yet the absence of university-trained physicians was not quite the unmitigated disaster he made it out to be. First, physicians like him tended to deal with only the small segment of society that could afford high medical fees. Second, some physicians obtained their European diplomas with very little formal study; for some institutions, a candidate could even send money and submit a thesis in absentia. And third, medicine was essentially a theoretical or academic subject at the great European universities, whereas the immediate need in the rugged North American colonies was for practitioners with hands-on skills.

The apprenticeship system was especially well suited to the needs of the colonists. As paying apprentices under established practitioners, aspiring young men learned how to interpret signs and symptoms, perform simple surgeries, and prescribe medicines. The apprenticeships could vary markedly in length, quality, and quantity. But seven years with a respected practitioner meant a lot in Boston or Philadelphia, where a graduate of the widely-accepted system would still be addressed as "doctor," even without the college degree.

In contrast to England, with its guilds and laws, there was no real regulation of physicians or surgeons in Britain's North American colonies prior to the 1760s.[7] Hence, others with less training also entered the highly competitive marketplace.[8] To quote William Smith from 1757: "The profession is under no kind of regulation. Any man at his pleasure sets up for Physician, Apothecary, and Chirurgen [surgeon]."[9]

Clergymen were among these other participants, and they had history on their side.[10] Men of the cloth had long participated in the healing arts, in part because illnesses had long been associated with sinning and demons, but also because they were willing to treat the poor. Reverend Cotton Mather, whose ideas helped to shape Franklin's life in medicine, once contended that preachers should play the leading role in colonial medicine because they were the most learned men in America. Opined Mather, "Tis an angelical connection when the ministers who do the pleasure of Christ shall also be the physicians and Raphaels unto their people."[11]

Historians estimate that approximately 10 percent of the practicing "physicians" in the colonies were trained as preachers when Mather penned these words in 1710.[12] Mather, however, was by no means typical of the group—he was one of the most important figures in colonial medicine.[13] He avidly read medical tracts, published letters and pamphlets, and tried new methods. He also wrote the first major treatise on medicine from North America, *The Angel of Bethesda*, which was completed in 1724 but not published in his lifetime. Nevertheless, some of Mather's writings were inundated with his deep religious beliefs about supernatural forces and prayer, which did not endear him to his more earthly contemporaries, including physician William Douglass, who assailed him for meddling in things he knew little about, and which bothered Franklin, whose approach to medicine was decidedly secular.

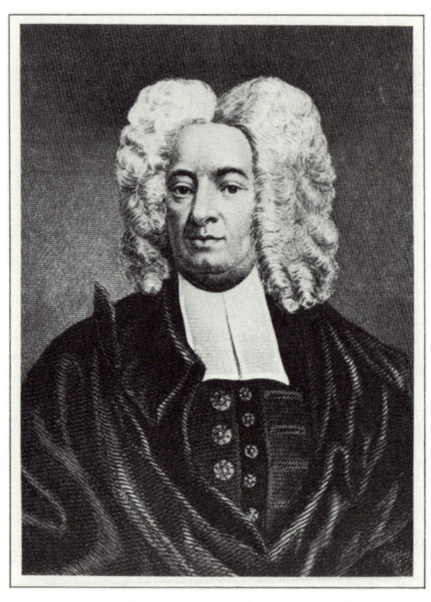

*The Reverend Cotton Mather (1663–1728) of Boston, a major figure in colonial medicine.*

Apothecaries also provided medical advice at this time.[14] For people with limited funds, going directly to a drug dispenser was one way to avoid paying an additional physician's fee. Astrologers likewise offered medical advice, a fact not lost on Franklin and the other almanac makers who were forced to deal with the pseudo-science.[15] And for hands-on procedures, midwives helped deliver babies, and barbers performed simple procedures, including bloodletting with their razors.

In addition to the marketplace healers who practiced for a living, many landowners, shopkeepers, farmers, trappers, and housewives took care of their own and tried to help their neighbors. George Washington gave medicines and routinely practiced the ancient art of bloodletting on his family and his slaves at Mount Vernon. Although he had some medical books, almost all of his medical knowledge was acquired by observation and from experience. Thomas Jefferson also took care of himself and his household, unless the matter required expert help.

In democratic America, even the most ordinary people, including a high percentage of women, felt that they had as much right to practice medicine as any physician, including the erudite Douglass. For these individuals, most diseases, bites, and injuries could be adequately treated with some basic medical knowledge, a few stock remedies, and a good dose of common sense. Whether in rural or urban areas, most medicine started in the home, as evidenced by the fact that self-help medical guides, including those that Franklin published, were among the best sellers of the day.

## THEORISTS AND PRAGMATISTS

Although the average citizen in Franklin's era cared little about academic debates concerning whether the hidden machinery of the body worked in one way or another, many broadly accepted treatments stemmed from highly speculative theoretical formulations. In this context, the ancient Greek theory of bodily fluids or "humors" was still very much alive at the bedside, although not necessarily in its original guise.[16]

The Greeks living more than two thousand years earlier had based their medicine on the idea that the body contains four basic humors: yellow bile, blood, phlegm, and black bile. They associated these fluids with the qualities hot and dry, hot and moist, cold and moist, and cold and dry, respectively. They contended that imbalances among the humors could make a person feel ill. Hence, the sick were treated with "opposites" to restore equilibrium. The continued use of heat and certain herbs that might make a patient with the chills feel warmer can be traced to this theory. So can drawing blood from feverish patients with flushed faces, signs that originally suggested an overabundance of this vital humor.[17]

The first significant challenge to humoral medicine emerged during the Renaissance. It was called iatrochemistry, which literally means "medical chemistry."[18] The iatrochemists, following the lead of Swiss physician Paracelsus, introduced a medicine based on the properties of sulfur (combustibility), mercury (vapor), and salt (solidity), while emphasizing such things as the chemistry of the blood and nerve "juices." Breaking with the past, they also introduced the strategy of treating some illnesses with poisons, which is something the Greek humoral theorists and their descendants would have shunned. The use of mercury and arsenic in mainstream eighteenth-century medicine can be traced to iatrochemical theories.

The newest medical theory in Franklin's day, however, was more mechanical.[19] It was stimulated by an increasing desire to break away from what seemed like alchemy to some learned individuals, and it embraced Newtonian physics with its emphasis on particles in motion. These physicians attributed signs and symptoms to such things as abnormally tight or flaccid nerves or abnormal vascular tension. The new objective, which was basic even to Mesmer's thinking, was to make sure matter flowed through the hollow tubes of the body as Nature intended and did not build up because of blockages to cause problems.

Distinctions between the three basic theories were not always sharp. Many academicians melded chemical and mechanical ideas together, and ancient Greek humoral ideas still made their way into newer theoretical conceptions. Differences of opinion surfaced, especially among the academicians and the medical elite, and resolving them was often impossible, because the internal changes associated with humoral, chemical, and mechanical theories could not be directly observed.

Still, whether it was to cool a fever, counteract a build up of "morbid matter," or alter the tone of the nerves, most physicians in Franklin's time carried pretty much the same weapons in their arsenals. Bleeding, cathartics, less potent laxatives, purges, blistering agents, and sweat-producing diaphoretics were very much in vogue. William Douglass, who was never at a loss for words, wrote that it was all "very uniform, bleeding, vomiting, blistering, purging, Anodyne, &c. If the illness continued, there was repetendi [repetition] and finally murderandi [murder]."[20]

For many already debilitated patients receiving the more demanding or "heroic" treatments, this had to have been the "Age of Agony."[21] But accepting the heroic therapies or the belief that pain was a sign that something powerful was at work was not the whole story. Less debilitating herbal medicines and alternative forms of healing were also important to the colonists. In this context, many pragmatic settlers were anxious to learn about the medicinal plants that might be growing in their backyards from the Indians.[22]

In North America, just about everyone accepted the fact that the natives who greeted the new settlers knew considerably more about treating bites from rattlesnakes and poisonous insects than did the ivory-tower academics thousands of miles across the ocean. In addition, many colonists believed that God provided a local remedy for each disease in every part of the world, including theirs, with its unique climate, terrain, flora, and fauna. The local Indians were a first source of information about the curative roots, barks, berries, and nuts in the region. Especially when the European cures did not work, theirs was valuable knowledge.

## FRANKLIN'S ENLIGHTENED MEDICINE

Given the state of the healing arts in the colonies, it should come as no surprise that Franklin would have strong interests in medicine and hygiene, even if he did not possess a college degree or have a medical apprenticeship. Instead, the surprise would have been if a man of Franklin's intellect, wide-ranging interests, love of natural philosophy, medical contacts, and legendary skepticism did not have a real interest in preventive medicine, epidemics, the disorders that affected his own body, therapeutics, and even the ravages of time.

What distinguished Franklin from the myriad other colonials who practiced or dabbled in medicine was that he approached clinical medicine with the mindset of an experimental natural philosopher. He skillfully designed experiments, collected data, kept careful records, and compiled tables to determine trends and outcomes. He also read voraciously, contacted authorities to solicit their opinions, and searched for historical antecedents. Franklin ran his printing business for eighteen years, and he conducted his famous "Philadelphia" electrical experiments, which included "capturing lightning" with a kite, for only six years. But he maintained his scientific approach to medicine from early on until his dying day.

Like most of his countrymen, Franklin was more interested in whether something worked than why, and he applied his pragmatism to his medicine. Throughout his medical life he avoided the metaphysics of the ancients and tended to shun the unanchored speculations of the academics that were circulating in his own time. He instead favored hard evidence based on repeated observations and experiments. His approach was that of an empiricist (from the Greek *emperia*, meaning trial or experiment). Of course, rationalism or reasoning was also extremely important to Franklin, but experiments, careful observations, and quantifiable results came first, reflecting changes that were hallmarks of the Enlightenment.

The term "Enlightenment" came forth in 1785, one year after Franklin put Mesmer's theory to the test. When Immanuel Kant was asked whether he thought he lived in an enlightened age, he answered: "No we are living in an age of enlightenment."[23] Kant's term for Enlightenment was *Aufklärung*, and what he was implying quickly caught on—not only among those who spoke German, but also among those who spoke English or French. The latter referred to the eighteenth century as the *siècle des lumières*, meaning the "century of light."

The Enlightenment is usually dated from about 1730 to 1790 in much of Western Europe, with a somewhat later start and a later finish in America.[24] The term itself can be problematic, because the timing, tone, and themes of the Enlightenment varied from country to country and even from city to city. The more pragmatic and secular Dutch, for example, were in many ways "enlightened" earlier than the British, Germans, or French. There were also distinct English, Scottish, and colonial versions of the Enlightenment. Within America, Franklin's adopted city of Philadelphia warmly embraced the intellectual and cultural ideals of the movement before Boston or New York.

Historians are in greater agreement about the fact that the seeds for the Enlightenment were planted well before Franklin was born in 1706. In the first half of the seventeenth century, Sir Francis Bacon wrote that it was time to sever ties with the "idols" of the past, meaning those metaphysical theories, unsubstantiated thoughts, and prejudices that might distort the truth.[25] Bacon's basic message was that the scope of human knowledge must now be extended "beyond the Pillars of Hercules," an allusion to what had once been a boundary of the known ancient world. This, he maintained, could be accomplished only by turning to detailed observations and experiments. The "Great Renewal" of learning, Bacon opined, must be based on the gradual accumulation of facts. Franklin would later refer to Bacon as a "prodigious genius," adding, "He is justly esteem'd the father of the modern experimental philosophy."[26]

Thomas Sydenham, who practiced medicine in England the second half of the seventeenth century, felt the same way about Bacon and his call for a fresh start.[27] "To escape the censure of the Great Bacon," Sydenham gathered case histories and accumulated a wealth of observable facts at the bedside about specific medical disorders. Although unable to put speculation totally in abeyance, most of Sydenham's "causes" remained fairly close to experience, and his theories were secondary to detailed observations. Sydenham's more empirical approach to clinical medicine drew adherents from his native England and from other parts of Europe.[28] His new approach to medicine was also exported to America, where it had a profound influence on Franklin.

The medical Enlightenment that blossomed after Sydenham died was based on a number of beliefs that he and Bacon valued highly. One of the most important was that the future of medicine must be based on careful observations, objective experiments, more sophisticated instruments, and above all, data. Another was that general laws would come from combining indisputable facts with solid reasoning. Exposing the errors, superstitions, and falsehoods of the past was basic to the Enlightenment, as was optimism about the future. The widespread belief was that there would soon be better ways of preventing some diseases and of treating others.

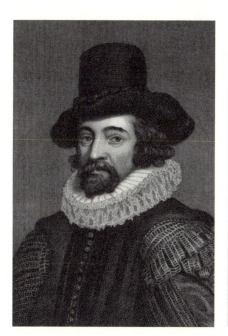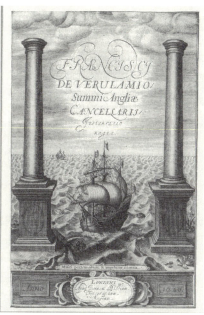

*Francis Bacon, Lord Verulam (1561–1626), and the cover plate of his 1620 treatise showing a ship going through the Pillars of Hercules, the known boundary of the ancient world.*

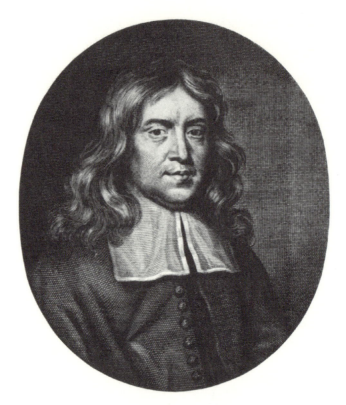

*Thomas Sydenham (1624–1689), the influential English physician who*
*applied Baconian philosophy to the practice of medicine. (Photo courtesy of*
*the University of California Press.)*

The medical Enlightenment evolved into a democratic undertaking, with ordinary citizens being recruited to search for truth alongside their more formally educated cousins. And it was an international venture, one in which national boundaries and even wars did not prevent people from communicating new ideas to each other. The ultimate humanitarian goal of the Enlightenment was to improve the lot of all people: men and women, young and old, and especially the poor and destitute who, through no fault of their own, could not help themselves.

Franklin's forays into medicine were inspired by the ideals of the Enlightenment, and without question he contributed significantly to the medical side of the movement. He was optimistic that experimental natural philosophy would lead to better disease prevention and medical care. He was deeply committed to the search for basic laws of nature that would be infallible and would put an end to superstition, quackery, and ignorance. He advocated accurate observations and careful experiments, and he built better instruments. Religious dogma, grandiose formulations, and the gripping tentacles of the past did not hold him back, and he was anxious to develop and share medical ideas with anyone, anywhere.

### "WHAT GOOD SHALL I DO THIS DAY?"

Franklin hoped that his medicine would "contribute to the relief of man's estate," to use Baconian language. Helping people in practical ways was always very important to him. In his *Autobiography,* which he started to write in England when he was well into his sixties, Franklin tied practical utility to his religious beliefs. Although this document is selective and clearly reflective of the image he wished to convey to others, he admitted that he was never one for organized religion with its dogma and mythology. Yet he also stated that he believed in God, and he proceeded to tell his readers that the best way he could think of to honor God was not in church, but with earthly deeds. In his words, "the most acceptable service to God was the doing good to man."[29]

Franklin also included this thought a number of times in his most famous publication, *Poor Richard's Almanack*. There we find: "The noblest question in the world is, *What Good may I do in it?*"[30] In a later edition of the *Almanack* he asked the question: "What is Serving God?" His answer: "'Tis doing Good to Man."[31]

Using Poor Richard as his mouthpiece, Franklin also expressed a closely related thought: "When you're good to others, you are best to yourself."[32] In other words, service to others is not just a way of honoring God; it is also an important step toward moral perfection.

Franklin's desire to do good for his community and to better himself were two goals he established early in life, after he read Cotton Mather's *Bonifacius: An Essay upon the Good*.[33] He would later sell some of Mather's books in his shop, and he would tell the famous cleric's son Samuel that his father "set a greater value on the character of a doer of good, than on any other kind of reputation; and if I have been, as you seem to think, a useful citizen, the public owes the advantage of it to that book."[34]

Franklin personally took on the "bold and arduous project of arriving at moral perfection" by listing thirteen virtues, beginning with Temperance and ending with Humility. Along with his resolution to pursue his listed virtues one at a time (he even drew up a checklist), he posed two questions—

one to be addressed in the morning and the other in the evening. Upon waking, he would ask himself, "What good shall I do this day?" And before retiring for the night, he would reflect, "What good have I done to-day?"[35]

Along with community service and moral perfection, Franklin also gravitated to medicine because he found it intellectually stimulating and loved the thrill of making new discoveries. Further, he liked to interact with the intellectual elite and doers in society, many of whom were respected physicians. But there is no reason to doubt that community service and moral perfection were very important to him, and that they were among the reasons why he was drawn to medicine and why he did so much in this domain.

## FRANKLIN'S MEDICINE AND ORIGINALITY

Franklin contributed to medicine in many ways. One had to do with improving personal hygiene and establishing regimens for healthy living. In this domain, preventive medicine, he strove to understand how a healthy body and a healthy mind could best be maintained or at least not abused. He looked very carefully at what he and other people ate and drank, the benefits of exercise, and the air people breathed. His writings about hygiene had roots in the past, but they also drew on the naturalistic observations and experiments he conducted.

Franklin was also involved in developing a better understanding of the nature of certain illnesses, trying to figure out how to prevent the onslaught of particular diseases, determining what might cure a disorder, and exposing quack remedies like mesmerism to the public. In this context, he studied and had reasoned opinions about many disorders, from simple colds to deadly smallpox.

Franklin's medicine also had an inventive component. He designed medical instruments for treating the sick and injured, and worked on new inventions to improve air quality in the home and workplace. Knowing that some physical conditions, such as those associated with aging, would not improve, he also developed prosthetic devices, such as bifocal glasses. Less well known is that he also invented a number of other aids for helping the lame and the aged, including a tool he called his "artificial arm" for grasping out-of-reach objects without having to climb a ladder.

Finally, the founding of institutions figured prominently into Franklin's medicine, and they stand among his proudest accomplishments. In this context, he was deeply involved with building hospitals for the poor and in improving existing facilities for treating the sick and wounded. He was also concerned with medical education in the colonies, and he played an important behind-the-scenes role in establishing the first medical school in North America.

Hence, Franklin's enlightened medicine has at least four components to it. The first is preventive medicine (hygiene). The second is illnesses and cures. The third is prosthetic devices and other inventions. And the fourth is institutions. But to what extent was he really original?

Franklin made a number of important, original contributions. But more often than not, he had an uncanny ability to catch on to something that another person might have said or written, to evaluate it, and to do more with it—provided it had practical utility and seemed worth the effort. Sometimes this meant collecting detailed observations and compiling statistics to confirm what he was hearing or reading. On other occasions, he followed through by conducting what medical researchers would now think of as clinical trials. Although some of his clinical investigations were on other people, he also performed or had others perform tests on his own body. When evaluating Mesmer's claims in 1784, for example, he served as a subject in a number of experiments to determine whether his ailing body was in any way susceptible to the alleged magnetic force.

Advancing an idea or a new finding also meant spreading the word orally and in letters. In this domain, Franklin communicated with leading physicians and sent written reports to journals and learned societies. Additionally, he presented important and timely medical material in his newspaper and almanac. And, as a printer, he printed select medical books and informative pamphlets written by others on his presses.

Franklin was a master of pithy medical sayings that would withstand the test of time, such as "Quacks were the greatest liars in the world, except for their patients."[36] But he was at his best when it came to getting other members of the medical community to look at ideas supported by impressive new findings. Moreover, he was never possessive of his own ideas.

Getting important backers and donations were also part of the picture, particularly when funding was needed for an important charitable project, such as a hospital in growing Philadelphia. When it came to supporting something good for the community, or for an overlooked segment of that community, Franklin had the rare ability to win endorsements from people with wealth and power. Of equal significance, he was capable of convincing working people, who might have only a few small coins in their pockets, to support worthy causes.

Thus, Franklin was at times original. But even when he was less than original, he was both a thinker, a man who readily picked up on good ideas and recognized the absurdity of bad ones, and a doer, a person who knew just how to get the job done. Remarkably well rounded, he used his talents adroitly in the field of medicine. This held true not just in Philadelphia, but in London, Paris, and other places as well.

# PART I
# THE COLONIST
# AND MEDICINE

CHAPTER 1

# Poor Richard's Medicine

Some of our Sparks to London town do go,
Fashions to see, and learn the World to know;
Who at Return have naught but these to show:
New Wig above, and new Disease below.

—*Poor Richard's Almanack*, 1734

$M$uch of what we know about Franklin's early life comes from the first part of his *Autobiography*. His father, Josiah, was an English religious "dissenter," who sailed for Boston with his wife, Anne, and three children in 1682. Strong and hard working, Josiah supported his family by making candles and soap in what was then a small city of 6,000 inhabitants. After Anne died bearing her seventh child in 1689, Josiah married Abiah Folger, and Benjamin was the eighth of their ten children. He was born on January 6, 1705, according to the Julian calendar. (When Parliament mandated a switch to the Gregorian calendar in 1752, his birthday changed to January 17, 1706, the date we celebrate today.)[1]

In his *Autobiography*, Franklin informs us that the fortune he made with his printing business enabled him to devote himself to his electrical experiments. Although he stops short of saying so, printing also played a significant role in drawing him into medicine.

As a printer of newsworthy information, Franklin had to be up to date on the epidemics that were ravaging or seemed poised to spread across the region. In addition, he had to know the latest medical advice for dealing with snakebites, and for preventing and treating dreaded diseases, such as smallpox and "intermitting Fever" (a term that usually meant malaria). To succeed as a printer, Franklin also had to have the medical knowledge to know which books were worth reprinting and which were not—and, of course, to decide whether it was worth gambling on a new book. Moreover, he needed to know and understand the needs of the physicians and the community they served. Thus, in a very real way, printing helped to educate Franklin about medicine, stimulate his interest in the healing arts, and serve as an important stepping stone into the field.

## FRANKLIN'S ENTRÉ INTO PRINTING

Franklin was the most intellectual of Josiah's children, which may be one reason why his father first thought that he should be trained for the ministry. Only after it became clear that this child's calling was not organized religion did Josiah transfer him from a Latin school to one that focused more on the practical arts. Franklin tells us: "I acquired writing pretty soon, but I failed in the arithmetic, and made no progress in it."[2] By age ten, his formal schooling was over.

Josiah now put his son to work in his own businesses, where he cut candlewicks, boiled soap, and poured hot wax into molds. It took a while before he fully recognized Benjamin's love of the printed word. "This bookish inclination at length determined my father to make me a printer," Franklin would later write, "though he had already one son (James) of that profession." He continued: "In 1717 my brother James returned from England with a press and letters to set up his business in Boston. . . . [I] signed the indentures when I was yet but twelve years old. I was to serve as an apprentice till I was twenty-one years of age."[3]

Franklin enjoyed learning the printer's art from his brother, with its typesetting, editing, and proofreading. At the same time, he furthered his education and began to sculpt the personality he wanted to present by reading books on mathematics, grammar, and philosophy. After completing Xenophon's *Memorable Things of Socrates*, he promised to express himself only "in terms of modest differences; never using, when I advanced any thing that may possibly be disputed, the words *certainly, undoubtedly,* or any others that give the air of positiveness to an opinion; but rather say, I conceive or apprehend a thing to be so and so . . . or *I imagine it to be so, if I am not mistaken.*"[4] These would be more than engaging personality traits; they would also serve Franklin well as a man of medicine.

In 1721 James decided to publish his own newspaper, the *New England Courant.* He let it be known that the new paper's purpose was to improve life in the commonwealth, a fact not lost on Benjamin, who sent a series of letters to the editor under the pseudonym "Silence Dogood." These letters made people think about issues that would become increasingly important to Franklin, including the need to help poor sick and injured citizens, and the personal and societal problems caused by excessive drinking.

Benjamin and James Franklin, however, did not always get along. Benjamin wrote that his brother "was passionate, and had often beaten me, which I took amiss; and, thinking my apprenticeship very tedious, I was continually wishing for some opportunity of shortening it."[5] The opportunity to leave surfaced when James ran afoul with the law for printing offensive remarks about the New England leadership and the mindless "religious knaves" that blindly followed their puritanical dictates. Fearing arrest, James slipped into hiding, had his name on the newspaper's masthead replaced with his brother's, and signed a document discharging Benjamin from his apprenticeship. Knowing that this was just a ruse, and that James now had no legal recourse if he ran away, Benjamin set off for New York in 1723.

Finding no employment in New York, and upon learning that there might be an opening for a printer in Philadelphia, Franklin continued south. His trip, already marred by rough seas, was made worse by a fever. "Having read somewhere that cold water drank plentifully was good for a fever, I follow'd the prescription," he would later write, adding, "Sweat plentifully most of the night, my fever left me."[6]

After a stop in Burlington, New Jersey, where he lodged with a practicing physician who shared his passion for books, he entered Pennsylvania with considerable ambition but only a few small coins in his pocket. Philadelphia had about 10,000 residents at the time, making it the largest city in colonial America. It also had the human and financial resources needed to move ahead of every other colonial city when it came to adopting the spiritual, intellectual, societal, educational, and humanitarian ideals that would soon characterize the Enlightenment.[7] In many ways, the city and its youthful new arrival were perfectly suited for each other.

Shortly after arriving, Franklin secured work with printer Samuel Keimer, who found lodging for him at the home of John Read. Once settled, Franklin began to seek the company of others who enjoyed reading, studying philosophy, and discussing ways to improve themselves and the city. As his circle grew, he met some of the more important people in the city, including Sir William Keith, the governor. Both Keith and Franklin agreed that the printers in the city were not particularly talented. Subsequently, over a glass of Madeira, Keith offered to help Franklin start his own printing business. The plan that emerged called for Franklin to go to London to buy his equipment.

Late in 1724, Franklin boarded the *London Hope*, only to discover that the letters of credit that Keith had promised him had never been written. The North Atlantic swells, combined with rain, sleet, and snowstorms, soon added to his growing anxiety. Upon arriving in London, with inadequate funds, he searched for a printing job and eventually found employment at Samuel Palmer's printing house. There he managed to meet some interesting people, who in turn introduced him to others, some of whom were in medicine. One such person was a surgeon by the name of Lyons, who "introduced me to Dr. Pemberton, at Batson's Coffee-house. He promis'd to give me an opportunity, some time or other, of seeing Sir Isaac Newton, of which I was extremely desirous; but this never happened."[8]

Franklin, who already had an appreciation for Newton's genius, was more successful when it came to meeting Sir Hans Sloane, who had apprenticed under Thomas Sydenham. Sloan was Physician-General to the British Army and president of the Royal College of Physicians. From 1727 to 1741 he would serve as thirteenth President of the Royal Society, following Newton, whose tenure had lasted twenty-four years. Sloane was also an avid collector of curiosities, and he invited Franklin to his house to see his collections, ultimately purchasing the unusual asbestos purse that Franklin brought with him from America, a piece that can now be found in the British Museum.

After about a year at Palmer's, Franklin moved on to John Watts's printing house, an even more impressive London establishment that employed nearly fifty printers. Here he impressed his fellow workers by being able to run up and down the stairs with two sets of heavy lead type, while others struggled with one. He left this establishment only after Thomas Denham, an engaging Quaker merchant from Philadelphia, agreed to send him home, if he would work in his dry goods store.

The two men headed back to Philadelphia during the summer of 1726. Franklin passed his time on the trip studying the ocean currents and marine life, and writing his personal doctrine for "regulating my future Conduct in Life."[9] Unfortunately, Franklin and Denham both became ill soon after they set foot in Philadelphia. Franklin suffered from a severe bout of pleurisy that made his breathing difficult. But unlike Denham, whose "distemper carried him off," Franklin slowly regained his strength. Once again in need of work, he returned to Keimer's printing shop, where he was used to train poorly skilled workers.

In 1728, at age twenty-two, Franklin finally opened his own printing establishment. It began as a partnership with Hugh Meridith, another young printer from Keimer's shop, whose father provided needed capital for the venture. As word of Franklin's printing skills spread, their new shop received orders to print all sorts of documents, including contracts for paper money that required great skill to produce.

A year later Franklin purchased Keimer's failing newspaper, which had just ninety subscribers when he bought it "for a trifle." He shortened its name to the *Pennsylvania Gazette* and, following in the footsteps of his brother James, gave the paper a more civic-minded orientation. The young printer did not, however, have James' combative personality, and he always tried to see and present both sides of an issue. "Printers are educated in the Belief," he wrote, "that when Men differ in Opinion, both Sides ought equally to have the Advantage of being heard by the Publick; and that when Truth and Error have fair Play, the former is always an overmatch for the latter."[10]

Franklin wrote that he "considered my newspaper, also, as another means of communicating instruction, and in that view frequently reprinted in it extracts from the *Spectator,* and other moral writers; and sometimes publish'd little pieces of my own."[11] In reality, he wrote most of the "little pieces" for the *Pennsylvania Gazette* in its early years, some of which dealt with pressing medical concerns.

## MARRIAGE AND MEDICAL OINTMENTS

Before he had sailed on his ill-fated trip to England, Franklin had courted Deborah Read, the daughter of John Read, his former landlord. "I had a great respect and affection for her," he wrote, "but, as I was about to take a long voyage, and we were both very young, only a little above eighteen, it was thought most prudent by her mother to prevent our going too far at present."[12] While stranded in England, he sent but a single letter to Debby and gave her no reason to believe that they would marry on his return, if he returned.

In his absence, Debby married John Rogers, a potter. The couple quickly separated—she "refusing to cohabit with him or bear his name, it being now said that he had another wife."[13] Also facing overwhelming debts, Rogers quickly ran off to the West Indies, where rumor had it that he died. Upon learning this, Franklin resumed his courtship of Debby and settled into a common-law arrangement with her in 1730, to avoid severe legal repercussions if Rogers were found to be still living.

Young, muscular, and virile, Franklin was lucky not to have contracted any sexually transmitted diseases while living in England. And having had intimate contact with some of the street women, he knew it. But to his disgrace and Debby's horror, in 1731 he had to inform his new wife that he had just become the father of an illegitimate son, William. The identity of the mother was never revealed and the boy was raised in the Franklin household.

John Read, Debby's father, had died several years earlier, and finances in

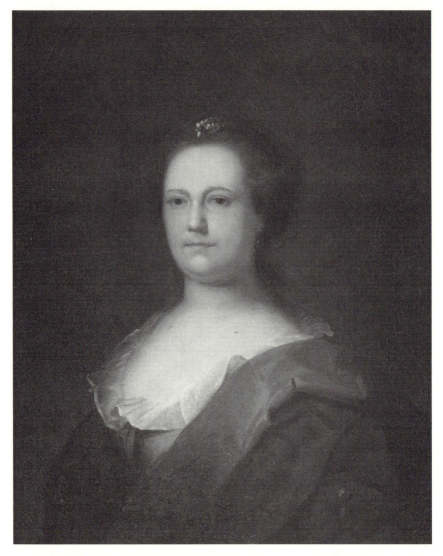

*Deborah Read Franklin (1704–1774). (Portrait attributed to Benjamin Wilson; image courtesy of the American Philosophical Society.)*

the Read household had been tight since his passing. Debby's mother, Sarah, however, managed to make ends meet by producing and selling homemade ointments with her daughter's assistance.[14] Now that Franklin had his own printing establishment, he helped out in two ways. First, since his shop on Market Street, above which he lived, was also a general store, he featured Sarah Read's homemade salves (along with thick blocks of Crown Soap from the Franklins in Boston) on the shelves.[15] Second, he wrote flyers and newspaper advertisements for the *Pennsylvania Gazette* to help sell her medicinal ointments.

A piece in his newspaper from August 19, 1731 reads:

The Widow Read, removed from the upper End of Highstreet to the New Printing-Office near the Market, continues to make and sell her well-known Ointment for the ITCH, with which she had cured [an] abundance of People in and about this City for many Years past. It is always effectual for that purpose, and never fails to perform the Cure speedily. It also drives away all Sorts of Lice in one or twice using. It has no offensive Smell, but rather a pleasant one; and may be used without the least Apprehension of Danger, even to a sucking Infant, being perfectly innocent and safe. . . . She also continues to make and sell her excellent *Family Salve* or Ointment, for Burns or Scalds (Price 1s. an Ounce) and several other Sorts of Ointments and Salves as usual.[16]

The "itch" was scabies, a nonfatal but very annoying disorder known since ancient times. It usually begins with itchy vesicles of clear fluid between the fingers.[17] The vesicles break open when scratched, spreading the problem to previously uninfected body parts. Shaking hands, sharing bedsheets, and coming in simple contact could also spread the itch.

Giovan Cosimo Bonomo and Diacinto Cestoni broke new ground in 1687 when they associated a tiny mite with the disorder.[18] The two Italian microscopists even drew a picture of the gnawing insect that dug into the skin to lay its eggs. They wrote that sulfur was "infallibly powerful to kill the Vermin lodged in the Cavities of the Skin."[19] Their reports were read by English physician Richard Mead, who translated them for English readers in 1703.[20]

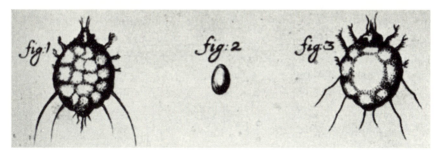

*The mite responsible for the itch as depicted by Italian microscopist Giovan Cosimo Bonomo in 1687. Left: dorsal view of* Acarus scabiei; *middle: egg; right: ventral aspect. (See* Medical Life, *44, 1937.)*

By Sarah Read's time, external treatments for the itch were being widely promoted, some of which were quack remedies. Notably, her own ointment contained sulfur, the agent shown to be effective by the Italians.

Franklin controlled the entire printing business by the time he printed this advertisement for the itch. He had decided to buy out Meredith, even if it meant acquiring a mass of debt. With his hard work, business skills, and common sense, he would now pay off his creditors and greatly expand his printing empire. He would also begin to print medical books.

## SELF-HELP MEDICAL BOOKS

The first medical tract published on North American soil that was specifically aimed at helping the settlers was a pamphlet by Thomas Thacher on how to deal with "Small Pocks, or Measles." This short, unoriginal work was published in 1678 and borrowed heavily from Thomas Sydenham. When Franklin opened his own printing shop, there were a few other small pieces from America. Yet, for all intents and purposes, medical books were still imported from Europe, sometimes at great expense.

Franklin was an astute businessman, and he recognized that just republishing European treatises on academic medicine would probably be unprofitable. He also knew that the colonists had unique health problems and that different medicinal plants grew in England and North America. For these reasons, and because it made economic sense, he began to print self-help medical books for his countrymen.[21]

In 1734, he published a new edition of *Every Man His Own Doctor: Or, The Poor Planter's Physician*.[22] Directing readers to "Medicines being chiefly of the Growth and Production of this Country" for easily diagnosed "Distempers incident to the Climate," it was "design'd for those who can't afford to dye by the Hand of a Doctor," and it was the first manual of colonial medicine printed in North America. Its author uncertain,[23] *Every Man His Own Doctor* could be purchased at Franklin's printing shop for the reasonable price of just one shilling. The demand for the manual was so great that the first printing quickly sold out; two more editions soon followed.[24]

The third edition of Thomas Short's *Medicina Britannica* was another self-help book, and it came off Franklin's press in 1751.[25] This book of more than four hundred pages included a preface and notes by John Bartram, the most respected botanist in the colonies (Linnaeus called him the greatest natural botanist in the world). Bartram told readers where many of Short's English plants or good substitutes for them could be found on American soil. He also gave directions for preparing medicines with local substitutes. As was the case for *Every Man His Own Doctor*, the Short-Bartram pharmacopoeia was directed at people who did not have access to professional care or ample resources to pay for such services.

## THE ALMANAC

The word almanac is derived from *al manakh*, Arabic for calendar. Andrew Boorde came forth with the first English almanac in the mid-1500s; there were hundreds a century later. The first almanacs published in America came off a press controlled by Harvard College in 1639. By Franklin's time, no publications in America, except for the Bible, were more widely read or more often consulted.[26]

Colonial almanacs could be found in all sizes and shapes during the early eighteenth century. They were advertised as guides to forecasting the weather, timing the tides, knowing when to plant seeds, and when to reap the bountiful harvest. They also gave dates for holidays, events, eclipses, and important meetings. Recipes, poems, jokes, essays and medical advice also found their way onto almanac pages.

Most almanacs followed a set pattern: an introductory statement, a dose of astrological prognostication, the year's calendar with all sorts of notes regarding tides, daylight, and weather, an assemblage of local material, and finally some anecdotes and short essays, which is where most hygiene and medicine appeared. How the latter subjects were treated varied considerably from one almanac maker to another—some emphasizing traditional medical advice, others folklore, and still others the occult.

Franklin's own entry into the lucrative almanac business was hastily prepared late in 1732, while his Philadelphia competitor Andrew Bradford was publishing five almanacs for other people. There was nothing particularly original in Franklin's product for the year 1733, but it was broader, more thoughtful, and decidedly wittier than the others, particularly when it came to dispensing philosophy about how to live a happier, more fulfilling, and healthier life. In his words: "I have constantly interspers'd *moral* Sentences, *prudent* Maxims, and *wise* Sayings, many of them containing *much good* Sense in *very few* Words, and therefore apt to leave *strong* and *lasting* impressions."[27]

Costing five pence, *Poor Richard's Almanack* (Debby called it *Poor Dick's*)

*Poor Richard,* 1733.

A N

# Almanack

For the Year of Chrift

# I 7 3 3,

Being the Firft after LEAP YEAR:

| *And makes fince the Creation* | Years |
|---|---|
| By the Account of the Eaftern *Greeks* | 7241 |
| By the Latih Church, when ☉ ent. ♈ | 6932 |
| By the Computation of *W.W.* | 5742 |
| By the *Roman* Chronology | 5682 |
| By the *Jewifh* Rabbies | 5494 |

*Wherein is contained*

The Lunations, Eclipfes, Judgment of the Weather, Spring Tides, Planets Motions & mutual Afpects, Sun and Moon's Rifing and Set-ting, Length of Days, Time of High Water, Fairs, Courts, and obfervable Days.
Fitted to the Latitude of Forty Degrees, and a Meridian of Five Hours Weft from *London,* but may without fenfible Error, ferve all the ad-jacent Places, even from *Newfoundland* to *South-Carolina.*

By *RICHARD SAUNDERS,* Philom.

PHILADELPHIA:
Printed and fold by *B. FRANKLIN,* at the New Printing-Office near the Market.

*The cover page of the first edition of* Poor Richard's Almanack. *(With permission of the Rosenbach Museum and Library.)*

quickly became an annual favorite in the colonies, appealing to all socio-economic classes. As word about it spread, it also developed a large following on distant shores. Whether it sold under the name *Poor Richard*, *Bonhomme Richard*, or *Le Pauvre Henri*, people could not get enough of it. Reminisced Franklin: "In 1732 I first published my Almanack under the name of Richard Saunders. It was continued by me about twenty-five years, commonly called Poor Richard's Almanack. . . . "I reap'd considerable profit from it, vending annually near ten thousand."[28]

Poor Richard was made out to be a lovable, sensible, and honest writer. In the first edition of "his" new almanac, Richard admitted to his readers that he wrote for two reasons. One was for "the publick Good" and the other was because "the Printer has offer'd me some considerable share of the Profits"—a fact known to his wife Bridget, who was always complaining about being excessively poor.[29]

Many maxims that filled the pages of the new publication were selected from anthologies of great literature and the Bible.[30] Poor Richard admits that he "pilfer'd" freely across countries, languages, and time. "Why then should I give my Readers bad Lines of my own, when good Ones of other People's are so plenty?"[31]

What made Poor Richard so appealing was how well he could modify his favorite hand-chosen "Scraps from the Table of Wisdom," so they would be more memorable, nourishing, and easier to digest.[32] In the words of Franklin biographer H. W. Brands: "Franklin thoroughly enjoyed adopting the guise of Richard Saunders. Where Franklin the businessman had to be circumspect, careful not to offend, Saunders the almanacker could be outrageous—indeed, the more outrageous the better. Franklin as Franklin had to hide his gifts to avoid inspiring envy; Franklin as Saunders could flaunt his wit, erudition, and general brilliance."[33]

Many of Poor Richard's maxims have stood the test of time, including: "Fish and Visitors stink in 3 days," "Diligence is the Mother of Good-Luck," "Well done is better than well said," "The worst wheel of the cart makes the most noise," "Success has ruin'd many a Man," "Little Strokes, Fell great Oaks," "The rotten Apple spoils his Companion," "God helps them that help themselves," and "Haste makes Waste."[34] It was even Poor Richard who commented that "Old Boys have their Playthings as well as young Ones; the Difference is only in the Price."[35]

## MEDICAL ASTROLOGY

Like the majority of almanac writers, Franklin presented the signs of the zodiac connected to a crude image of a man right after the introductory remarks in his almanac. The image depicted how the twelve constellations ("houses") governed twelve corresponding parts of the anatomy. Leo, for example, was associated with the heart, whereas Scorpio, with its tail, regulated the genitals. Known as the "Zodiac Man," "the Anatomy," or by other names, these images were common at the time. They were used along with the geometrical relationships of the heavenly bodies ("aspects") and known powers of each (Mars, for example, was the "Master of Disorders") in medicine.

While astronomers tracked the movements of the stars and planets, astrologers concentrated on the physical and mental effects of those movements. The art began with the Babylonians, was developed by the Greeks and Romans, and was further extended by the Arabs. It soon permeated all facets of European life.[36] Even Sir Walter Raleigh wrote: "If we cannot deny but that God hath given virtue to springs and fountains, to cold earth, to plants and stones, minerals and to the excremental parts of the basest living creatures, why should we rob the beautiful stars of their working powers?"[37]

Raleigh went on to write about specific virtues of the heavenly bodies. By his time it was thought that there were ideal astrological times for picking medicinal herbs and administering them to the sick, and propitious times for more physical interventions. After all, the moon controlled not just the tides but all things moist. This included the blood—a factor not to be overlooked when bleeding a patient. The moon also governed the brain, thought to be the moistest organ in the body. This association led to the terms "lunatic" and "moonstruck" for those whose brains did not seem to work quite right.

Astrology was clearly in decline by Franklin's century. But, especially among the uneducated, stargazing and personal fortune telling were not yet dead. Franklin knew this, which was why he did not follow the example set by Cotton Mather, who had chosen to exclude all heathenish material from the almanac he assembled.

Mather, like just about everyone else, did not doubt that the phases of the moon and nearness of the sun could influence the tides and affect the weather. This was objective, legitimate, "natural" astrology, and it was backed by solid science. What Mather could not accept was "judicial astrology"—the belief that astrologers could accurately predict personal actions and life events. To

count, that the Buyer of my Almanack may confi-
der himfelf, not only as purchafing an ufeful Uten-
fil, but as performing an Act of Charity, to his
poor  *Friend and Servant*     *R. SAUNDERS.*

## The Anatomy of Man's Body as govern'd
### by the Twelve Conftellations.

The Head and Face

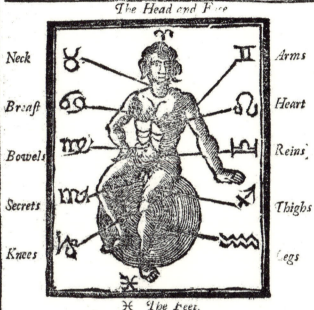

| | |
|---|---|
| *Neck* | *Arms* |
| *Breaft* | *Heart* |
| *Bowels* | *Reins* |
| *Secrets* | *Thighs* |
| *Knees* | *Legs* |

℣ The Feet.

*To know where the Sign is.*

First find the Day of the Month, and againft the
Day you have the Sign or Place of the Moon in
the 5th Column. Then finding the Sign here, it
fhews the part of the Body it governs.

### The Names and Characters of the Seven Planets.
♄ Saturn, ♃ Jupiter, ♂ Mars, ☉ Sol, ♀ Venus,
☿ Mercury, ☽ Luna, ☊ Dragons Head and ☋ Tail.

### The Five Afpects.
☌ Conjunction, ✶ Sextile, ☍ Oppofition, △ Trine,
□ Quartile.

### Common Notes for the Year 1733.

| Golden Number | 5 | Cycle of the Sun | 6 |
|---|---|---|---|
| Epact | 25 | Dominical Letter | G |

*The "Anatomy" as depicted in Franklin's almanac. (With
permission of the Rosenbach Museum and Library.)*

Mather, the stars and planets might affect the seasons and even bodies, but not matters related to free will and the human soul. Some occasional successes in judicial astrology, he contended, were just lucky guesswork; others suggested pacts with the Devil.[38]

Franklin had no intention of endorsing astrology either, but his reaction was more suited to his own personality and legendary sense of humor: he chose to poke fun at the absurd stargazers. In doing so, he again followed in the footsteps of his brother James, who had used "Poor Robin" to lampoon astrology in the almanac he published. Jonathan Swift, who had published a masterful hoax under the name "Isaac Bickerstaff" at the expense of London astrologer John Partridge, had taken this same approach.

Franklin thus decided that he would have Poor Richard use astrology to predict the moment of death of one of his most important rivals in the competitive almanac business, Titan Leeds. In the almanac's first issue, Poor Richard tells his readers that "inexorable Death, who was never known to respect Merit, has already prepared the mortal Dart," and that Leeds will die "on Oct. 17, 1733, 3 ho. 29 m P.M." The time of death, he emphasized, will be "at the very instant" when Mars, Sol, and Mercury align—not some nine days later at the time of the eclipse (about eleven o'clock), when "my good Friend" Leeds was predicting his own demise.[39]

In the next issue of the almanac, Poor Richard reported back that family matters kept him from being with Leeds, so he was not sure when Leeds died or even if he died. Nevertheless he thought he had departed this world, based on some uncharacteristically nasty comments about his own person in his latest almanac. Tongue-in-cheek, Franklin continued the game by having Poor Richard refute Leeds's claim that he was still alive.[40] His comments about the wonderful powers of astrology outdid anything his rival could write back, and his mockery of the pseudo-science continued to amuse readers for several more years.

In his own way, Franklin was able to have his cake and eat it too. He maximized sales of his almanac by including the Anatomy for those readers that demanded it. And by employing gentle humor, he helped dismantle one of Bacon's great false "idols" without offending anyone except, of course, Titan Leeds.

Interestingly, Titan Leeds was not one for judicial astrology either, but with the hope of selling almanacs to more marginal segments of society, he too had chosen to include the Anatomy in his publications. In the 1725 edition of *The American Almanack*, he openly admitted: "Should I omit to place this figure here, My book would hardly sell another Year."[41] Like Leeds, Franklin was smart enough to realize that economic survival required giving the public at least some of what it wanted, albeit his way.

## HYGIENIC AND MEDICAL ADVICE

As a philosopher for all seasons, Poor Richard had his share of earthly opinions about health, diseases, and medicine. Most often he emphasized disease prevention and advice for living a long and active life. Here the onus was on the individual to take care of his or her body by avoiding gluttony, drunkenness, and one's passions. Additionally, he provided conventional and folk remedies for the sick, knowing that not everyone would follow his ideas for preventing disease, and that certain illnesses might still strike people who took good care of themselves.

Poor Richard's most famous saying about preserving health would have to be "Early to bed and early to rise, makes a man healthy, wealthy and wise."[42] But he wrote considerably more about eating and drinking in moderation, and he was not alone. Proper food and fluid intake had been associated with good physical and mental health since ancient times, and no one in the eighteenth century doubted that poor diet and excessive drinking could result in disease, or that moderation was the key to good health.[43] As had been put in a thirteenth-century Latin poem on health: "If you lack doctors, these three will be doctors for you: a cheerful mind, rest, and a moderate diet."[44]

Prudence was the key to preserving health, advised John Locke, who had studied medicine at Oxford and was a devoted follower of Thomas Sydenham. With dietary moderation reflecting a triumph of reason over the emotions, many nonmedical writers also embraced and promoted this thought. In this context, Poor Richard warns: "He that spills the Rum, loses that only; He that drinks it, often loses both that and himself." And then more poetically: "Life with Fools consists in Drinking; with the wise Man, Living's Thinking." He also states: "Eat few Suppers, and you'll need few Medicines," "Eat to live, and not live to eat," "A full Belly makes a dull Brain," and "To lengthen thy Life, lessen thy Meals."[45]

To some of his most sophisticated readers, a few of Poor Richard's maxims on eating and drinking might have been identifiable from earlier publications. "Many dishes many diseases." for example, appeared with embellishment more than a hundred years earlier in Henry Peacham's *The Complete Gentleman* as "Many dishes, many diseases, dulleth the mind and understanding, and not only shorten but take away life."[46] Other sayings, however, may have come across as quite new.

Poor Richard even devoted several pages to the "Rules of Health and Long Life" and associated "Rules to find out a fit Measure of Meat and Drink" in the 1742 edition of his almanac.[47] His message for longevity remained a regimen of moderation. In fact, he even linked temperance to piety.

Franklin's colonial sage continued to drive home the benefits of not overeating or overdrinking in later editions of his almanac, sometimes by including a brief sketch of a highly regarded person who lived a moderate, sober life. Martin Luther, who was "remarkably temperate in meat and drink," was described in this way in 1749. After mentioning him, Poor Richard continued: "Cicero says, *There was never any great man who was not an* industrious *man;* to which may, perhaps be added, *There was never any* industrious *man who was not a* temperate *man:* for intemperance in diet, abates the vigour and dulls the action of mind and body."[48]

Reminding us that "We are not so sensible of the greatest Health as of the least Sickness,"[49] Poor Richard included numerous entries on avoiding specific diseases in the twenty-five volumes of the almanac. One reads: "To avoid Pleurisies, &c. in cool weather; Fevers, Fluxes, &c. in hot; beware of Over-Eating and Over-Heating."[50] And with regard to sexually transmitted diseases, Poor Richard's advice has a modern ring to it: "Against Diseases here, the strongest Fence, Is the defensive Virtue, Abstinence."[51]

Poor Richard did not always show great respect for paid practitioners of the healing arts. In fact, he became so critical of and sarcastic about the medical profession that some of his loyal fans prayed that the witty sage would stay healthy and not be smitten by a dreaded disease requiring professional medical care. They feared for what might happen to him, because he had written, "God heals, and the Doctor takes the Fees" and "There's more old Drunkards than old Doctors."[52] Adding fuel to the fire, he also wrote, "He's a Fool that makes a Doctor his Heir" and "Beware of the young Doctor and the old Barber."[53]

Richard Saunders had a serious message behind his witty health and medical sayings, and not all were presented in a humorous way. He was not trying to be funny when he advised: "Don't misinform your Doctor nor your Lawyer" and "It is ill Jesting with a Joiner's Tools, worse with a Doctor's."[54] Similarly, he was very serious when he wrote the one-liner that best characterizes what Franklin would conclude in his numerous campaigns against quackery, including his assessment of Mesmerism: "He's the best physician that knows the worthlessness of the most medicines."[55]

In addition to his many aphorisms, when Franklin heard or read about a new cure that seemed to have potential, he considered including it in *Poor Richard's Almanack*. For example, after reading John Tennent's *Essay on the Pleurisy*, he published some lines about the Virginian's cure.[56] It called for bleeding and three spoonfuls of "Seneka Rattle-Snake Root," which the local Indians had long been using for poisonous snakebites. Tennent reasoned that, much as the blood became viscous after rattlesnake bites, the same might be happening with pleurisy. He tried rattlesnake root on a few pleurisy patients during the winter of 1734–1735, thought they improved, and decided to write an essay on the cure. In advertising the 1740 edition of his almanac, Franklin even used the "infallible cure" as a sales tool. "As the Plant is very plainly described . . . and as the Method of using it is particularly laid down, it is not doubted but this Almanack may be a Means of saving the Lives of Thousands."[57]

After the almanac was expanded as *Poor Richard Improved* in 1746, lengthier pieces of preventative and therapeutic advice began to appear. For example, the following entry on dealing with bedbugs, then a common source of infections, was read by purchasers of the 1750 almanac: *"Bed-Bugs,* by some called *Chinces,* because first brought from China in East-India Goods, are easily destroy'd, Root and Branch, by boiling Water, poured from a Tea kettle into the Joints, &c. of the Bedstead, or squirted by a Syringe, where it cannot well be poured. The old Ones are scalded to Death, and the Nits spoilt, for a boil'd Egg never hatches. This done once a Fortnight, during the Summer, clears the House."[58]

In 1756, Poor Richard presented some "Recipes" for "the Health of the Body." He included short pieces on heartburn, skin burns, and dysentery, and somewhat longer passages for the "Dry-Gripes" and the "Augue or Intermitting Fever." The Dry-Gripes was one of several older terms for lead poisoning, and "Intermitting Fever," as noted at the beginning of this chapter, signified malaria, a disease marked by dramatic swings in body temperature. The almanac advised treating the latter disorder in the following way: "Take one Ounce of good Peruvian Bark, finely levigated; make it into an Electuary with Treacle or Molasses, mixing therewith twenty or thirty Drops of Laudanum; take this at about six or eight Doses two or three Hours apart, washing it down with a Glass of Madeira or red Wine. If any thing like the Jaundice, or Yellowness about the Eyes remains, chew Rhubarb a few Mornings."[59]

While he was residing in Philadelphia, Franklin heeded much of Poor Richard's sound advice for treating diseases. And he maintained a healthy body and a sound mind by eating and drinking in moderation. He also kept his body in excellent physical shape by exercising, following another important rule for healthy living, as we shall see in the next chapter.

CHAPTER 2

# In Praise of Exercise

I had from a child been ever delighted with this exercise [swimming],
had studied and practis'd all Thevenot's motions and positions, [and]
added some of my own.

—*Autobiography of Benjamin Franklin*

Despite his emphasis on staying healthy in addition to becoming wealthy and wise, Poor Richard says almost nothing about the importance of exercise. Yet Franklin, like other well-read people in the eighteenth century, knew that some exercise should be a part of any regimen for maintaining good health. In fact, although Franklin is usually portrayed as an overweight man reading or writing behind a desk, he was an expert swimmer, lifted weights, and tried to make exercising a part of his daily routine.

Franklin exercised from youth into old age, often setting a striking example for others to follow. Unsurprisingly, he tried to approach exercising, even in his formative years, with the mindset and creativity of an experimental natural philosopher. And although Poor Richard remained surprisingly silent about the need to abandon an old and comfortable chair, his accomplished publisher found other means to spread the word on the subject.

## SWIMMING, SCIENCE, AND HEALTH

Throughout his life, Franklin looked upon swimming as the best of all exercises for several reasons. It kept one fit by using many muscles, was a means of keeping clean, and was thoroughly enjoyable. Whether in a lake, a river, or an ocean, or whether one swam alone or with other people, swimming was the ideal exercise.

Yet very few people knew how to swim at the start of the eighteenth century. This was true not only for the large numbers of farmers and shopkeepers that practiced their trades on land, but also for the crews on military ships and even for most men who whaled and fished for a living. Historians

Lawrence Brockliss and Colin Jones note that "frequent immersion in water was socially and medically frowned upon. Even aristocrats washed infrequently, for body odour was considered a protective cocoon and sexual stimulant."[1]

Franklin, who would help to change this negative opinion about swimming, learned to handle himself in the water when he was very young. He went with his boyhood friends to Boston Bay and the neighborhood ponds and, weather permitting, waded or jumped in. But he was also bigger and more muscular than the other boys his age, and unlike his childhood friends, he was already thinking about useful new tools and inventions that could be used by people drawn to the water. "When I was a boy," he relates,

I amused myself one day with flying a paper kite; and approaching the bank of a pond, which was near a mile broad, I tied the string to a stake, and the kite ascended to a very considerable height above the pond, while I was swimming. In a little time, being desirous of amusing myself with the kite, and enjoying at the same time the pleasure of swimming, I returned; and, loosing from the stake the string with the little stick which was fastened to it, went again into the water, where I found, that, lying on my back and holding the stick in my hands, I was drawn along the surface of the water in a very agreeable manner. Having then engaged another boy to carry my clothes round the pond, to a place which I pointed out to him on the other side, I began to cross the pond with my kite . . . with the greatest pleasure imaginable.

Franklin concluded this short narrative: "I have never since that time practiced this singular mode of swimming, though I think it not impossible to cross in this manner from Dover to Calais." He added wryly, "The packet boat, however, is still preferable."[2]

Franklin described this episode from his childhood to a French physician-friend, Jacques Barbeu-Dubourg, who had written to him about learning to swim.[3] His correspondent did not know how to swim and could find little on the subject in Diderot's otherwise authoritative *Encyclopédie*. To learn more, he asked Franklin to answer ten pages of questions about swimming, ranging from the ideal water temperature to what the ancients had written on the subject. Replying from London, Franklin did his best to make swimming sound like fun, provide clear answers to his friend's questions, and recommend additional sources of information. He even told Barbeu-Dubourg that, while still a lad in the colonies, he came up with the idea of using paddles on his hands and feet to move through the water with greater efficiency.

"When I was a boy," he explained, "I made two oval palettes, each about ten inches long, and six broad, with a hole for the thumb, in order to retain it fast in the palm of my hand. They much resembled a painter's palettes. In swimming I pushed the edges of these forward, and I struck the water with their flat surfaces as I drew them back. I remember I swam faster by means of these palettes, but they fatigued my wrists. I also fitted to the soles of my feet a kind of sandals; but I was not satisfied with them, because I observed that the stroke is partly given by the inside of the feet and the ankles, and not entirely with the soles of the feet."[4]

Thus, even while growing up in Boston, Franklin was thinking about swimming fins and leg flippers, not to mention kites for water travel. But more than just thinking about the water, he had become a serious student of the art of swimming, which was why Barbeu-Dubourg solicited his opinions. In fact, Franklin was so serious about it that, in 1726 when he was a strapping lad of twenty, he even considered becoming a professional swimming instructor.

Franklin had sailed to London to buy printing equipment at the time, only to find that his backer, Governor Keith, never sent the needed letters of credit. Having no money of his own, he was forced to take jobs to pay for his food and lodging, which he did at Palmer's and then Watts's printing houses. He tells us in his *Autobiography* that he had made some friends there, including a book lover and linguist named Wygate.

One day he and Wygate decided to travel to Chelsea. It was there, on the banks of the Thames on an unusually nice day, that Wygate asked Franklin to show some "gentlemen from the country," who had joined them, what he could do in the river. The request did not come out of thin air. Franklin had already taught Wygate and a friend of his how to swim proficiently in the river. And from knowing what we do about Wygate, who "had been better educated than most printers," Franklin might have done so in a fairly scientific way. Franklin tells us that, "At the request of the company, whose curiosity Wygate had excited, I stripped and leaped into the river, and swam from near Chelsea to Blackfryar's, performing on the way many feats of activity, both upon and under water, that surpris'd and pleased those to whom they were novelties." He continued: "I had from a child been ever delighted with this exercise, had studied and practis'd all Thevenot's motions and positions, added some of my own, aiming at the graceful and easy as well as the usefulness. All these I took this occasion of exhibiting to the company, and was much flatter'd by their admiration."[5]

The distance from Chelsea to Blackfriars on the Thames River was about two miles, so the exuberant twenty-year-old would have shown off for some time before finally emerging from the water. Clearly, Franklin was exceptionally skilled and had great endurance. But just who was Thevenot, the writer he had read "from a child" and whose work served as his point of departure, allowing him to claim that he had invented some new motions and positions?

Melchisédec de Thévenot was a brilliant man who had attracted other intellectuals to his home in France for informal discussions about various subjects, most involving natural philosophy. The meetings he organized eventually led to the formation of the Académie Royale des Sciences, an organization that would later honor Franklin with a distinguished foreign membership. Among Thévenot's personal interests was swimming. He popularized the breaststroke and was the author (in French) of *The Art of Swimming Illustrated by Proper Figures with Advice for Bathing*, a landmark publication that illustrated various swimming strokes and exercises.[6] Thévenot completed his manual just before he died in 1692, and Franklin's wording suggests he read it before leaving Boston. Unfortunately, Franklin does not tell us exactly what he did above and beyond what he found in the treatise—only that he demonstrated a few motions or strokes "of my own."

Just a few months after showing Wygate what he could do in the Thames, Sir William Wyndham, a friend of Jonathan Swift, asked Franklin to teach his sons to swim before they sailed for the Continent. Franklin explained: "He had heard by some means or other of my swimming from Chelsea to Blackfriar's, and of my teaching Wygate and another young man to swim in a few hours. He had two sons about to set out on their travels; he wish'd to have them first taught swimming, and proposed to gratify me handsomely if I would teach them. They were not yet come to town, and my stay was uncertain, so I could not undertake it." He added, "From this incident I thought it likely that, if I were to remain in England and open a swimming school, I might get a good deal of money; and it struck me so strongly, that, had the overture been sooner made me, probably I should not so soon have returned to America."[7]

Franklin continued to impress people with his knowledge of swimming and his skills later in 1726, while heading home from his ill-fated, printing equipment buying trip to England. When the wind and seas permitted, he dove off the ship and swam laps around it. In the journal he kept of his lengthy voyage home, he recorded: "This morning we had a fair breeze for some hours, and then a calm that lasted all day. In the afternoon I leaped overboard and swam around the ship to wash myself."[8] Franklin was not foolhardy. A later journal entry reads: "I was determined to wash myself in the sea to-day, and should have done so had not the appearance of a shark, that mortal enemy of swimmers, deterred me."[9]

Franklin was aware of the unique dangers of ocean swimming. He also knew that swimming in rivers and lakes could be perilous—especially if a person lacked experience, fatigue easily, or suffered leg cramps. With this in mind, he later spelled out advice for all swimmers, above and beyond the age-old adage of looking before leaping, based on what he had read and his own experiences.

One of his suggestions concerned what to do when beginning to tire, if simply coming out of the water was impossible. He recommended that the swimmer should "turn himself sometimes on his back, and to vary in other respects the means of procuring a progressive motion."[10] Another was how to handle muscle cramps. Here he wrote that "when he is seized with the cramp in the leg, the method of driving it away is, to give the parts affected a sudden, vigorous, and violent shock; which he may do in the air as he swims on his back."[11]

Franklin was also concerned that some exuberant swimmers who may not know better might jump into frigid water on a very hot day. He wrote: "During the great heats of summer there is no danger in bathing, however warm we may be, in rivers which have been thoroughly warmed by the sun. But to throw one's self into cold spring water, when the body has been heated by exercise in the sun, is an imprudence which may prove fatal." He even cited a real-life example: "I once knew an instance of four young men who, having worked at harvest in the heat of the day, with a view of refreshing themselves, plunged into a spring of cold water. Two died upon the spot, a third the next morning, and the fourth recovered with great difficulty."[12] As long as one proceeds cautiously, Franklin advised, "the exercise of swimming is one of the most healthy and agreeable in the world. After having swam for an hour or two in the evening, one sleeps coolly the whole night, even during the most ardent heat of summer."[13]

Franklin never viewed age as a barrier to swimming. In a letter written in the 1760s, he explained to Oliver Neave: "I cannot be of the opinion with you that 'tis too late in life for you to learn to swim." Therefore, "as your new employment requires your often being on the water, of which you have such a dread, I think you would do well to make the trial." He then told his friend how to gain confidence and overcome his fear that the water will not support him, without using corks or bladders for support:

The practice I mean is this. Chusing a place where the water deepens gradually, walk coolly into it till it is up to your breast, then turn round, your face to the shore, and throw an egg into the water between you and the shore. It will sink to the bottom, and be easily seen there, as your water is clear. It must lie in water so deep as that you cannot reach it to take it up but by diving for it. . . . Then plunge under it with your eyes open, throwing yourself towards the egg, and endeavouring by the action of your hands and feet against the water to get forward till within reach of it. In this attempt you will find that the water buoys you up against your inclination; that it is not such an easy thing to sink as you imagined.

Continuing, he told Neave that he would "feel the power of the water to support you, and learn confidence in that power; while your endeavours to overcome it and reach the egg, teach you the manner of acting on the water with your feet and hands, which action is afterwards used in swimming to support your head higher above the water, or to go forward through it."[14] The rest of Franklin's letter to Neave presents seven mental "particulars" for Neave to consider before even entering the water, with the hope that they will add to his confidence as he learns to swim. One is that the body as a whole is lighter than water, and therefore not about to sink. And another is that a swimmer can float on his back with his head straight back and, with the help of some small hand actions, still not submerge his face.

Franklin deemed the material he mailed to Neave so worthwhile that he decided to share it with the public. First, he included it in the fourth edition of his *Experiments and Observations on Electricity*, which came out in 1769.[15] He then published it as "Useful Hints for Learning to Swim" in *Gentleman's Magazine*, a periodical with a large and varied readership.[16]

## INSTITUTIONALIZING EXERCISE

Before he published his treatise on swimming, but after he had contemplated becoming a swimming instructor, Franklin proposed making exercising a regular activity in some of the Philadelphia institutions he created or helped create. One was his Junto, the club that he started for self-improvement and community betterment.[17] Another was his institution for higher education, the Academy of Philadelphia, which he designed as a secular institution, in contrast to the other colleges in the colonies, which were all still seminaries.

Franklin laid out his vision for the academy in his *Proposals Relating to the Education of Youth in Pennsylvania,* which he distributed to backers and other interested parties in 1749. Most of the document dealt with the courses that would be offered, including writing, history, and mathematics, and administrative issues, such as hiring faculty and a headmaster. But there was also a section on keeping the students at the academy fit and healthy. After all, Franklin reasoned, sick students miss classes. And more positively, a healthy body makes for a sharp mind.

With these thoughts in mind, Franklin proposed "That the boarding scholars diet together, plainly, temperately, and frugally." And "That to keep them in Health, and to strengthen and render active their Bodies, they be frequently excercis'd in Running, Leaping, Wrestling and Swimming, &c."[18]

Two footnotes accompanied the last sentence. The first cites Milton's *Tractate of Education,* in which it is proposed "that an Hour and a Half before Dinner should be allow'd for Exercise." It also cites Turnbull, who wrote, "Corporal Exercise invigorates the Soul as well as the Body. . . . For this, and other Reasons, certain hardy Exercises were reckoned by the Ancients an essential Part in the Formation of a liberal Character; and ought to have their Place in Schools where Youth are taught the Languages and Sciences."[19]

The second footnote cites John Locke, who had studied medicine with Thomas Willis, Richard Lower, and Robert Boyle in Oxford, and then received additional bedside training from Thomas Sydenham. Locke is best remembered today for stating that we gain knowledge entirely through our senses (that there are no innate ideas), and that ideas are formed by associating sensory impressions with each other—a process that often works but can sometimes give false impressions and lead to mistaken beliefs.

Still, as important as Locke was in helping people to understand the origin of ideas, what drew Franklin to Locke in this context was the Englishman's personal interest in swimming and ancient history. Locke had been a part of Thévenot's circle, and he had written about swimming in a treatise on education. This treatise began as a lengthy correspondence between Locke and Edward Clarke, a wealthy landowner and distant relative. Clarke had been using Locke as a medical advisor, and he asked for his advice on child rearing and education.[20]

In these matters, Locke was not in the mainstream. He believed that boys and girls should not only be brought up with the same learning, but that both should engage in outdoor exercises in all sorts of weather to promote better health. With this philosophy, Locke responded to one of Clarke's letters with the suggestion that science should be an integral part of a child's education—and so should swimming.

Franklin wrote: "Tis suppos'd that every Parent would be glad to have their Children skill'd in *Swimming* if it might be learnt in a Place chosen for its Safety, and under the Eye of a careful Person. Mr. Locke says . . . in his *Treatise on Education*; 'Tis that saves many a Man's Life; and the Romans thought it so necessary, that they rank'd it with Letters; and it was the common Phrase to mark one ill educated, and good for nothing, that he had neither learnt to read nor to swim; *Nec Literas didicit nec Natare.*'"[21]

Thus, Franklin had his share of reasons for wanting to include swimming and other forms of exercise in his school's curriculum. And, as he traveled and gained fame, he picked up followers. One was Erasmus Darwin, who was familiar with Franklin's writings on science and health, including his treatise on swimming, and who met with Franklin several times while Franklin served as a colonial agent to England. As a physician, Darwin found merit in swimming for exercise and health, and although terribly overweight, he learned to swim in the rivers near his Litchfield home. Even after Franklin's death, he continued to campaign for adding swimming and other forms of exercise to school curricula. He advised schoolmasters to make sure that their students were allowed a few hours each day for playing ball, ice skating in winter, and swimming in summer.[22] And he emphasized that exercising was just as important for physical and mental health in women as it was for men.

### MATCHING DIFFERENT FORMS OF EXERCISE

Franklin, with his muscular six-foot body and broad chest, did more than just swim. He also lifted weights, rowed, and occasionally sailed to build up his stamina and to preserve his health during his years in the colonies. His jobs also provided him with considerable exercise. He traveled long and hard as a representative of Pennsylvania, and made numerous trips in his position as a colonial postmaster. He was on his feet, in the saddle, and at the oars more than his plump popular image would suggest.

In subsequent years, beginning with his first diplomatic trip to England in 1757, he found less opportunity to exercise, especially outdoors. But knowing the importance of staying in good physical and mental shape, he arranged to take at least one lengthy trip each year, usually during the summer months. In 1766, for example, he wrote to the Pennsylvania Assembly: "I acquainted you that I was about to make a Journey for the Establishment of my Health. I accordingly went to Pyrmont, where I drank Waters some Days; but relying more on the Air and Exercise of Travelling, I proceeded to Hanover . . . and thro' Treves to Holland."[23]

Five years later, he told Debby about a trip that he had just made to Birmingham (where he met Erasmus Darwin), Sheffield, Leeds, and Manchester. In his words: "My Journey has been of use to my Health, the Air and Exercise have given me fresh Spirits, and I feel now exceedingly well."[24] And two months later: "I continue pretty well, but find more Exercise necessary to preserve my Health, and therefore am about to make the Tour of Ireland."[25]

To Franklin, not exercising represented the real danger. But was taking an occasional long trip sufficient? While pondering this question and his own heavy workload, he asked himself some challenging questions: Precisely how many hours or minutes of exercise do we really need per day? Can various forms of indoor and outdoor exercises be equated? And is time spent the best way to equate different forms of exercise?

After thinking the matter through, he concluded that the amount of exercise a person needs should not be measured in just minutes or hours. Although he would long maintain that walking "is an excellent thing for those whose Employment is chiefly sedentary,"[26] he knew that taking a nice walk on a pleasant summer day was not the same as trying to cover the same terrain while being battered with snow and a blustery winter wind. Moreover, because some forms of exercise, such as weight lifting, can take place indoors, it did not make sense to compare exercises in terms of distances traversed. The key, he concluded, had to be in the amount of heat generated by the body during the activity. Today we would be more likely to talk about the number of calories burned, yet there is no question that Franklin had already come to this remarkable conclusion.

Just when Franklin realized this, and whether he might have read something of the sort in the literature, is hard to say. The one thing that we know for sure is that he put his revelation on paper in 1772. His letter was sent to his son William, then Royal Governor of New Jersey.[27] Franklin wrote that he was happy to learn that William had made a resolution to exercise more frequently. Knowing from Poor Richard that promises are easier to make than deeds are to perform ("*Saying* and *Doing* have Quarrel'd and Parted"),[28] as well as how hard it is for even the best of men to stick to an exercise program, he told him, "I hope you will steadily perform it." He then explained why he should stick with it, again sounding very much like Poor Richard, who did not have great confidence in the medical profession: "It is of the greatest importance to prevent diseases," he stated, "since the cure of them by physic is so very precarious."[29]

Franklin wrote that he had arrived at his theory through experimentally verifiable observations. The most significant passage in the letter reads:

In considering the different kinds of exercise, I have thought that the *quantum* of each is to be judged of, not by time or by distance, but by the degree of warmth it produces in the body: Thus, when I observe if I am cold when I get into a carriage in a morning, I may ride all day without being warmed by it, that if on horse back my feet are cold, I may ride some hours before they become warm; but if I am ever so cold on foot, I cannot walk an hour briskly without glowing from head to foot by the quickened circulation. . . . There is more exercise in *one* mile's riding on horseback, than in *five* in a coach; and more in *one* mile's walking on foot, than in *five* on horseback; to which I may add, that there is more in walking *one* mile up and down stairs than *five* on a level floor.

Franklin further told William that he liked the idea of running up and down stairs "when one is pinched for time," because it compacts "a great quantity of exercise in a handful of minutes." He also praised weight lifting as another form of exercise that one could engage in when the weather was bad. By the use of dumb bells, "I have in forty swings quickened my pulse from 60 to 100 beats in a minute, counted by a second watch; And I suppose the warmth generally increases with quickness of pulse."[30]

## THERAPEUTIC EXERCISE

To Franklin and others at the time, exercising was more than just a way of preserving health. Physicians also maintained that it could be therapeutic for those who were ill. This sort of thinking was in accord with the writings of the Hippocratic physicians and their intellectual descendants. Thomas Sydenham, for example, recommended exercising to fight melancholy, hysteria, hypochondriasis, and other disorders characterized by lethargy and fatigue.[31] In effect, he viewed it as a stimulant.

Sydenham often advised simple walking or some running (for young men), but he was most fond of horseback riding. Others agreed. In a lecture on hysteria, a physician at the Edinburgh Infirmary stated: "I had an account of a lady who on the slightest threatening of a fit was immediately placed on horseback and obliged to ride pretty hard. . . . This always prevented the further progress of the paroxysms and at length performed a cure."[32]

While Franklin was still in Philadelphia, horseback riding was even being recommended for the "West-India Dry-Gripes," a painful colic caused by lead ingestion. Franklin even published physician Thomas Cadwalader's essay on treating the disorder in 1745. Cadwalader wrote: "To complete the Cure, let the Patient, as soon as able, use constant and moderate Exercise on Horseback . . . for the Fibres of the Mesentery and Intestines having been with the long Pains much weakened and relaxed, are by this Means brought to recover their proper Tone, and resume their former Oscillations, so as to shake off and expel the morbific Impurities." He also told his readers that because "Perspiration is very much increased in Riding, it is of vast Advantage not only in this, but in almost every Chronical Disease, by driving the noxious Humours from the Center to the Circumference, and expelling them through the Ducts of the *Milliary Glands*."[33]

Franklin's own letters show he also recommended exercising therapeutically. Like Sydenham, he thought it was best for lethargic disorders, such as melancholia, where a stimulant made intuitive sense. For example, while in France he repeatedly chastised his neighbor, Madame Brillon, who was on occasion depressed, for not exercising. "You do not take enough exercise to keep yourself well," he scolded her. "I advise you to take a walk every day for an hour, in your beautiful garden if the weather is good, otherwise in your house. Or, if you don't have sufficient leisure, take a more strenuous but shorter kind of exercise, and the result will be the same. You can do that by going up and down the steps of your garden or your house for a quarter of an hour every day before dinner."[34]

Franklin's exercise prescription was straightforward and he took his own advice, even in his senior years. John Adams, in his diary for the year 1782, states: "Dr. Franklin, upon saying the other day that I fancied he did not exercise so much as he was wont, answered, 'Yes, I walk a league every day in my chamber; I walk quick, and for an hour, so that I go a league; I make a religion of it.'"[35]

During the fall of 1787, at age eighty-one, Franklin told the Comte de Buffon, "By observing Temperance in Eating, avoiding Wine and Cyder, and using daily the Dumb Bell, which exercises the upper part of the Body without much moving the Parts in contact with the Stone, I think I have prevented its *Increase*."[36] He had expressed the same thought about his painful bladder stone to his French friend Louis Guillaume Le Veillard that spring.[37]

These letters reveal a great deal about Franklin and his lifelong commitment to exercise as therapy and as a means of preserving health. Nevertheless, the most telling example about Franklin's dedication to exercise took place in France just a few years earlier. Despite his deteriorating heath and advanced age, Franklin made his way down to the Seine near his residence in Passy to give swimming lessons to a boy of about fourteen who accompanied him down the hill, his grandson Benjamin Franklin ("Benny") Bache. Franklin did not just wade into the shallows to shout out a few words of advice to his grandson. The most celebrated American in France, who at times could hardly move on land, jumped into the river and swam from one side to the other, and then back again, to his own and the boy's delight.[38]

# CHAPTER 3

# The Smallpox Wars

By this account it appears, that in the way of [smallpox] Inoculation there has died but one patient in 267, whereas in the common way there has died more than one in four.

—Benjamin Franklin, 1759

In 1772, Benjamin Franklin responded to some flattering words from his sister Jane Mecom about his young grandson, Benny Bache, who was then just three. While writing back about this "uncommonly fine boy," his thoughts shifted to his son Franky, "now dead 36 years, whom I have seldom since seen equal'd in every thing, and whom to this Day I cannot think of without a Sigh."[1]

Francis Folger Franklin passed away in 1736, when he was four years old, and his death broke the hearts of his parents. He had been their only child after six years of marriage, and Benjamin and Deborah were not sure they could have another child, much less one with so much promise. He was, as his parents had inscribed on the original stone that marked his grave, "The Delight of all that knew him."

Franky was a victim of smallpox, a disease with a predilection for young children and one all too common during the colonial period. What made his death so noteworthy was that his father, who was becoming well known in Philadelphia, had been advocating inoculation as a means of preventing such tragedies. Thus, some cynics began to insinuate that Franklin was not a man of his word; that he preached one thing but practiced another. Equally disheartening, other faultfinders were convinced that inoculation either killed Franky or failed to give him the protection he needed.

The gossip and insinuations clearly put Franklin on the defensive. He had to "sincerely declare" to the public that Franky "was not inoculated, but receiv'd the Distemper in the common Way of Infection." But, he added to his one paragraph notice in his *Pennsylvania Gazette*, "Inoculation was a safe and beneficial Practice," and explained, "I intended to have my

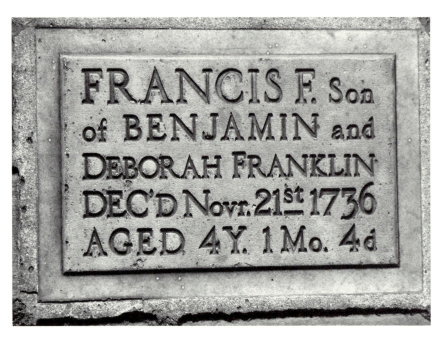

*Stone currently marking the Philadelphia grave of Francis Folger Franklin, who died from smallpox at age four.*

Child inoculated, as soon as he should have recovered sufficient Strength from a Flux with which he had long been afflicted."[2]

Franky's death clearly weighed heavily on his father's mind for the rest of his life. In the third part of Franklin's *Autobiography,* which was written in 1788, he reflected: "In 1736 I lost one of my sons, a fine boy of four years old, by the smallpox, taken in the common way. I long regretted bitterly, and still regret that I had not given it to him by inoculation. This I mention for the sake of parents who omit that operation."[3] If anything positive came from Franky's death, it was the resolve and determination of his father to convince other parents that they owed it to themselves and to those they loved to inoculate their children as soon as possible.

Franklin's leadership role in the inoculation wars, even before Franky's death, would involve his printing press and writing skills as tools to sway public opinion. Moreover, it would lead him to collect statistics on survival with and without inoculation, and it would put him in contact with some of the most important men of medicine in the colonies and leading physicians in England.

## THE SPECKLED MONSTER

No one really knows precisely when smallpox first emerged, because some epidemics suggestive of mild smallpox might well have been chickenpox or some other disease. Many historians believe that smallpox probably appeared with the first agricultural settlements in northeastern Africa about 12,000 years ago, although some think it is a newer disease and point to its birth in Asia or the Middle East.[4] Soldiers that had been stationed in North Africa probably first brought the disease to Europe in 710, and Crusaders a few hundred years later also carried it home.

An early term for smallpox was *variola,* from the Latin word *varius,* meaning spotted, or *varus,* meaning pimple. Initially this term was applied rather broadly, but during the eleventh century *variola* began to be applied specifically to smallpox. At about the same time, the Anglo-Saxons also began to use the term *poc* or *pocca* to refer to the sacks, bags, pustules, or pouches that appeared on the skin. During the fifteenth century, syphilis began to show itself in Europe. Because it was associated with larger pus-filled blisters, the English began to distinguish between the *great pockes* of syphilis and the *small pockes*.[5]

Although smallpox was not associated with high mortality when it first appeared in Europe, mortality rates began to rise during the fifteenth century. Some epidemiologists speculate that this might have been due to a change in virulence of the virus or even to the advent of a new strain.[6] Just what transpired is unclear, but smallpox acquired several nicknames as death tolls increased from 1 percent to over 20 percent. One of the most telling was "the speckled monster."

In 1562, Queen Elizabeth I contracted the virus, and it left her bald and deeply scarred for the rest of her life. Queen Mary was not as fortunate, and she succumbed to the disease in 1694. Smallpox was not just a disease of royalty. When the Portuguese and Spaniards sailed to the Americas, they brought the speckled monster with them, where it was even deadlier than in Europe. There were about 2,500,000 natives when the Spaniards began to build their sugarcane plantations in Hispaniola early in the 1500s. Within a decade, the population was a fraction of what it had been. At about the same time, Cortez and his 600 soldiers annihilated millions of Aztecs, not so much with their swords, but by inadvertently spreading smallpox.

The Indian populations in North America fared little better. The once formidable coastal Indians were so weakened by the disease that the new settlers encountered little more than token resistance when they staked their claims to the land.[7] To many of the pioneers and their leaders, including the devout Mather family, smallpox was an avenging angel sent by God to destroy soulless heathens. But in addition to killing nine of ten coastal Indians, it also killed many immigrants and their particularly vulnerable children.

During Franklin's youth, Americans, like their counterparts in Britain, recognized that the disease usually begins with a high fever and some non-specific symptoms, which could include chills, splitting headaches, joint pains, cramping, vomiting, backaches, and general malaise. Some recognized that these symptoms might follow exposure to a sick person, but only after a delay of about two weeks. A few days later, the fever would temporarily abate and pink spots would begin to appear on the face. The small spots would then spread over the body, covering it with pea-sized blisters.

Everyone knew that the disease was more likely to kill the very young and very old. As for the people who survived the ordeal, the lucky ones would be left permanently scarred; those not so lucky, or about 15 percent, would also be blinded. The only good thing that could be said was that those who managed to beat the speckled monster would not have to fight it again.

## THE 1721–1722 EPIDEMIC AND INOCULATION

Boston was a city of just over 10,000 people in 1721, when fifteen-year-old Benjamin Franklin witnessed what a smallpox epidemic could do. The disease was transported to Boston by men aboard the *Seahorse*, a British naval vessel from the Tortugas in the West Indies. This was not, however, Boston's first smallpox epidemic. There were others in 1648–1649, 1666, 1678, 1690, and 1702. During the seventeenth century, about 60 percent of the new immigrants contracted smallpox and at least 10 percent succumbed to it, despite quarantine laws dating back to 1647.[8]

The colonists were hampered by the fact that they did not understand what caused smallpox. Some clerics blamed it on the wrath of God and the forces of darkness. Others pointed to putrid airborne substances ("miasmas") escaping from the earth. Still others hypothesized that a faulty body or some impurity from the mother's blood could be behind it.

Nevertheless, the New Englanders knew they had a choice to make when smallpox began to appear in their communities. They could flee to the countryside, which about 10 percent did, or stay, try to protect themselves, and hope for the best. Those choosing to stay held rags soaked with vinegar over their noses, plugged their nostrils with tobacco leaves, dangled bags of camphor from their necks, and even smeared foul-smelling tar on their faces, hoping to ward off the smells of illness and death. Isolating the sick made sense, and fumigating their sheets, garments, and even letters with dense smoke was also deemed protective.

Unfortunately, there was no effective cure for those who still caught the disease. But this did not stop desperate citizens from seeking medical help and trying all kinds of remedies. Dietary changes, bleeding, vomiting, laxatives, and medicines concocted with soap, mercury, and other ingredients were given. Some colonists even tried to "draw out" the fever by wrapping the sick in blankets and placing them near roaring fires. Others turned to cooling.

Some colonists purchased medicinal herbs, one theory being that the shape, color, or some other features of the plant, its flowers, or its seeds signified that it could combat smallpox. Astrology sometimes entered the picture, because it was believed that a controlling heavenly body might further give clues about the needed plant. Since smallpox was a "lunar" disease, lentils and rapeseed, which reminded people of spots on the moon, were tried. For those who preferred treating with opposites, there were also hot and dry "solar" plants, which they were told could counteract the cold and moist lunar disorders.[9]

Given the terror associated with smallpox and the inability of even the most learned physicians to treat it effectively, any promising new weapon against the disease had to be considered seriously. In 1721, while New Englanders braced themselves for the worst, the seemingly bizarre concept of acquiring immunity by exposing oneself to smallpox scabs that had fallen off was new and just beginning to receive attention in England.[10]

On January 5, 1700, Joseph Lister of the East India Company had written to Dr. Martin Lister of the Royal Society to tell him about a Chinese practice called "planting the heavenly flowers." It involved collecting smallpox scabs, drying them, and then blowing them into the nose to produce a mild case of smallpox and then immunity. Although Lister's report was interesting, the English remained content with their own flower gardens.

The Royal Society subsequently received a few letters about inoculation as practiced in Constantinople. These letters described how dried scabs were placed in cuts on a person's arm. The word inoculation actually derives from the Latin *in oculare*, for "giving eyes." And much like gardeners who took the "eyes" from some plants, such as potatoes, to start new ones, the Turks had learned how to plant smallpox scabs under the skin relatively safely.

One communicator of this procedure was Emanuele Timoni, an Italian physician to English diplomats in the Turkish Empire. Timoni had studied medicine at Padua and Oxford and was a Fellow of the Royal Society. Another was Dr. Jacob Pylarini, also a Padua graduate. Their letters were published in the *Philosophical Transactions of the Royal Society* in 1714 and 1716, respectively, but they had no immediate impact.[11]

Attention began to increase, however, after Lady Mary Wortley Montagu returned from Constantinople during the spring of 1721.[12] She had gone there in 1717 with her husband, the newly appointed British ambassador to the Sublime-Port. Two weeks after arriving, she wrote a letter to a friend in England, telling her about the operation.[13] She stated that women skilled in the technique were invited to inoculation parties and came with a "nut-shell" of dry scabs—enough to treat about fifteen people, usually children. Going from one person to another, they open a vein with a large needle and inserted as much of the infectious material as would go onto the head of the needle. The procedure was repeated a few times, after which the wounds were bound and the treated individuals were isolated from those without immunity. The operation resulted in a mild form of smallpox, but the sick emerged less scarred and with lifelong immunity.

Disfigured from her own bout with smallpox, having lost a brother to it, and fearing the worst for her own children, Lady Mary had her five-year-old son Edward inoculated far from her native England on March 19, 1718.[14] After returning home, and with smallpox raging in London, she asked English surgeon Charles Maitland to inoculate her four-year-old daughter.[15] Maitland had traveled with the family to Constantinople, and he performed the first inoculation in England in April 1721.

Caroline of Anspach, the Princess of Wales and future queen of George II, was a friend of Lady Mary, and she now took up the cause. Along with Maitland and some royal physicians, she approached George I and asked him to free six inmates doomed to be hanged at Newgate Prison, if they would accept inoculation. Their inoculations were performed that summer, and they were successful. After more experiments, including one involving eleven children in a London orphanage, Caroline had her own daughters inoculated, setting a well-publicized royal example.

The Reverend Cotton Mather did not know that inoculations were beginning to be performed in England when he called for them in Boston in 1721. News traveled very slowly across the ocean at that time. But two things led him to favor inoculation. First, William Douglass, the Scot who did not have a high regard for Boston's medical practitioners, had shown him the Timoni and Pylarini reports.[16] And second, Mather had learned that inoculation was also practiced in the Eastern Sahara from his servant Onesimus; a fact he confirmed by questioning other slaves and traders. Cotton Mather was so excited after acquiring this important information from such an unexpected "authority," that he even wrote a letter to the Royal Society in 1716. Why, he asked, were the English not practicing inoculation? Mather even stated that he would introduce the practice the next time smallpox threatened New England.

True to his word, Mather did his best in June 1721 to encourage the physicians of Boston to begin inoculating.[17] Nevertheless, only one of the ten physicians then practicing professionally took up the cause. That individual was Zabdiel Boylston, who had been trained as a medical apprentice.[18] The sole Boston physician having a European degree at this time was Douglass, and he had a low regard for Boylston as a physician, in part because of his lack of academic training.

Boylston, a smallpox survivor, inoculated his thirteen-year-old son and two black servants later that June. This was still before the colonists had learned about Lady Mary and the London inoculations. But it was after there seemed to be no hope of stopping the raging Boston epidemic (the guards were even removed from the doors of the houses of infected people). After the operation seemed to work on his first cases, Boylston transplanted scabs under the skin of others. The selectmen of the city were appalled and tried to stop him, while irate citizens rioted and even threatened to lynch him.[19]

Prominent among the opposition was Benjamin Franklin's brother James, the owner of the *New England Courant*. James argued that the procedure was dangerous for the individual and even worse for the community. But beneath the surface, his stance also reflected how he felt about Cotton Mather and the gripping tentacles of his church. He was not one to forget that Mather had supported the courts that condemned innocent people to the gallows during the Salem witchcraft trials of the 1690s, and he knew that Mather still believed that the devil and his forces of evil were behind all mishaps. To James and his associates at the *Courant*, Cotton Mather was a religious extremist who had no business dabbling in medicine—a man who had to be curtailed.[20] As might be expected, Mather did not take the assaults in the *Courant* lightly. He shot fiery salvos back using emotionally and morally charged rhetoric, such as "Satanic Fury" and "Malicious and Murderous," and accusing "the wicked printer and his accomplices" of blasphemy, debauchery, and libel.

At the time, many physicians were as frightened of the new procedure as they were of the disease. William Douglass, who was never one to be silent, argued that inoculation demanded more study with names and vital information and stricter enforcement to protect the community from the spread of the potentially deadly infection. He knew that some inoculated patients were venturing out or receiving visitors before their scabs fell off, putting others at risk. Many laymen, particularly the poor and those who viewed inoculation as human tinkering with God's divine plan, were even more terrified of inoculation than were their physicians. Public concern about inoculation would become so intense that rioting would break out over the issue in some communities.[21]

## GOING BY THE NUMBERS

Simple statistics began to be used in the eighteenth century to support arguments that might have been based solely on impressions in the past. They allowed natural philosophers to check reckless speculations and to shore up or reject ideas based solely on logic. Tables and percentages were also used to support legislation and bolster public opinion. The question of whether inoculation was worth the risk, at least to the individual, began to be assessed statistically soon after the procedure made its debut in Boston.

Cotton Mather and Boylston led the way.[22] They informed the Royal Society that, of the approximately three hundred people inoculated during the 1721 Boston epidemic, approximately one in sixty died, whereas the mortality percentage was higher than one in six for those who caught the disease in the natural way. Boylston personally inoculated 242 persons, only six of whom died, probably because they had been infected prior to the procedure. In contrast, he calculated that the epidemic killed 844 of the 5,889 non-inoculated people who contracted smallpox naturally.

Boylston was made a member of the Royal Society for his efforts, joining Cotton Mather, who had become the first American member of the elite organization prior to the epidemic. Nevertheless, the statistics presented by these two pioneers, like those that would follow, would tell only part of the story. Whether inoculating some people might also endanger others was another matter, and one much more difficult to assess.

Boylston's counterpart in England was Thomas Nettleton, a physician who collected statistics on the epidemic that swept through his part of Yorkshire in 1722. Nettleton surveyed how many people were inoculated in his region and how they fared relative to those who contracted smallpox in the natural way. He found that only one person of the 61 who had been inoculated died, whereas 20 percent of those not inoculated succumbed to smallpox. To Nettleton, who compared what he was doing to "the Merchant's Logic" in a business decision, it was clear where "the Balance Lyes."[23] Nettleton sent his material to physician James Jurin, secretary of the Royal Society, and the two men began a correspondence. Late in 1722, Jurin published Nettleton's Yorkshire findings in the Royal Society's *Philosophical Transactions*.[24] Jurin also asked other physicians to send statistics to him, while personally analyzing the London bills of mortality.

The statistical evidence, along with the letters and pamphlets that followed, motivated some people in the British Empire to have themselves inoculated.[25] Yet success still depended on three things: further spreading the word, helping those who could not afford the procedure, and making sure it was done properly.

## ENTER FRANKLIN

Young Benjamin Franklin was silent on the inoculation issue while he was in Boston, perhaps not knowing who was right, perhaps not wanting to get in trouble with his brother. Once he had his own printing press in Philadelphia, however, he did not hesitate to express firm opinions in public. With his uncanny ability to latch on to a good idea that had been put into circulation, he quickly grasped the advantages of collecting and presenting actual statistics: "Opinions are continually varying, where we cannot have mathematical evidence of the nature of things," he once wrote.[26] And with a determination to present more mathematical proof that inoculation really does work, he entered the arena, collecting, sharing, and reporting survival statistics, and then referring to inoculation as God's gift to suffering humanity.

One of Franklin's first published statements involving statistics appeared in the *Pennsylvania Gazette* during the spring of 1730. He informed his readers: "We hear from New-England, that the Small-Pox spreads in divers parts of the Country. There is an Account published of the Number of Persons inoculated in Boston in the Month of March, amounting to Seventy-two; of which two only died, and the rest have recovered perfect Health. Of those who had it in the common Way, 'tis computed that one in four died."[27]

He also sent statistics to friends and family members in distant localities, expecting them to spread the word. For example, during the summer of 1731 he penned a letter to his sister Jane Mecom in Rhode Island. "We have had the small pox here lately, which raged violently while it lasted," he wrote. "There have been about fifty persons inoculated, who all recovered, except a child of the doctor's, upon whom the small pox appeared within a day or two after the operation, and who is therefore thought to have been certainly infected before."[28]

The physician behind the Philadelphia inoculations at this point in time was John Kearsley, sometimes regarded as the father of medicine in Pennsylvania. Kearsley hoped to set an example for others by inoculating himself and the students apprenticed to him, who included John Redman, Thomas Bond, Phineas Bond, Lloyd Zachary, Thomas Cadwalader, the elder William Shippen, and John Bard. Franklin would soon collaborate with these distinguished Philadelphians on various civic projects, including the establishment of Pennsylvania Hospital.

Franky died from smallpox while Franklin was compiling statistics showing that inoculation was effective. In 1742, six years after this tragic event in his life, Debby gave birth to a healthy daughter. Four years later, Sarah, better known as Sally, was successfully inoculated, to the relief of her parents.

William Vassall, who had just moved to Boston from Philadelphia, was one of the people who asked Franklin for some of his statistics the year Sally was inoculated. "By the best Informations I have been able to procure, and which I believe are pretty near the Truth," Franklin responded, "between 150 and 160 Persons (mostly Children, the Small Pox having gone thro' this place twice within these 15 Years) have been inoculated since the 10th of April last, when the Distemper began to spread here; of which Number one only died. . . . Of the Rest who recovered or are on the Recovery, none have had so much as one dangerous Symptom."[29]

Franklin informed Vassall that the one child who died did not succumb from the inoculation. But he was concerned that many citizens were still not recognizing the value of the operation, in part because the latest epidemic was so mild that few people died. With this on his mind, he added: "Our Physicians however agree, that those who have taken the Infection in the Common Way here, have not generally had the Distemper so light as those that were inoculated."[30]

Franklin even told Vassall how he might inoculate himself using the colonial postal system he had done so much to improve. "As to your going to New York to be inoculated, perhaps such a Journey is not quite necessary," he wrote, since . . . a dry Scab or two will communicate the Distemper by Inoculation. . . . And such might be sent to you per Post from hence, cork'd up tight in a small Phial."[31] Showing his breadth of knowledge on the subject, Franklin closed his letter with a short remark about the Chinese method of inoculation, which had been described to the Royal Society in 1700 by Joseph Lister. "And I have somewhere read, that the Chinese actually preserve Scabs from a healthy Person for the Purpose, tho' their Manner of Inoculation is different from ours."[32]

Four years later, in 1750, Franklin exchanged letters with Samuel Johnson, who held a doctorate from Oxford and was a candidate to head Franklin's newly formed Academy of Philadelphia.[33] While Johnson was weighing the pros and cons of moving to Philadelphia, Franklin informed him that yet another smallpox epidemic was starting in the city. He warned him that he should definitely be inoculated "for greater safety."

Later in that year, a more notable exchange took place. Franklin had been in contact with Dr. Adam Thompson, who was born and trained in Scotland but settled in Philadelphia in 1748. Thompson was touting a better way to prepare the body for inoculation.[34] He had begun to work on his safeguards in 1738, and his recommendations evolved into a two-week regimen. Key features included a light diet, bleeding, purging, and a combination of two agents thought to act as antidotes against smallpox "poisoning," mercury and antimony.

Thompson wanted permission to give a public lecture in Philadelphia on his new technique, and Franklin helped by securing a large lecture hall for his speech.[35] The talk took place in November 1750, only to create a storm of protest. Some listeners thought his methods too severe. But even more were incensed by his condescending contention that most American medical practitioners were so poorly educated that laws should be passed to allow only qualified physicians to inoculate.

Thompson's words about limiting the practice of inoculation must have been disturbing to Franklin. After all, he had just informed Samuel Johnson how to do it himself. Nevertheless, Franklin wanted to be fair and to give both sides full access to his press. Hence, he first published Thompson's *Discourse on the Preparation of the Body for the Small-Pox*.[36] Then he published various objections to Thompson's ideas, including a rebuttal by physician John Kearsley. Not quite finished, he printed Thompson's rejoinders.

Franklin came forth with more statistics after the debate, some of which went to William Douglass, the Boston physician who had been violently opposed to the procedure in 1721.[37] Douglass had asked Franklin for the latest Philadelphia statistics when Boston's eighth smallpox epidemic started in 1752. Not blind to the data he had already seen, he was now willing to promote the operation, provided the patient was kept in strict isolation until the scabs fell off.

Franklin informed Douglass that the latest epidemic had been particularly severe. One-third of the population had contracted smallpox naturally, and at least 10 percent had died. In contrast, there were few deaths among those who had been inoculated. The statistics confirmed yet again the effectiveness of the procedure against a disease that no medicine seemed able to cure.

What Franklin did not tell Douglass was that smallpox was slowly becoming endemic in Philadelphia. The problem was that inadequate laws and weak enforcement were permitting recently inoculated people to mingle with the masses before it was safe, much as Douglass feared. Inoculation was still a two-edged sword: a gift to some, a curse to others.

## POOR RICHARD AND THE SPECKLED MONSTER

Poor Richard, like his publisher, was not passive about smallpox prevention. In 1737, a few lines of his poetry touted inoculation as "Life's great Preservation."[38] But it was not until thirteen years later that Poor Richard really showed his readers just how learned he had become, and precisely why he was so biased on this issue.

"On the 17th of this Month, 1722," he told his loyal readers,

the Princesses Amelia and Carolina, were inoculated for the Small Pox, after the Experiment had been tried for the first Time in England on some condemned Malefactors. The Example of the Court was soon followed by many of the Nobility and Gentry, and Success attending the Practice, 'tis now grown more common in many Parts of Europe. Tho' at first it was reckoned by many to be a *rash* and almost *impious* Action, to give a Distemper to a Person in Health, . . . it now begins to be thought *rash* to hazard taking it in the common Way, by which one in seven is generally lost; and *impious* to reject a Method discovered to Mankind by God's good Providence, whereby 99 in 100 are saved.[39]

Poor Richard also summarized a report from Charles-Marie de La Condamine, explorer, chemist, and follower of Newton: "Monsieur Condamine, a French Academician, who, in 1744, made a Voyage from Peru, down the River Amazones, thro' the Middle of South America [to determine whether the earth was a sphere], reports, that a few Years before, the Small-Pox getting among the Indians, full half of those taken sick were carried off by it: Which a Portuguese Missionary observing, and having met by Chance with an Account of Inoculation in a News Paper, he try'd it on great Numbers of his Indian Disciples, and preserved them all."[40]

Poor Richard did not tell his readers how to inoculate themselves using his master's postal system. But his many verses, histories, and short entries showed his many faithful followers that there was only one sensible course to choose, and it was not being passive or trying to run away.

## THE POOR

Franklin did not abandon his inoculation campaign after he was asked to go to England in 1757 by the Pennsylvania Assembly. Rather, he expanded his horizons and began to press for inoculations in Europe as well as in his homeland. In addition, he showed an increasing concern for the poor—the group least likely to undergo inoculation because they could not afford to miss going to work while being kept in isolation.

The need to support smallpox charities for the poor was a recurrent theme in *Gentleman's Magazine*, which was founded by Edward Cave in 1731 to disseminate the latest political, scientific, and medical information.[41] Cave usually avoided taking a stand when material was controversial; he was much more likely to publish letters from people with different opinions and to stand back. But he and his medical editors came out in favor of inoculation.

In 1752, a piece from him or one of his staff members stated: "Why will the inhabitants of Great Britain risk their lives with this most dreadful, shocking disease, when they may, almost to a certainty, escape it with eyes and features, I mean by Inoculation."[42] Cave also urged the magazine's readership not to think about individuals but about whole communities, including those at the bottom of the ladder that could not afford the procedure. Franklin regularly read and occasionally published material in *Gentleman's Magazine*, and he embraced this philosophy even before he sailed to England in 1757.

Soon after settling in London, Franklin met William Heberden, a distinguished member of the Royal College of Physicians. The two men discussed smallpox inoculations among the masses, both in England and America. England had gone through its most extensive and deadly outbreak of smallpox in 1752, and it followed the previous epidemic by just six years. The odds of still another deadly "visitation" were already high and increasing daily.

Franklin wanted to be proactive, especially with the poor, and he pushed Heberden to write a brief pamphlet. The result, *Some Account of the Success of Inoculation for the Small-Pox in England and America Together with Plain Instructions, by Which Any Person May Be Enabled to Perform the Operation and Conduct the Patient through the Distemper*, was published in 1759.[43] In his four-page introduction to this twelve-page pamphlet, Franklin had a few facts wrong, such as the date of one epidemic. But these errors did not detract from what Heberden and he had set out to accomplish.

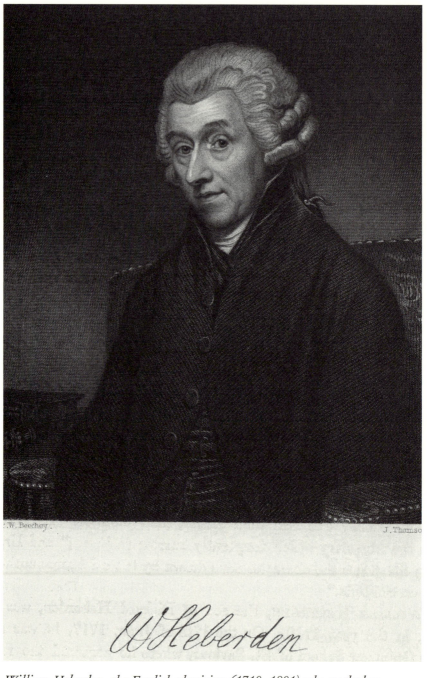

*William Heberden, the English physician (1710–1801) who worked on smallpox inoculations with Franklin.*

Franklin began by describing how most Bostonians opposed inoculation until statistics repeatedly showed it could save lives. To drive the point home, he provided a table of statistics from North America. Of those Americans who were not inoculated and came down with the disease, more than 10 percent died. In contrast, only 1 percent of those that had been inoculated died from smallpox. He also presented statistics gathered from the London Smallpox and Inoculation Hospital, the charitable institution that was founded in 1746 to treat and prevent the disease.[44] There were 6 deaths among the 1,601 persons inoculated at the hospital, but 1,002 deaths among the 3,856 smallpox patients not inoculated. "By this account it appears, that in the way of Inoculation there has died but one patient in 267, whereas in the common way there has died more than one in four," explained Franklin. The message in simple words that everybody could understand was unmistakable.[45]

After presenting these compelling statistics, Franklin turned to the monetary issues that for too long had acted as a barrier. He commented on how a surgeon may charge more money than could be spared. Then he promised that Heberden's contribution, which would follow, would show parents how to inoculate themselves and their children step by step at minimal expense.

Heberden hesitated putting his name on the pamphlet, not seeing a reason to take personal credit. But Franklin was insistent on divulging his name. As a printer, he knew how best to reach the public and he was sure that Heberden's fame would greatly increase the likelihood of their pamphlet being read. If people would just read what was written, he reasoned, "surely parents will no longer refuse to accept and thankfully use a discovery GOD in his mercy has been pleased to bless mankind with."[46]

True to the ideals of the Enlightenment, the two contributors then absorbed the expenses involved with the pamphlet's publication. Franklin personally sent 1,500 copies to David Hall, who was running his printing operations in Philadelphia, with instructions to distribute it free to the needy. He also sent copies to Jonathan Williams, Sr., for distribution in Boston, and to relatives, friends, and acquaintances elsewhere, in the hope that they would share it with others.

Thomas Moffatt, who lived in Newport, Rhode Island, received one of the pamphlets. Although hardly a skilled writer, he sent a note back to Franklin. "I return you thanks for sending me Dr. Heberdens method of inoculating the small pox of which perhaps to you it may not be necessary to say that it bears every mark of Judgment candour and benevolence," were his grateful words.[47]

## CONSEQUENCES

Franklin's sustained efforts to fight smallpox, even while in England, can be associated with multiple effects. One was that more organizations were now established to help inoculate the poor. In 1774, he helped raise money for a new organization in Philadelphia, the "Society for Inoculating the Poor Gratis." Eight physicians, including Thomas Bond, helped with the inoculations and, following the example set in London, Philadelphia soon had its own "Inoculating Hospital."

A second tangible consequence of Franklin's good work was a greater willingness of people from higher socioeconomic classes to be inoculated. In America, this group included delegates to the First Continental Congress, which met in Philadelphia in 1774. Many well-to-do Europeans, including a good number of Franklin's friends in Britain, also heeded his advice, and those with children inoculated them as soon as it was safe.[48]

Franklin's campaigning also helped change the course of the American War of Independence. But, as pointed out by historian Elizabeth Fenn, even with another smallpox epidemic raging at the time the war started, the battle against smallpox in the army neither started off well nor came easily.[49] George Washington was initially prevented from inoculating his troops and, by the end of 1776, approximately ten times as many soldiers died from smallpox (the worst offender) and other diseases than from battle wounds. Equally discouraging, the fear of contracting smallpox was making it difficult to enlist new recruits. The poor health of the Continental Army gave a distinct advantage to the British, who made sure their fighting men had immunity.

Following a series of disasters, the program to inoculate all susceptible men in the Continental Army and all new recruits finally began in 1777. It was received enthusiastically by the soldiers and their officers. Franklin was in France when he received the letter that informed him: "Our Troops have been under inoculation from the Small Pox with great success." The letter continued: "It will frustrate one Cannibal Scheme of our Enemies who have constantly fought us with that disease by introducing it among our troops."[50] Both Washington and Franklin believed that the British employed biological warfare from 1775, when they first occupied Boston, through the epic battle at Yorktown in 1781.[51]

Not mentioned by Franklin was the fact that smallpox-infected blankets had previous been used to protect the settlers in Western Pennsylvania from hostile Indians. During Pontiac's Rebellion in 1763, Sir Jeffrey Amherst, then commanding general of the British forces in North America, gave Colonel Henry Bouquet permission to distribute scab-infested blankets to the natives.[52] The Indians who took the blankets became sick and then spread the disease by sneezing and coughing. The result was an epidemic that ended the uprising.[53]

## BEYOND INOCULATION

Today, the person most likely to be associated with smallpox prevention is Edward Jenner, who made his mark just after Franklin died.[54] Jenner's contribution was *vaccination* (*vacca* means cow in Latin), an improvement over *variolation* (the use of human material). By collecting information on milkmaids and dairy farmers in England, and by conducting careful experiments, he showed that exposure to cowpox could give people immunity against human smallpox without the risk of spreading a potentially deadly disease.

Jenner's publications were landmarks in medicine, but he did not write the opening chapter in the inoculation story, and his work had no effect on the epidemics and wars that claimed so many lives and changed the course of history during the turbulent eighteenth century. In this regard, what Lady Montagu, Cotton Mather, and Zabdiel Boylston managed to do prior to Jenner was important. So were the efforts of Thomas Nettleton and James Jurin in England, and Benjamin Franklin of Philadelphia, who successfully campaigned for inoculation by collecting more statistics and spreading the word with the help of pervasive pens and powerful printing presses.

# CHAPTER 4

# The Citizen and the Hospital

This Building by the Bounty of the Government, and of many Private Persons, was Piously Founded for the Relief of the Sick and Miserable.

—Benjamin Franklin's inscription for cornerstone of Pennsylvania Hospital, 1756

On February 10, 1752, American cultural and medical history was made in Philadelphia. That day, two patients, Margaret Sherlock and Hannah Shines, were admitted to the temporary building that would be used until construction could be completed on a recently approved new building for the city's Pennsylvania Hospital. This institution would be the first major civilian hospital in the colonies for needy men and women. It would become a haven for physically sick or injured patients, Margaret Sherlock being the first such patient, and for the mentally ill, of which Hannah Shines was the first.

Benjamin Franklin did not come up with the idea for the new hospital. That honor belongs to Philadelphia physician Thomas Bond. At the time, a major movement was under way in Europe to build hospitals for the sick-poor. Philanthropic citizens in England and Scotland were deeply involved in the movement, and they provided shining examples of what could be done for suffering humanity. Franklin, like Bond, was aware of what was happening abroad. To his credit, he recognized the importance of Bond's floundering proposal and played the leading role in securing funding for the charitable project, thereby making it a reality.

Before even starting on the hospital project, Franklin had immersed himself in a number of other institutional projects for the public good: his Junto, Library Company, and American Philosophical Society. These efforts, like his campaign for inoculation, stemmed from his philosophy to do good for his community and his drive to better himself. But in addition to citizenship and self-betterment, they brought him into contact with many talented and influential people. Some of these people became his friends, others provided him with information for his newspaper, and still others helped him to become more financially secure with lucrative printing contracts and civil service appointments. Of equal importance, some of his earlier institutions had clear ties to medicine, which helped him to appreciate how important a hospital could be for his adopted city.

## THE JUNTO

When Franklin sailed home from London in 1726, he looked for a club to improve himself and life in general in Philadelphia. Not finding one, he founded a club a year later, basing it on Cotton Mather's neighborhood benefit societies. But whereas Mather's societies in New England had deep religious overtones, Franklin's new club was decidedly secular. Franklin first called his small group the Leather Apron Club, since it was initially composed of twelve young artisans and tradesmen. It included a copier of deeds, a surveyor, a shoemaker, a mechanic, a clerk, and some friends from the printing trade. The group first met on Friday evenings at a local alehouse. Later the club became known as the Junto.

"The rules I drew up," Franklin tells us, "required that every member, in his turn, should produce one or more queries on any point of Morals, Politics, or Natural Philosophy, to be discuss'd by the company; and once in three months produce and read an essay of his own writing, on any subject he pleased. Our debates were to be under the direction of a president . . . without fondness for dispute, or desire of victory."[1]

The Junto went over a list of "Proposals and Standing Queries" at every meeting, some of which pertained to health and medicine. In order to help maintain the health of the membership, the suggestion was made "That once a month in Spring, Summer and Fall the Junto meet of a Sunday in the Afternoon in some proper place cross the River for Bodily Exercise."[2] A greater number of the group's queries, in contrast, were more involved with practical medicine than with personal hygiene and prevention. One read: "Have you or any of your acquaintance been lately sick or wounded? If so, what remedies were used, and what were their effects?"[3] Another raised a deep moral question: "Is it justifiable to put private Men to Death for the Sake of publick Safety or Tranquility, who have committed no Crime? As in the Case of the Plague to stop Infection."[4]

With questions such as these, it is easy to understand why Franklin called his Junto "the best school of philosophy, morality, and politics that then existed in the province."[6] It proved so successful that it led to several smaller Juntos, each headed by one of the original members, and it resulted in several more visible colonial institutions. Among its offspring were the Library Company and the American Philosophical Society, both of which also helped to change the medical landscape by dispersing information and stimulating the development of new ideas.

## THE LIBRARY COMPANY

The idea of "clubbing our books to a common library" first emerged in Franklin's mind in 1730.[6] But although the pooling idea was well received, the Junto members, being mainly tradesmen, did not own a large number of books. Not one to abandon a good idea, and understanding the power of grouping resources, Franklin proposed a circulating subscription library that would not be restricted to Junto members.

Franklin described the origin of the Library Company as follows: "I pro-pos'd to render the benefit from books more common, by commencing a public subscription library. I drew a sketch of the plan ... by which each sub-scriber engag'd to pay a certain sum down for the first purchase of books, and an annual contribution for increasing them. So few were the readers at that time in Philadelphia, and the majority of us so poor, that I was not able, with great industry, to find more than fifty persons, mostly young tradesmen, willing to pay down for this purpose, forty shillings each, and ten shillings per annum. On this little fund we began."[7]

It did not take long before some of Thomas Sydenham's medical books were on the shelves, along with other medical and philosophical tracts. In addition, the Library Company acquired animal specimens, fossils, and pieces of equipment, including globes and a telescope. "The library afforded me the means of improvement by constant study," wrote Franklin, "for which I set apart an hour or two each day, and thus repair'd in some degree the loss of the learned education my father once intended for me."[8] With obvious pride in what he was able to achieve, he stated: "This was the mother of all the North American subscription libraries, now so numerous. . . . These libraries have improved the general conversation of the Americans, [and] made the common tradesmen and farmers as intelligent as most gen-tlemen from other countries."[9]

## THE AMERICAN PHILOSOPHICAL SOCIETY

The notion of a national society for exchanging useful knowledge fol-lowed several years later. John Bartram, a self-educated farmer who started a botanical garden near Philadelphia in 1728 and then became a world-famous botanist, might have been the first Philadelphian to envision an inter-colonial society.[10] In a letter to Peter Collinson in London, which was probably written in 1739, he asked the English Quaker and natural philosopher what he thought about an American academy that would bring "ingenious & Curious men" together for the "study of naturale secrets[,] arts & scyances." Collinson, however, was not enthusiastic, thinking the colonists not yet ready for such a society.

Bartram was discouraged only temporarily, because a few years later he shared his vision with Franklin, who concluded that the time was right. Franklin then used his formidable persuasive skills to institutionalize Bartram's idea. In 1743 he wrote and published *A Proposal for Promoting Useful Knowledge Among the British Plantations in America*.[11] It began with some words about the drudgery of settling the new colonies now being a thing of the past. And it called for "One Society be formed of Virtuosi or ingenious Men residing in the several Colonies, to be called the American Philosophical Society."

The proposal "to improve the common Stock of Knowledge" for "the Benefit of Mankind in general" was personally distributed by Franklin and Bartram. A year later, the American Philosophical Society had its core group and began meeting in Philadelphia.[12] It promoted discourses on a wide variety of subjects, including, as stated in the original plan, the discovery of "New Methods of Curing or Preventing Disease."

This subject was of particular interest to Thomas and Phineas Bond, brothers and the two Philadelphia physicians in the founding group. And since this topic included medicinal plants, it was also of special interest to John Bartram and John Tennent, who was a corresponding member from Virginia. Cadwallader Colden, who had practiced medicine in Philadelphia but now lived in New York, was also drawn to the society by the medical theme. In fact, he had been thinking about an "arts and sciences" society even before Bartram, as revealed in a communication dated 1729 to William Douglass in Boston.[13] Despite the enthusiasm of Franklin, Bartram, Colden, and several others, however, the American Philosophical Society got off to a rocky start. Franklin complained to Colden that "The Members of our Society here are very Idle Gentlemen, they take no pains."[14] For all intents and purposes, the organization was dead by 1747, although Franklin, then its secretary, preferred the term "dormant."

In 1767, while Franklin was in England, Thomas Bond resurrected the society and two years later it merged with the newer American Society for Promoting Useful Knowledge. At the time, the two groups overlapped in their objectives, but their members differed in politics, religion, and social status. Franklin was made president of the united "American Philosophical Society, held at Philadelphia, for Promoting Useful Knowledge," and Thomas Bond was elected vice president. John Bartram, the hunter and gatherer of America's botanical assets, and since 1764 Botanist to the King, remained an active member of the reorganized society, which became increasingly important on the world stage.

Thus, Franklin's Junto, Library Company, and American Philosophical Society all had ties to medicine. But to most Philadelphians at mid-century, Franklin's most significant institutional project in the medical sphere was the highly visible Pennsylvania Hospital.

## THE VOLUNTARY HOSPITAL MOVEMENT

Pennsylvania Hospital, founded on January 23, 1751, is usually regarded as the first permanent, public hospital established for the care of needy sick civilians in the English colonies.[15] Prior to this date, almshouses and work-houses took in sick paupers, but their primary concerns were to provide shelter and sustenance, not medical care, for men and women who could not take care of themselves.[16]

In addition, there were pest houses and lazarettos, which were located away from the cities on such places as Spectacle Island (Boston), Bedloe's Island (New York), and Fisher's Island (Philadelphia). These structures for the "distempered," however, were erected only to isolate infected individuals from the larger, vulnerable community that demanded protection. They were not set up to heal.

To be fair, some British Colonial facilities that deserved to be called hospitals existed prior to 1751, but they were so small, short-lived, or poorly documented that very little is known about them.[17] In 1612, for example, the sick and the lame on the James River were put in a separate structure. But we know nothing more about this small "Hospitall" in Virginia that might have been burned to the ground during an Indian uprising.

By the middle of the eighteenth century there was a growing need for facilities in the colonies to serve the physically sick who had nowhere else to turn, and the insane who were wandering the streets. This humanitarian need and growing burden to society was greatest in the rapidly growing coastal cities. It reflected the increase in immigration to America and included an increasing number of men and women without families, friends, or tangible resources.

Between 1730 and 1750, Philadelphia had grown by 33 percent to some

15,000 residents, making it the second largest city (behind London) in the British Empire and one of its most important commercial ports. Although the number of sick poor is impossible to estimate, this segment might have grown even faster than the general population, negatively affecting the image, social order, and economics of the city.[18] With its philanthropic Quaker population, civic-minded leaders, and businessmen, no city in America was more aware of its poor and how they affected the economy. And with some of the best doctors in the colonies, no city could match the human resources Philadelphia could provide for restoring impoverished men and women to health and productivity.

The idea for a proper sick house was discussed at a Friends' monthly meeting as early as 1709, but nothing came of it. When the idea rose again four decades later, the model for what should be done came from the growing voluntary hospital movement in Britain.[19] Reflecting the evolving concerns and social values of the Enlightenment, the hospital movement went hand in hand with the building of charity schools, orphanages, almshouses, and better prisons.

Robert Nelson, a Puritan writer and philanthropist, was a key figure behind what transpired in England. In 1715, he published his *Address to Persons of Quality and Estate*.[20] It called for hospitals for the incurable and for other facilities to treat the major "distempers of the body," which in his mind included consumption, dropsy, and rheumatism. He felt that building new hospitals would save thousands of lives, while providing subjects for "useful experiments" that might advance medicine.

Nelson's publication brought attention to the poor in need of medical help, and to the idea that hospitals would be good for the public at large. And he was not alone. John Bellers, an English merchant, also played a part in the movement.[21] His proposal also called for well-staffed hospitals to treat the sick poor, and he too linked teaching and research to the venture. He thought that free hospitals would provide physicians with much needed post-mortem material, a right rarely obtained in private practice.

The Westminster Infirmary was the first of the major British voluntary hospitals to provide the poor-sick with "food and physick." It opened in London in 1720, and more voluntary hospitals soon sprung up in London, Bath, Liverpool, Exeter, and Winchester. All were organized by concerned citizens and backed by large individual benefactors or groups of philanthropic subscribers. Assisting the sick in this way was viewed as an act of Christian charity, although such actions also enhanced the prestige of the donor, unless that person chose to remain anonymous.

With limited resources, the managers of the new voluntary hospitals did their best to distinguish between the sick poor worthy of services and the lower sort who did not deserve help. The bias was clearly to treat injured or ill workers, as well as sick mothers with dependent children. The overseers were decidedly less interested in helping alcoholic men and prostitutes, who tried to take advantage of the shelter, food, and care that was offered.

## THE EDINBURGH INFIRMARY

In retrospect, it was a facility in Scotland, more than any other British voluntary hospital, that Thomas Bond, Franklin, and other enlightened Philadelphians looked up to and hoped to emulate on American soil. Founded in 1729, the Edinburgh Infirmary treated worthy charity patients with physical or mental illnesses, and reduced the welfare rolls by allowing many of these people to become productive again.[22] It was also a leading institution for practical training and bedside medical education. And unlike the voluntary hospitals in London, it served a city comparable in size to Philadelphia.[23]

In a letter dated January 3, 1760, to Sir Alexander Dick, president of the College of Physicians of Edinburgh, Benjamin Franklin wrote: "It may give you and my good Lord Provost some Pleasure, to see that we have imitated the Edinburgh Institution of an Infirmary in that remote Part of the World. Thus they that do good, not only do good themselves, but by their Examples are the Occasion of much Good being done by others."[24]

Franklin was unable to visit the Edinburgh Infirmary prior to involving himself with Pennsylvania Hospital. His first trip there took place in 1759. But a number of Philadelphia physicians and civic leaders had visited Edinburgh and had been corresponding with Scottish physicians. In addition, reports were appearing in *Gentleman's Magazine* about what was transpiring at the Edinburgh Infirmary and with other British voluntary hospitals.[25] In 1741, for example, the periodical published "A View *of the many* peculiar *Advantages* of a Public Hospital." It concerned the new Devon and Exeter Hospital, but its message was much broader:

A *Public Hospital* is the only *certain* way of relieving the Poor-Sick; who are frequently neglected and over-looked at their own Homes; . . . It is the most *safe* and *eligible* manner of doing it; because the Care and Neatness as well as the Simplicity and Regularity of the Diet with which the Poor are kept in an Hospital, do all contribute much sooner to their Recovery, than their own way of living; . . . The *Expense* of relieving a great Number of Sick Persons in any Hospital, bears no proportion to *that* of assisting them at their respective Homes; . . . It opens a channel for *private* Charities. . . . It *prevents* most of the Evils that are common to the *Poor,* by administering an *immediate* Support in the time of Sickness; . . . It provides for the Relief and Comfort of Multitudes who are *unable* to be at the Expense of Advice or Physick . . . and are of the Diligent and Industrious sort, which is a most useful and valuable part of society. . . . It preserves them from the ill Usage of *Quacks* and *Imposters* . . . [and] it is of infinite Use to *all other* Persons, by furnishing the *Physicians* and *Surgeons* with more experience in *one* Year, than they could have in *ten* without it.[26]

Thomas Bond, who was born in Maryland in 1713, fully understood the benefits that a new hospital would bring to Philadelphia. Details of Bond's own medical training are scant, but it is believed he entered medicine as an apprentice and made his first pilgrimage to Europe in 1738, after he had practiced medicine in Philadelphia for several years.[27] Bond seems to have spent about fifteen months in England, where he visited several hospitals and spoke with physicians, and in France, where he spent time at the Hôtel Dieu, the famous Paris hospital. And although he did not get to Edinburgh, his younger brother Phineas studied medicine there.[28] After Thomas Bond returned to Philadelphia, he engrossed himself in private practice and served as port inspector for contagious diseases. He also joined with Franklin on several projects. He suggested medical books for his Library Company, was involved with establishing the Academy of Philadelphia, and was among the founding members of the American Philosophical Society. With his background, clinical practice, and philanthropy, Thomas Bond was ideally positioned to recognize the need for a public hospital in Philadelphia—one that would do more than the small Philadelphia Almshouse that was established two decades earlier. But when the idea for a charity hospital entered his mind in 1750, he lacked the skills to attract needed financial backers.

## FUNDING AND BUILDING THE HOSPITAL

It was under these circumstances that Bond approached Franklin for help with his proposed project, which, he admitted, was "not well understood." Franklin described what transpired, although without his usual modesty. "At length, he came to me with the compliment that he found there was no such thing as carrying a public-spirited project through without my being concern'd in it," he wrote. "'For,' says he, 'I am often ask'd by those to whom I propose subscribing, Have you consulted Franklin upon this business? And what does he think of it? And when I tell them that I have not . . . they do not subscribe, but say they will consider it.'"[29] Franklin further relates that he "enquired into the nature and probable utility of his scheme, and receiving from him a very satisfactory explanation, I not only subscrib'd to it myself, but engag'd heartily in the design of procuring subscriptions from others."[30]

Franklin's means for "procuring subscriptions" were so ingenious that they still elicit smiles from professional fundraisers. He effectively used his *Pennsylvania Gazette* to convince the citizens how much the poor really needed a hospital, and how important it was for the people in the region to be recognized as good Samaritans. In his words: "I endeavoured to prepare the minds of the people by writing on the subject in newspapers, which was my usual custom in such cases, but which he [Bond] had omitted."[31] Second, he drafted a petition to the Pennsylvania Assembly that thirty-three upstanding citizens signed. Third, he wrote and distributed a pamphlet to present the hospital plan in more detail to interested backers, whose financial support was critical. Finally, he called for matching funds from the government, a fundraising tool that did not appear to have been used before, at least not in America.

For Franklin, matching funds meant going to the Pennsylvania Assembly and convincing its representatives to promise £2,000 for the project, contingent on an equal amount being raised from the citizenry. Thinking such an enormous sum would never be raised, the rural members of the Assembly, who were not particularly enthusiastic about the project, voted for the proposal, many wanting just to look charitable. The representatives from Philadelphia, in contrast, were more strongly in favor of the project, knowing it would be located in their city, where it was most needed.

As it turned out, the doubting Thomases from rural Pennsylvania grossly underestimated how positively the citizens in and around Philadelphia would respond to the project. Following the lead of some significant donors, men and women from all social classes opened their purses and gave what they could. Contributors believed they were giving twice as much, "since every man's donation would be doubled," as Franklin put it. In brief, once Franklin threw his full support and creative fundraising methods into the Pennsylvania Hospital project, what had once been just a kindly physician's lofty dream became brick-and-mortar reality.

After funding was assured and twelve managers were elected, negotiations began with the Penns, the proprietors of the Province of Pennsylvania, who lived in London. The managers hoped for an outright gift of a suitable plot of land for a new building. The Penns endorsed the project, but sent the befuddled managers a contract for a piece of land that was less than ideal, with stipulations they were unwilling to accept. The fact that the site offered by the Penns was near a swamp was particularly discouraging, since every-one believed that individuals living or working near bogs and marshes faced a greater risk of contracting dangerous fevers and other diseases. This fear was based on the notion that airborne "miasmas" permeated these salubrious regions, especially during the warmer months.[32] In the eighteenth century, the term "malaria" literally meant bad air.

After more negotiations and delays that took the frustrated managers into 1754, plans for the building were finally able to move forward. The managers purchased almost an entire block on the southwestern outskirts of the city for £500. It would be here that the new hospital would be constructed.

Two years before this land was even purchased, however, the sick and maimed of the poorer class began to line up for services at an inner-city house that served as temporary hospital quarters. The first patients were admitted in 1752, and Thomas Bond performed the first surgery, a leg ampu-tation, later that year. By the spring of 1753, more than sixty worthy patients had been treated at the temporary facility, and there were more applicants than the building could handle.

The chief architect-engineer for the new building was Samuel Rhoads, a member of Franklin's American Philosophical Society and one of the twelve hospital managers. Rhoads had worked closely with the medical staff on the hospital's design. Given the serious financial constraints, his plan called for

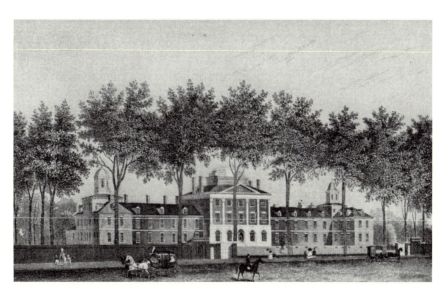

*An engraving of the Pennsylvania Hospital as it appeared around 1800.*

the hospital to be constructed in three phases. The east wing of the elegant new hospital was constructed first, and it opened during the winter of 1756. Franklin composed the inscription for the cornerstone, and Thomas Bond and he designed the hospital's seal. (The west wing opened in 1796, and the center wing with its surgical amphitheater opened in 1804.)

Franklin did everything he could to make sure the hospital had sufficient revenues for day-to-day services. Never at a loss for ideas, he promoted the use of charity boxes, like those found at places of worship. A coin box was put at the entry to the hospital, and each of the twelve hospital managers was handed his own tin box with "Charity for the Hospital" printed in gold letters on it.[33] Although the individual contributions varied in size, they were considerable when combined, much like the funds pooled to buy books for his Library Company.

In addition to these monies, Franklin helped to write bylaws that required each apprentice to pay the hospital 34 shillings per year to cover expenses. And to conserve money while also helping patients regain a good work ethic, Franklin backed Rule 15, which read: "Such patients as are able shall assist in nursing others, washing and ironing the Linen, washing and cleaning the Rooms, and other such Services as the Matron shall require."[34]

## MEDICINE AT THE HOSPITAL

Three established physicians volunteered to help at the new hospital. Two, as might be expected, were the Bond brothers, and the third was Lloyd Zachary. None accepted fees and all even purchased drugs with their own funds, until "the charitable Widows, and other good Women of Philadelphia" stepped forth to help with the costs of the medicines. The widows also donated linens, surgical dressings, and other items, setting an example for other citizens to follow.

The hospital rules specified who could be treated. Although the institution was built for "The relief of the sick poor and for the reception and cure of lunaticks," the managers could allow other patients to be admitted—provided empty beds were available and a family member or a sponsor would be willing to cover the expenses associated with the room, meals, and medical services. Still, the rules made it clear that the hospital would not serve the physically incurable or the dying. These people, however worthy, belonged at home, in almshouses, or elsewhere. Also excluded were people with certain infectious diseases, including smallpox and yellow fever, for fear that they would infect others.

Rules to get rid of disruptive patients, meaning those men and women of right mind who should know better, were also enforced. Expulsion could result from swearing, cursing, drinking, acting indecently, gambling, or begging for money. To lessen the chances that unruly patients would even be admitted, character references from the proper sort had to be presented to the hospital staff prior to an admission.

Medicine was practiced in a traditional manner on the patients who met these standards. The physicians looked at their bodies, monitored what went in and came out, and tried to provide nourishing foods. The patients were given vegetables, grains, dairy products, fowl, meat, and fish. Wine, beer, cider, and rum were also offered, the belief being that alcoholic beverages, in moderation, may be beneficial to health. Following the European model that was popular at the time, the so-called heroic therapies were employed when needed. Hence, patients at Pennsylvania Hospital were bled, purged, and sweated to remove suspected poisons and excesses, and to open up suspected blockages. On occasion, native cures and folk medicine were also practiced at the bedside.

Dr. Benjamin Rush, a major figure in American medicine whom Franklin helped early in his career, reminisced years later about Pennsylvania Hospital's start. He wrote that "When our late illustrious fellow citizen Dr. Franklin walked out from his house to lay the foundation stone of the Pennsylvania Hospital, he was accompanied by the late Dr. Bond and the managers and physicians of the Hospital. On their way Dr. Bond lamented that the Hospital would allure strangers from all the then provinces in America. 'Then,' said Dr. Franklin, 'our institution will be more useful than we intended it to be.'" In his next sentence, Rush told the managers that Franklin was right, "particularly in the relief our Hospital has afforded to persons deprived of their reason from nearly all the states in the Union."[35]

Indeed, the new hospital quickly became a center for treating the sick and injured, not just in Philadelphia but for surrounding regions and provinces. And it garnered an excellent reputation for humane care for the mentally ill, who were nonetheless not treated well by today's standards. Early on, some insane patients were chained with leg locks, manacled, or kept in straitjackets, as was done in Britain's mad hospitals. Moreover, they tended to be housed in the worst cells, the rationale being that the mad seemed more beast-like, and therefore less sensitive to cold and other stressful environmental conditions.[36]

Equally disheartening, curious members of the outside community were at first allowed to wander the hospital wards freely. Although most visitors meant well—especially those who wanted to see how people they knew were being treated or how their donations were being used—a few deliberately teased, mocked, and tormented the mentally ill for sheer entertainment. The situation again paralleled what was taking place in the public madhouses in Britain, most notably at Bedlam, where the hospital managers were hesitant to lock the gates, believing that having company would be therapeutic and would result in more coins in the charity boxes.[37] Greater sensitivity would not emerge until later in the eighteenth century.

## AN ACCOUNTING

In 1754, Franklin published a forty-page report on what had been accomplished since Pennsylvania Hospital's start in 1751, largely to generate more funding.[38] In *Some Account of the Pennsylvania Hospital* he presented a description of the institution's brief history and copies of its most important early documents. Franklin, ever concerned about financing, placed a contribution form at the end of his account. Surprising even him, it elicited £2,000, some from subscribers thousands of miles away.

Franklin's report included a list of admissions and, consistent with the strategy he was using to promote smallpox inoculations, some eye-catching statistics. Between February 1752 and May 1753, "there were Sixty-four Patients received into the Hospital, afflicted with Lunacy, and various other Disorders, which required the Conveniences of such a Place; of which Number Thirty-two were cured and discharged, and some others received considerable Relief. We likewise report, that we have visited the Hospital, and find a considerable Number of distemper'd Patients there, who are well taken Care of." Thus, concluded Franklin, "the Whole appears to us to be under very regular and good Management, and likely to answer the original design."[39]

Although only minimal records were kept in the eighteenth century,[40] it is clear that the hospital treated a large number of people from the start. Between 1751 and 1773, the hospital physicians saw about four hundred patients a year and dealt with a wide variety of injuries and illnesses. On any given day, an attending physician might treat a leg fracture, an ulcer, a gunshot wound, and a burn. Head, neck, and back injuries were frequent, since the city received a large number of ships, and hundreds of manual laborers were employed on its docks. In addition, there were patients with rheumatism, palsies, tremors, and seizure disorders. And then there were the mad patients, for decades the largest subgroup in the hospital.

A year after his *Account* came out, Franklin, who had been on the hospital's board and served as its secretary from 1751 to 1752, was elected president of the board. He served from 1755 to 1757, and his duties included overseeing the admissions and releases. Trying to do everything he could for the worthy poor, he even wrote some short pieces for his *Pennsylvania Gazette* to help these patients receive community support and employment upon discharge.

Franklin's actual presence at the hospital ended in 1757, when the Pennsylvania Assembly sent him to England to help settle a dispute over taxation with the Penns. Before he sailed, the directors asked him to use his connections and good name to solicit donations in Europe. With his do-good philosophy, America's foremost philosopher, civil servant, and fundraiser probably did not have to be asked. While in Europe, he retold the history of Pennsylvania Hospital to anyone who was interested, collected cash donations for the institution, and secured books for its medical library. He also met with foreign hospital administrators, who eagerly shared their own ideas about improving hospital care and fundraising with him. And to his credit, he and John Fothergill were even able to obtain an Act of Parliament and a favorable decision by the Lord Chancellor of England making the hospital a recipient of the proceeds of the defunct Pennsylvania Land Company-an act that increased the hospital's coffers by several thousand pounds.

When Franklin died in 1790, his last will and testament gave Pennsylvania Hospital the right to collect and retain all outstanding debts still owed to him. The hospital managers graciously declined the gift, knowing how difficult it would be to find living debtors and then to collect enough money to make their efforts worthwhile. Further, thanks in good measure to Franklin's involvement with the hospital over a span of almost four decades, the charitable institution he helped to establish had reasonable financial resources. It even had the funding to start construction on its second wing, which was now needed to treat the sick in the still expanding coastal city.

# CHAPTER 5

# Electricity and the Palsies

I never knew any Advantage from Electricity in Palsies that was
permanent.
—Benjamin Franklin, 1758

We have seen that Franklin was a collector, disseminator, and printer of
medical information, and a publicist willing to involve himself in worthy
causes. He was concerned with preventative medicine and dealing with
infectious diseases at the individual level, with discussing medical ethics and
discussing new information in small groups, such as his Junto and American
Philosophical Society, and with building physical institutions to serve public
health needs, as exemplified by the landmark Pennsylvania Hospital.

From what has been covered so far, it would be easy to develop the miscon-
ception that Franklin was not personally involved with treating patients or
with actually conducting experiments to determine whether certain treatments
worked. But there was a hands-on therapeutic side to Franklin's medicine that
was tied to his commitment to Baconian science and to the experiment as the
best way to advance knowledge. Nowhere is this clearer than in Franklin's
desire to determine whether electricity, the force he understood better than
anyone else at the time, might help the sick and injured.

## ELECTRICITY BEFORE FRANKLIN

In 1600, William Gilbert, physician to Queen Elizabeth I, coined the word
"electricity," deriving it on the Greek term for amber *(elektron)*, a resin long
known to attract feathers and straw when rubbed. But it was not the scientific
study of amber that opened new vistas in Franklin's century. Rather, it was a
later seventeenth-century technological development: the advent of fric-
tional machines that could create electrical sparks on demand.[1]

Otto von Guericke in Magdeburg, Germany, built the first static electricity
machine. In 1672 he described how he rotated a large sulfur globe on a spindle and rubbed it to attract and repel small objects, sometimes with sounds

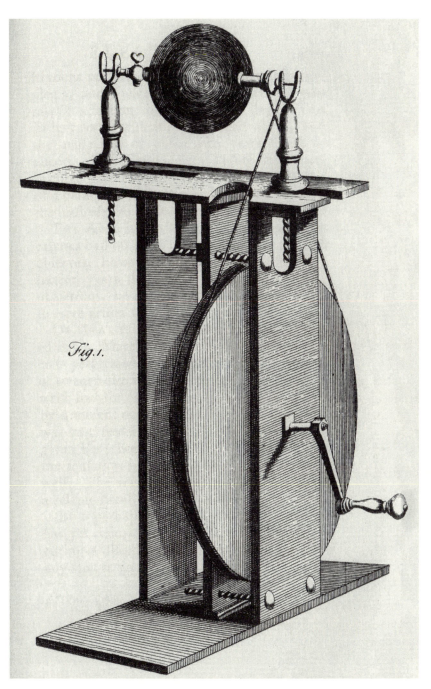

*Francis Hawksbee's electrical machine. (Illustration in Joseph Priestley's* History and Present State of Electricity, *3rd ed., vol. 1 [London: Bathurst and Lowndes, 1775].)*

and sparks.[2] Francis Hawksbee, curator of experiments for the Royal Society, took the next step early in the eighteenth century. He invented even better electrical machines from glass and used them to generate sparks, make thin pieces of brass "dance," and even light up a nearby globe.[3]

A third important pioneer was Stephen Gray, who showed that electricity from static machines could be transmitted over threads and wires.[4] Gray also demonstrated that the human body could be electrified safely. His classic experiment involved suspending a boy from a ceiling with silk cords and rubbing a glass tube near his feet. The boy would not be endangered, but he would then attract feathers and brass strips to his body, and crackling sparks could even be drawn from him, to the delight of onlookers.

After the Leyden jar was invented in 1746 by Pieter van Musschenbroek, a Dutchman Franklin would later meet, working with electricity became much easier.[5] Made of glass, covered with foil, and filled with water or lead shot, the jar could store a charge and release it on demand. Jean-Antoine Nollet, the official court electrician to Louis XV, demonstrated what the Leyden jar could do before amazed royal onlookers at Versailles. Nollet wired 180 grenadiers together and showed how the soldiers would leap into the air in unison when the circuit to a fully charged jar was completed. Delighted by his achievement, he extended the experiment to a human chain of more than seven hundred hand-holding monks from the Couvent de Paris.

## FRANKLIN'S INTRODUCTION TO ELECTRICITY

The first time Franklin witnessed a demonstration with man-made electricity was in 1743, just before the Leyden jar was invented. While visiting Boston, he paid to witness a private showing of its wonders from Archibald Spencer, who had come over from Edinburgh.[6] Many years later, he wrote: "Dr Spence[r] . . . show'd me some electric experiments. They were imperfectly perform'd, as he was not very expert; but being on a subject quite new to me, they equally surpris'd and pleased me."[7] Franklin encouraged Spencer to visit Philadelphia, where he advertised the Scotsman's "Course of Experimental Philosophy" in the *Pennsylvania Gazette* and served as his ticket agent. William Black and John Smith, who attended the lecture-demonstrations, tell us that one of Spencer's demonstrations involved "Sparks of Fire Emitted from the Face and Hands of a Boy Suspended Horizontally, by only rubbing a Glass Tube at his Feet."[8]

Although Spencer piqued Franklin's interest in electricity, Peter Collinson was the person who radically changed his life with it. Late in 1746, Collinson

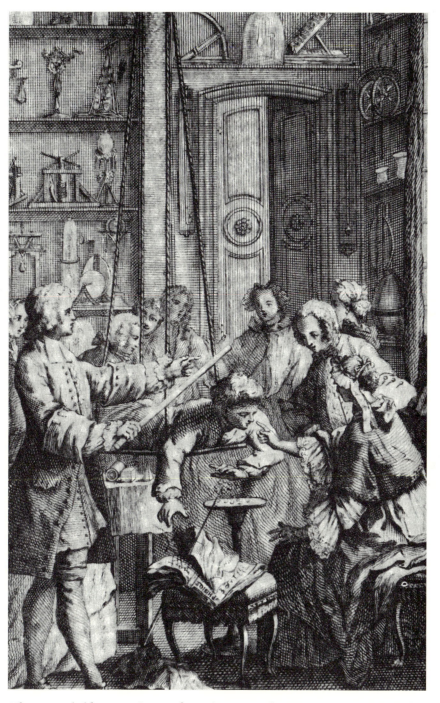

*The suspended boy experiment of Stephen Gray. (From Jean-Antoine Nollet's* Essai sur l'Electricité des Corps *[Paris: Guerin, 1746].)*

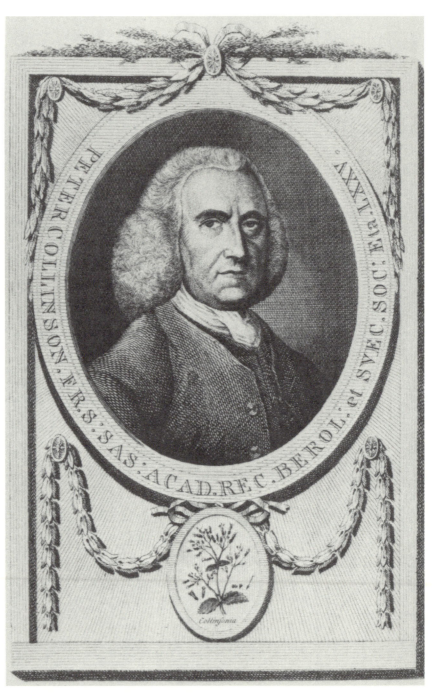

*Peter Collinson (1694–1768), London agent of the Library Company, who sent Franklin and his friends some electrical equipment.*

shipped Franklin's Library Company a gift of a three-foot glass tube with instructions on how to rub it to obtain sparks that could set spirits or oil on fire. He also sent a review article on electricity from *Gentleman's Magazine*—gifts to his friends in America.[9]

It did not take Franklin long to immerse himself in electrical experiments. "Your kind present of an electric tube, with directions for using it," Franklin informed Collinson in 1747, "has put several of us on making electrical experiments. . . . For my own part, I never was before engaged in any study that so totally engrossed my attention and my time as this has lately done . . . I have, during some months past, had little leisure for any thing else."[10] By this time, Franklin had local glassblowers making additional tubes, and he had purchased all of Spencer's instruments. Thomas Penn, who had been generous to the Library Company in the past, also pitched in. "Our honourable Proprietor enabled us to carry those Experiments to a Greater Height, by his generous Present of a complete Electrical Apparatus," Franklin noted.[11]

The "several of us" Franklin alluded to in his 1747 letter to Collinson were Philip Syng, Jr., a silversmith, Thomas Hopkinson, a merchant and lawyer, and Ebenezer Kinnersley, an unemployed Baptist minister. All were "amateurs"; the pursuit of science in colonial America was almost entirely in the hands of individuals who did not study natural philosophy in college. For Franklin, Syng, Hopkinson, and Kinnersley, the intellectual challenge, the thrill of making a new discovery, and being a part of the brotherhood of natural philosophers was motivation enough.

Franklin became so enthused about the amazing powers of electricity and what he was discovering that, in 1748, he entered into an agreement with David Hall, his foreman at the printing shop. Hall would run the shop and give him £673 up front and a payment each year, keeping the rest for himself. Franklin thus retired from running his printing business and moved with his wife to a new house on the corner of Race and Second Streets. With his highly successful almanac and investments in printing businesses from New England to the Caribbean, Franklin had become one of the wealthiest tradesmen in America. And he was anxious to engage in "Philosophical Studies and Amusements" and to converse with "ingenious and worthy men" in a manner befitting a successful gentleman.

Soon after replicating some published studies, Franklin's group had its first important new discovery. Points, they discovered, are much better than balls and "blunts," not just for throwing off sparks but also for attracting the "electrical fire." This revelation, first made by Thomas Hopkinson, led Franklin to

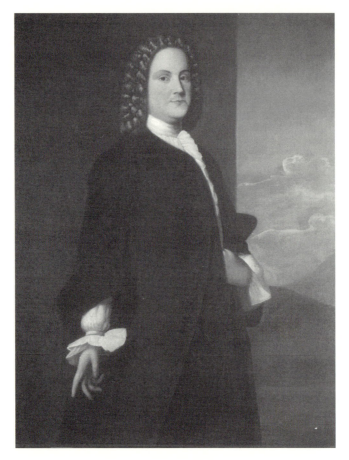

*A young Benjamin Franklin dressed to convey the image*
*of a successful, young gentleman. (Portrait by Robert*
*Feke, circa 1748; image courtesy of the Harvard*
*University Portrait Collection, Bequest of Dr. John*
*Collins Warren, 1856.)*

the pointed lightning rod. In a March 1750 letter to Collinson, he wrote: "From what I have observed on experiments, I am of the opinion that houses, ships, and even towns and churches may be effectually secured from the stroke of lightning by their means: for if . . . there should be a rod of iron 8 or 10 feet in length, sharpen'd gradually to a point like a needle . . . the electrical fire would, I think, be drawn out of a cloud silently, before it could come near enough to strike."[12]

Collinson shared Franklin's letter with members of the Royal Society and published it in *Gentleman's Magazine* to enlighten the public. At the time, many people were still associating thunder and lightning with supernatural forces. All through Europe and in the colonies, church bells would be rung during thunderstorms to "repel the demon," to use the words of Thomas Aquinas. Franklin knew that many people had been killed by lightning while ringing church bells during storms, and he decried the ridiculous superstition, telling one of his correspondents, "it was now time to try some other trick."[13] And with his pointed lightning rod, which he bequeathed without financial gain to humankind, he effectively redirected thinking away from the supernatural and showed that experimental natural philosophy could have significant utilitarian benefits.

Franklin also realized that the theory of electricity then in vogue had serious problems. The prevailing idea was that there are two opposing types of electricity, called vitreous and resinous, because one is associated with glass and the other with amber. Not so, Franklin reasoned. Instead, there is probably only one type of electricity composed of extremely subtle particles. An object will be "plus" or "electricised positively," he wrote, if it has an "over quantity" of the electrical matter, whereas it will be "minus" or "electricised negatively" if it has an "under quantity." He further opined that Nature prefers an equilibrium condition. He then used his new theory to explain attraction and repulsion, why there are "Thunder Strokes," and even how "Mr. Musschenbroek's wonderful bottle" worked.[14]

One of the most debated issues at the time was whether lightning and static electricity are identical. In 1749, Franklin drew up a list of twelve clear similarities, such as "Giving light" and "Swift motion."[15] But, he wondered, could lightning, like artificial electricity, charge a Leyden jar? To answer this and related questions, he designed an experiment with an iron rod that would rise high into the air above a steeple, and a sentry box that would house a man who would be able to draw sparks from the base of the rod.[16] Franklin felt he could not immediately conduct the experiment himself, because construction of the tall steeple on Christ Church in Philadelphia was still not completed.

Thomas-François d'Alibard, a Frenchman who read Franklin's description of the "critical" experiment, was the first person to capture lightning in this way.[17] He then graciously gave Franklin full credit for proving that lightning and artificial electricity are the same, except in quantity. Louis XV, who witnessed a replication of the landmark experiment, even sent a letter to the Royal Society of London praising the American whom he had never met.

Franklin did not know what had transpired in France when he suddenly realized that he could also capture electricity with a specially rigged kite. His famous kite experiment probably took place in June 1752, and how he

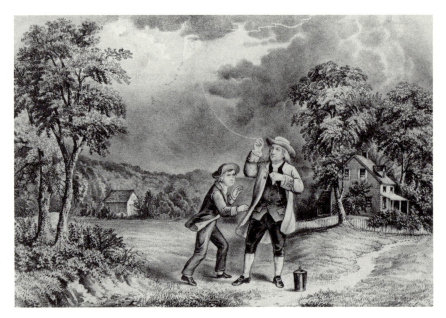

*The Currier & Ives depiction of Franklin's kite experiment. William is shown as a small boy, although he was about twenty at the time.*

captured electricity from the heavens with a child's toy was made public a few months later.[18]

By this time, Peter Collinson had given Edward Cave, the owner and editor of *Gentleman's Magazine*, a number of Franklin's letters for publication in the periodical. Cave, however, was so impressed that he opted for a freestanding pamphlet in 1751 that bore the title *Experiments and Observations on Electricity, Made at Philadelphia in America*.[19] The pamphlet included Franklin's findings on points, his new theory of electricity, the lightning rod, directions for the sentry box experiment, meteorological explanations, and much more. The eighty-six page book also introduced many new words into the vocabulary, including plus and minus, positive and negative, electrical shock, electrician, charging, discharge, electrical battery, armature, brush, conductor, and condenser.[20] It went through five editions by 1774 and was a best seller for a book of its type.

Franklin was now regarded as first among electricians in the world. Immanuel Kant called him "the new Prometheus," and Joseph Priestley referred to him as "the father of modern electricity."[21] Franklin's biographer Carl Van Doren, however, might have put it best when he wrote: "He found electricity a curiosity and left it a science."[22]

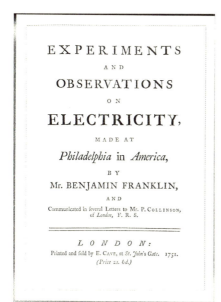
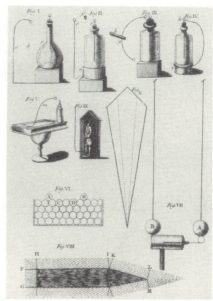

*Left: The cover of Franklin's famous pamphlet on electricity. Right: a page showing Leyden jars and some experiments, including the sentry box (middle left) for capturing electricity from the sky.*

## THE ROAD TO MEDICAL ELECTRICITY

The idea of using powerful shocks to treat paralyses, epilepsy, and a host of other physical problems originated in antiquity with electric fish.[23] Catfish with electric organs can be seen in stone tablets made by the ancient Egyptians, and electric rays, called torpedoes, can be observed in classical Greek pottery. Whether the Egyptian and Greek healers used their shocks therapeutically is uncertain, but the electric ray was certainly used during the height of the Roman Empire. Legend has it that Anteros, one of Nero's freed slaves, stepped on a torpedo while walking on a beach. Although he initially suffered an excruciating cramp, the pain he had long endured from what might have been gout miraculously disappeared. Upon hearing the story, Scribonius Largus, an imperial physician in the first century, began to use the torpedo to treat painful disorders, discovering that the treatment could really provide some relief. Roman physicians who followed even attempted to treat paralyses with torpedoes, probably because the shocks could induce violent muscular contractions, even in the lame. And at the time of the Middle Ages in Europe, Avicenna and Averrhöes, two Middle

Eastern physicians, treated headaches, melancholy, vertigo, and seizures by placing the electric fish on the affected part. Nevertheless, electric fish were never really a part of mainstream medicine, because they were too difficult to catch and keep alive, and it was impossible to control the shocks they seemed to emit.

About the time that Franklin was introduced to electricity, the idea of medical uses for electricity began to reemerge in Europe, but not with shocks from fish. Johann Gottlob Krüger, a professor in Halle, Germany, told his students that "all things must have a usefulness: that is certain. Since electricity must have a usefulness, and we have seen it cannot be looked for either in theology or in jurisprudence, there is obviously nothing left but medicine." Krüger then hypothesized that "the best effect [of electricity] would be found in paralyzed limbs."[24]

Krüger's words were published in 1744, the year in which his student Christian Gottlieb Kratzenstein set out to test them. Kratzenstein worked with two patients who could not move their fingers. He found that gentle electrification allowed one to overcome a contraction in her little finger and the other to play his harpsichord again. He described these cases in some letters and then included them in a monograph published in 1745.[25] Joseph Priestley called Kratzenstein's writings "the first account I have met with of the application of electricity to medical purposes."[26]

Kratzenstein's early successes were with arthritic patients, not people paralyzed by strokes or brain injuries. But two years later, the Abbé Nollet used the newly invented Leyden jar to apply electricity to, and draw sparks from, the affected body parts of three brain-damaged paralytic patients.[27] Although the Abbé saw some potential for medical electricity at the time, his optimism slowly waned after working with brain-damaged soldiers at the Hôtel Royal des Invalides in Paris.

Nevertheless, others became wildly optimistic about the new therapy. One such person was Giovanni Francesco Pivati, a Venetian who added camphor, opium, and other medicines to his glass tubes and Leyden jars, or had his patients hold medicines while being electrified. Although Pivati claimed miraculous cures, the Abbé Nollet was doubtful and traveled to Italy in 1749 to investigate these assertions, only to conclude that the highly touted cures were solely due to imagination.[28] Franklin, who closely followed the debate, sided with Nollet. He told American physician Cadwallader Colden that, after "Reading in the Transactions the Accounts from Italy and Germany, . . . I was persuaded they were not true."[29]

Positive and negative reports on shock treatments without the combined use of medications now began to flood into various publications. In one report from Switzerland, readers were informed that a locksmith, who had been paralyzed in one arm by an accident that occurred fifteen years earlier, was able to return to work.[30] But others disagreed, pointing out that the cure did not last.[31] With medical electricity open to anyone who could obtain an apparatus, even established practicing physicians found it impossible to ascertain what was true from what was wishful thinking.[32]

One theory behind the electrical treatment was that constrictions and blockages of the nerves and blood vessels could impair function, as could increases in the density of internal fluids.[33] In the 1745 *Gentleman's Magazine* article that Peter Collinson sent to Franklin, we read: "It has already been discover'd, or believ'd to be so, that electricity accelerates the movement of water in a pipe."[34] The suggestion that electricity could make sluggish fluids less turgid was backed up by the statement that electricity had now been shown to cause blood to flow more freely from a cut vein, and to enhance the pulse.

The possibility that the nerves might function by electricity was also beginning to circulate at this time. And it fueled the related idea that applying electricity might be able to stimulate a slow machine or jump-start one that was not working. With the potential to be beneficial in several ways, the author of the 1745 *Gentleman's Magazine* article found several reasons to be optimistic. "There are hopes for finding a remedy for the sciatica or palsy" were his closing words.[35]

Of course, not everyone was driven by theory. Franklin's first concern was that no harm must come from the treatment; his second was with the outcome. For the pragmatic Philadelphian who understood the potential of careful experimentation, the matter was straightforward. Assuming it could be administered safely, does electricity really improve the patient's condition, or is it just another quack remedy?

## PALSY AND STROKE

In Franklin's day a "palsy" might signify the "common paralytic disorder," meaning a stroke. But it might also be used for "the shaking palsy," the old term for Parkinson's disease, or for a unilateral facial palsy of unknown cause, a condition later called Bell's palsy. Under the broad umbrella term palsy we might also find cases of hysterical paralyses, and patients "paralyzed" with advanced joint or arthritic diseases, like those treated by Kratzenstein.

The various palsies just mentioned can exhibit different changes over time, adding to the confusion. A palsy resulting from a massive stroke could leave a person hemiplegic for the rest of his or her life, no matter how treated, whereas the facial problems associated with Bell's palsy would probably remit within a few months. Parkinson's disease and the stiffness associated with arthritic problems would worsen over time. As for the hysteric, that person's palsy would most likely wax and wane with the stresses of everyday life.

In this context, Bohemian physician Joannes Baptist Bohadsch deserves some praise. In a paper published in 1751, while Franklin was seeing palsy cases of his own, Bohadsch at least warned: "Every species of palsy does not arise from the nerves being either obstructed or compressed." Bohadsch was preparing people for the possibility that electricity might not work in every case of palsy. But, he added, "of all other distempers the hemiplegia seems most properly the object of electricity."[36] In other words, he was most optimistic about electrical treatment of paralysis resulting from stroke.

## THE CASE OF JAMES LOGAN

One of Franklin's first patients was James Logan, an eminent Quaker who had been educated in Ireland and came to the New World in 1699 as secretary to the first proprietor of Pennsylvania, William Penn.[37] Logan stayed on after Penn returned to England and became a successful businessman, making considerable money in the fur trade. And as a respected public figure, he was put in charge of Indian affairs and served as chief judge of Pennsylvania's Supreme Court.

Logan's favorite pastime was natural philosophy, and he was a first-class scholar who could read Latin, Hebrew, Greek, French, Italian, and even Arabic. He might have been the only colonist at the time who had read all of Newton's *Principia*. He wrote on mathematics, astronomy, botany, and optics, and several of his papers were published in the *Philosophical Transactions of the Royal Society*.

Logan's concern for the public welfare, his library of some three thousand books, and his thirst for knowledge were among the reasons Franklin was drawn to him, despite their thirty-nine-year age difference. Franklin actively sought Logan's advice about acquisitions for the Library Company and deferred to him on many civic issues. Logan, in turn, chose Franklin to publish some of his books. He even confided to Peter Collinson that Franklin is "certainly an Extraordinary Man, one of a singular good Judgment, but of Equal Modesty."[38]

In 1739, Logan suffered a stroke that partially affected his right side. He slowly recovered his memory and hand for writing, although his painful rheumatism compounded his problems when it came to his mobility. The event took place before electricity was being used medically and before Franklin began to study it.

Some eight years after his first stroke, Logan became interested in electricity and in Franklin's electrical experiments. In a letter dated February 23, 1747, he explained to Franklin: "Yesterday was the first time that I ever heard one syllable of thy Electrical Experiments, when John Bartram surpriz'd me with the account of a Ball turning many hours about an Electrified Body, with some other particulars that were sufficiently amazing."[39] He told Franklin he was now reading Francis Hawksbee, having actually seen his electrical apparatus in 1710. "But," Logan added as only a Quaker could, "your own Experiments in my judgment exceed them all. I could therefore wish as soon as it can suit thee that thou wouldst step up hither bringing an Account with thee."[40]

Near the end of 1749 and early in 1750, Logan suffered one or more strokes that left him paralyzed, speechless, and helpless. In retrospect, it is highly likely that he ruptured another branch of the middle cerebral artery, the so-called artery of stroke, on the left side of his brain. Damage to this artery typically causes paralyses and sensory losses on the right side of the body, in addition to a loss of fluent speech, a condition known today as a Broca's aphasia or motor aphasia.

Logan was familiarizing himself with medical electricity when stricken, and Franklin was called to help. Logan's biographer, Frederick Tolles, writes of the "Quaker virtuoso" that "The old man even allowed him to administer electric shock treatments for palsy of his right side."[41] Franklin's letters confirm that he helped with Logan's treatment, supplying both advice and equipment. One letter dated December 16, 1749 reads: "I send you herewith a new French piece on electricity, in which you will find a journal of experiments on a paralytic person. I will also send you Neal on Electricity, and the last *Philosophical Transactions*, in which you will find some other pieces on the same subject. If you should desire to see any of the experiments mentioned in those pieces repeated, or if any new ones should occur to you to propose, which you cannot well try yourself, when I come to fetch the apparatus they may be tried. I shall be glad to hear that the shocks had some good effect on your disordered side."[42]

Franklin left it up to Logan, the Quaker's personal physicians, and others in his household to follow through on a day by day basis. But he did not have high hopes, and his pessimism grew over the ensuing months. On June 28,

1750, he wrote to Cadwallader Colden: "My good old Friend Mr. Logan, being about three Months since struck with a Palsy, continues Speechless, tho' he knows People, and seems in some Degree to retain his Memory and Understanding." He then told Colden, "I fear he will not recover."[43]

Franklin had good reason to be worried. The electrical treatments did not have any lasting beneficial effects and Logan continued to grow progressively weaker. James Logan, the man who envisioned Philadelphia blossoming into the Athens or intellectual capital of the colonies, passed away with his family gathered about him in 1751.

## THE CASE OF JONATHAN BELCHER

Jonathan Belcher, a colonial governor of New Jersey. was "stricken with the palsy" in 1750, while attending commencement at the school he founded, the College of New Jersey (later to become Princeton University).[44] Belcher was sixty-eight at the time and, although free from pain, he became indecisive and weak in political matters afterward.[45]

Quite likely, given the word "stricken," Belcher had "the common paralytick disorder." Nevertheless, and perhaps in addition to having a stroke, he might have suffered from or developed Parkinson's disease.[46] The confusion stems partly from the fact that Belcher's body was thereafter described as "tremulous." In addition, records from July 1752 inform us that "his paralytic affection has so far increased that for 18 months he has not been able to hold a pen"—words suggesting that what he had might have been progressive.[47] Belcher was no longer able to walk by himself three years later, also suggestive of Parkinson's disease, which may begin with tremors and progress to a gradual stiffening that can confine individuals to their chairs and beds.

Belcher received advice from Colonel Brattle "relative to his tremulousness" in 1751.[48] He also contacted Dr. Thomas Cadwalader, his personal physician, asking him for his opinion about trying electrotherapy for his palsy.[49] Cadwalader did not reply immediately, preferring to discuss his case with several medical colleagues, including Drs. James McGraw, Thomas Greame (whose daughter would be courted by Franklin's son William), and William Brattle. All eventually agreed that electricity was safe and worth trying.

Upon receiving the news, Belcher responded that, "If my Country man Franklin will be so good and obliging as to come and make the Operation himself I think to venture upon it in Moderation."[50] Franklin had been Belcher's printer at the time and had visited him in New Jersey. Corresponding through Joseph Warrell, the attorney general of New Jersey, Franklin was told of the situation and consented to help. In one of Belcher's letters to Franklin in 1751, he expressed thankfulness to Franklin for his willingness "to come hither and make the Operation on me your self."[51]

This plan was scrapped when pressing governmental concerns in Pennsylvania made it impossible for Franklin to travel to New Jersey. Nevertheless, some electrical equipment with specific instructions for its use could be sent by coach to Burlington. Belcher appreciated the offer of the equipment, writing: "I find my Self obliged for your kind Intention to have made an Electrical Operation upon me at Burlington had your Affairs allow'd your coming. . . . And I take thankful notice of your readiness to send me an Electrical Apparatus with the particular directions how to use it which I shall be glad of as soon as you can conveniently send it."[52]

Unfortunately, the apparatus was shattered in transport. Belcher broke the news to Franklin on December 18, 1751: "the box with the Electrical Apparatus came to my hands the 16: Currant and I am sorry to Inform you that when I came to open it the Glass Globe was broke all to pieces. . . . This is a great misfortune. . . . I have tried to get another at New York without Success."[53]

Belcher sent yet another letter to Franklin on January 20, 1752, explaining that the Reverend Aaron Burr was able to use what remained of the apparatus. Burr was Belcher's close friend, a minister of the First Presbyterian Church, the second president of the College of New Jersey, and the father of the more famous Aaron Burr, who killed founding father Alexander Hamilton in a duel. He lectured in natural philosophy and was acquainted with electricity. There were no details of how many shocks were given per session, nor how strong they were, nor where they were applied, but Belcher did inform Franklin that the treatments were not having the anticipated effects: "Sir, I wrote you a few lines the 18th: of last month telling you of the misfortune that had befell your Electrical Globe. I have however made some use of the rest of the Apparatus and with Mr. Burr's assistance have been electrifyd several times but at present without any alteration in my Nervous disorder. As Mr. Burr has another Apparatus as yours and lends it to me I think to go on with the Operation some little time longer."[54]

Jonathan Belcher, like James Logan, did not recover from his palsy, or perhaps palsies, although he continued his treatments for some time. He died in 1757 and his close friend Aaron Burr delivered his funeral oration.

## FRANKLIN'S REPORT ON THE PALSIES

Franklin never published the Belcher or Logan cases, or any detailed case studies involving stroke victims. But he amassed enough material from these two cases, plus an unknown number of others, to present a good summary of how he fared with palsy patients. His synopsis of what had transpired in the colonies was written in 1757, the same year the Pennsylvania Assembly sent him to England.

The person who pushed Franklin to inform others about his experiments and results with medical electricity was John Pringle, a Scot who had become

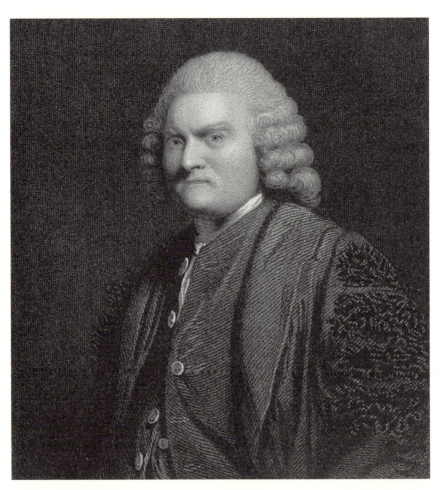

*John Pringle (1707–1782), distinguished physician, member of the Royal Society, and close friend of Benjamin Franklin.*

a major figure in the Royal Society.[55] On December 15, 1757, about three weeks after Franklin was formally inducted into the Royal Society (he had been elected a member in 1756), Pringle read some communications to the membership. One was "An Instance of the Electrical Virtue in the Cure of a Palsy" by Patrick Brydone, and it involved a woman who was cured of hysterical paralyses.[56]

This report generated an animated discussion about the electrical cure for the palsies, coming on the heels of two reports by Cheney Hart, whose electrical treatments failed to cure a woman with a "wasted" paralytic arm, but helped another with a painfully contracted "rheumatic" hand.[57] With heads spinning from the different outcomes, Pringle asked Franklin to comment on his results from America. Franklin's report to the Royal Society was dated December 21, 1757, and it appeared in the *Philosophical Transactions* in 1758. Beginning in 1774 it was also included in updated editions of Franklin's own *Experiments and Observations on Electricity*.[58]

Dealing only with his paralytic cases, Franklin began: "Some Years since, when the News papers made Mention of great Cures perform'd in Italy or Germany by means of Electricity, a Number of Paralytics were brought to me from different Parts of Pensilvania and the neighboring Provinces, to be electricis'd, which I did for them, at their Request." He then mentioned his method, which "was, to place the Patient first in a Chair on an electric Stool, and draw a Number of large strong Sparks from all Parts of the affected Limb or Side. Then I fully charg'd two 6 Gallon Glass Jarrs . . . and I sent the united Shock of these thro' the affected Limb or Limbs, repeating the Stroke commonly three Times each day."

Turning to his findings, Franklin at first seemed optimistic: "The first Thing observ'd was an immediate greater sensible Warmth in the lame Limbs that had receiv'd the Stroke than in the others; and the next Morning the Patients usually related that they had in the Night felt a prickling Sensation in the Flesh of the paralytic Limbs, and would sometimes shew a Number of small red Spots which they suppos'd were occasion'd by those Pricklings. The Limbs too were found more capable of voluntary Motion, and seem'd to receive Strength."

An example was presented to illustrate the observed changes, although the patient was not named. "A Man," explained Franklin, "who could not, the first day, lift the lame Hand from off his Knee, would the next day raise it four or five Inches, the third Day higher, and on the fifth Day was able, but with a feeble languid Motion, to take off his Hat." He went on to state that "These Appearances gave great Spirits to the Patients, and made them hope a perfect Cure." But he then explained to the members of the Royal Society that he could "not remember that I ever saw any Amendment after the fifth day: Which the Patients perceiving, and finding the Shocks pretty severe, they became discourag'd, went home and in short time relapsed." His closing words in this revealing paragraph were: "I never knew any Advantage from Electricity in Palsies that was permanent."

Franklin could have ended his letter at this point, but felt he had to address why some patients exhibited transient improvements. He brought up two factors: exercise and high expectations. But not wanting to be dogmatic or speculative, he chose his words carefully: "And how far the apparent temporary Advantage might arise from the Exercise in the Patients Journey and coming daily to my house, or from the Spirits given by the Hope of Success, enabling them to exert more Strength in moving their Limbs, I will not pretend to say."

## THE CASE OF DEBBY FRANKLIN

Franklin never changed his mind about the ineffectiveness of electricity as a treatment for the common paralytic disorder. Nowhere is this more apparent than when his wife became a stroke victim.

Debby Franklin experienced her first stroke in 1768, and it appeared to be in her left cerebral hemisphere. Sally, who was with her at the time, penned a letter to London to inform her father about it. Although she let him know that her mother seemed to be improving, Franklin sought confirmation. He wrote back to Debby herself: "I rejoice to hear you so soon got over your late Indisposition, but am impatient for the next Packet which I hope will bring me that good News under your own hand."[59]

Two weeks later, he received a letter from Thomas Bond. The physician behind the Pennsylvania Hospital project had noted some improvement, but was not optimistic. He explained: "Your good Mrs. Franklin was affected in the Winter with a partial Palsey in the Tongue, and a sudden Loss of Memory, which alarmed us much, but she soon recovered from them, tho her constitution in general appears impaired. These are bad Symptoms in advanced Life and Auger Danger of further Injury on the nervous System."[60]

Just how badly Debby was affected is evident from her letters. Although she had never been a good speller or grammarian, her sentences had a logical flow and whenever she spelled "Elicktresatecy" or ended her letters "your a feck shonet Wife" Franklin had known exactly what she meant. But what she was now trying to convey had become considerably more difficult to decipher; there were problems maintaining a thought, a loss of logical flow, worse spelling, and obvious confusion. Consider this sentence, penned in a letter to her husband dated November 1769: "I muste tell you as well as I Can my disorder was for this reason my distres for my dear Bebbeys mis-forten and hers being removed so far from her friend and such a helples famely and before I had got the better of that our Cusin Betsey macum was taken ill and so much distrest so soon that aded to my one dis satisid dis-tressed att your staying so much longer that I loste all my resey lushon and the verey dismall winter bouth Sally and my self live so verey lonley that I had got in so verey low a Staite and got into so unhapey a way that I cold not sleep a long time."[61]

Debby attributed her stroke to psychological factors. The winter had been long and hard, making her feel lonely and depressed. She had also been under considerable tension trying to take care of the household while her husband was away. Unable to cope, she managed to explain that she lost her appetite, her ability to sleep, and her "resolution"—"I was not sick I was only more to bair aney more and so I fell down and cold [illegible word] not get up agen indead it was not aney sicknes but two much disquiit of mind."[62]

Medical advice came from some of the best practitioners of the day. Franklin passed along recommendations from John Pringle (since lost), and she also received guidance from physician Cadwalader Evans, who had just seen Franklin in England. At home, Thomas Bond and Benjamin Rush tried to care for her. "Dr Bond to cume and supmited to be Bleeded," she wrote in one of her letters, pleading for her husband's help.[63]

Although Debby seemed to hold her own for a while, she suffered mem-ory problems and became remiss in her record keeping. Her slovenliness in money matters even triggered a regrettable scolding from her husband in England. "I know you were not very attentive to Money-matters in your best Days," Franklin insensitively lashed out, "and I apprehend that your Mem-ory is too much impair'd for the Management of unlimited Sums without Danger of injuring the future Fortune of your Daughter and Grandson."[64]

Debby's last surviving letter to her husband was dated October 29, 1773. "Our youngest Grand Son is the finest child as a live," she told him, the ref-erence being to Sarah's five-month-old boy, William Bache. But then she lamented: "it is so dificall to writ. . . . I Cante write aney mor."[65]

Franklin did not sail home after receiving Debby's letters, even though his diplomatic mission was effectively over. Instead, he sent several notes inquiring why Debby was no longer writing. "It is now a very long time indeed since I have had the Pleasure of a Line from You," he informed her in May 1774.[66] And four months later: "It is now nine long Months since I received a Line from my dear Debby."[67]

The winter of 1774–1775 Debby suffered another stroke, much as Thomas Bond had predicted. Sarah's husband Richard Bache sent a letter to his father-in-law on December 17 to brace him for the possibility that she would not survive. On December 24, 1774, Bache wrote that Deborah Read Franklin had continued to deteriorate and, "without a Groan or even a Sigh, she was released from a troublesome World."[68]

The fact that Franklin did not head home after Debby's first stroke could have been due to several factors. One was the importance of his diplomatic mission. But another, not to be overlooked, was that he knew there was little even the best trained eighteenth-century physician could do for a stroke victim. In the latter context, his silence on trying medical electricity looms significant. If Franklin had changed his mind about electricity for stroke patients, he almost certainly would have asked Cadwalader Evans or another of his physician friends who knew how to apply electricity to try it on his ailing Debby. But he never brought up this possibility. And equally significantly, neither did those physicians who knew him and were trying so hard to help his disabled wife.

Franklin's last statement about medical electricity for stroke victims, dated 1788, was still pessimistic. The inquirer was Mather Byles, the nephew of Cotton Mather who inherited his immense library and had been instrumental in getting Harvard College to grant Franklin his first honorary master's degree. In 1787, Byles had asked Franklin whether electricity might cure his palsy. For more than a year, Franklin did not write back—perhaps because he had been too busy with other matters, perhaps because Byles had been a Tory sympathizer during the Revolutionary War. "I wish for your sake," he finally informed Byles, "that Electricity had really prov'd what at first it was suppos'd to be, a Cure for the Palsy."[69]

## GROWING DOUBTS AND ENTHUSIASTIC CLAIMS

After Franklin presented his colonial material in 1757, several influential practitioners began to express doubts about medical electricity as a cure for the common paralytic disorder. One was William Heberden,[70] who had written a pamphlet with Franklin to promote smallpox inoculations among the poor. Another was John Wesley, the founder of the Methodist Church, who wanted to help sick bodies in addition to saving immortal souls. In his *The Desideratum: Or Electricity Made Plain and Useful,* published in 1760,

Wesley admitted that electricity was not quite the cure he at first thought it would be for paralyses. And in making his statements, we can find words that show the strong influence Franklin had on him. After presenting the case of a man who seemed to have been successfully treated by another electrotherapist for a paralytic stroke, Wesley added: "I have not yet known any Instance of this Kind. Many *Paralytics* have been helped: But, I think, scarce any *Palsy* of a Year standing has been thro'ly cured."[71]

Yet neither Franklin nor Wesley was able to stop the flood of exaggerated claims about medical electricity that appeared in the second half of the eighteenth century. In Britain, *Gentleman's Magazine* overflowed with communications touting it for all sorts of illnesses and physical disorders. In France, more than twenty-five articles on curing paralyses with it appeared between 1750 and 1780 in just one periodical, the *Journal de Médecine*. In Germany, an encyclopedia published in 1777 included more than one hundred pages of references on medical electricity, many having to do with curing paralyses.[72]

Although Franklin, ever the careful experimentalist, had good reason to question the reports dealing with the common paralytic disorder, he never argued that electricity should be abandoned altogether. For some types of patients, as we shall now see, Franklin was decidedly more optimistic about the electrical cure.

CHAPTER 6

# Electricity, Mental Disorders, and a Modest Proposal

About this time there was a great talk of the wonderful power of electricity. . . . Accordingly I went to Philadelphia, the beginning of September 1752, and apply'd to B. Franklin, who I thought understood it best of any person here.

—C.B.

Franklin recognized that a medical treatment that may not work with the common paralytic disorder might still be beneficial with other disorders. This chapter examines Franklin's use of medical electricity with hysteria and melancholia, two conditions that were viewed very differently in the eighteenth century than they are today.

## HYSTERIA'S UNUSUAL HISTORY

Hysteria has been associated with different ideas at different points in time.[1] Today it is called a conversion disorder, because it involves motor and/or sensory system problems that do not appear to have a physical basis, and therefore are attributed to the mind.

Although modern practitioners approach hysteria as a psychological or psychiatric disorder, in ancient Egypt, Greece, and Rome, hysteria was considered a physical disorder, just like a cold or an attack of gout. But unlike these disorders, hysteria was characterized by one very unusual feature—the ancients were convinced that it targeted sexually unfulfilled women.

The basic idea was that the uterus could dry up in such women, making it light enough to float upward. The very word *hystera*, from which hysteria is derived, means "womb" in Greek. By worming its way through the body in search of moisture, the ancients thought, the displaced uterus put pressure on other internal organs. The result might be choking, anxiety, seizures, or other problems, depending on where it went and lodged. Marriage was highly recommended for hysterical women, but aromatic fumigations, tight bandages, and massages were also prescribed.

Hysteria remained a disorder of women during the Middle Ages and into the Renaissance, although it was more likely to be associated with demons, divine punishment, and occasionally with witchcraft. Consequently, prayer was one frequent course of action. Paintings from this time period depict the possessed making trips to churches and shrines, where priests would pray for them and exorcise demons from their bodies. The idea of demoniac possession was only partially overcome by the start of the eighteenth century. Cotton Mather, for one, remained a believer. But Mather's medicine was only partly based on the supernatural, and he suggested combining prayer with more earthly "physic" to treat individuals afflicted with hysteria.

In contrast to the devout Mather, Franklin and his more secular contemporaries preferred to view hysteria as a medical problem having nothing to do with demons. Yet speculative theory was not out of the picture. His contemporary George Cheyne, who sought a mechanical explanation for all diseases, wrote about blockages that could not be seen.[2]

The logic of the day was fairly simple. Just as a diseased body could affect reasoning and disrupt a once healthy mind, a sick mind could wreck havoc with the body and cause real physical changes. After all, stressed most physicians at the time, strong protracted emotions and disordered thinking could alter the natural flow of juices in the nerve tubes, the mobility of the spirits to and from the brain, and even the tension of the fibrous nerves. The emotions could also alter the viscosity of the blood, throw the internal organs of the abdomen into violent commotion, and cause vapors from poorly digested food to rise and poison the upper body. Hence, it was important to keep one's emotions and disruptive thought processes in check.

Accepting the possibility that the health of the mind could affect the well-being of the body, John Wesley made three very interesting statements in his best-selling *Primitive Physic,* which first appeared in 1747:

1. The passions have a greater influence on health, than most people are aware of.
2. All violent and sudden passions dispose to, or actually throw people into, acute diseases.
3. The slow and lasting passions, such as grief and hopeless love, bring on chronical diseases.[3]

George Baker, one of the physicians Franklin interacted with in London, similarly contended "that the violent passions of the mind are capable of exciting various disturbances in the human machine is a fact, which can admit of no doubt."[4] To eighteenth-century physicians, the body was just as much at the mercy of the mind as the mind was of the body.

Hysteria remained a female malady in the mid-eighteenth century, but not because it was still a disease of the womb. Instead, females were seen as more emotionally labile and prone to fantasy than males. In addition, women were thought to have weaker constitutions and more fragile nerves. Social factors also began to enter the picture. Pampered well-to-do women, especially those who could not cope with the unnatural stresses of city life, were thought to be most vulnerable to hysteria. Notably, the disorder was rare among their hard-working country cousins, who awoke early to milk the cows, feed the herds, and harvest the produce.

Stimulants were recommended for treating hysteria in Franklin's day. It did not matter whether the practitioner still believed in humoral theory, in iatrochemistry, or in the mechanical doctrines that emphasized faulty bodily passages, blockages, and viscous humors. Hysterical women were given tonics, blisters, bitters (to stimulate appetite), warm baths, red meat, and even wine and opium (both considered stimulants in low doses). In addition, exercising was highly recommended, particularly brisk walking or an hour or more of good horseback riding.

Late in the 1740s, electricity became another therapeutic option. As electrotherapist Richard Lovett put it, electricity has "a mighty Tendency to accelerate the Motion of the Fluids in general, and of the Blood in particular." Immediately after quoting Lovett, John Wesley added: "and to pervade the finest Arteries and Nerves, to dilate their obstructed or contracted Orifices; as well as to restore the Tone of any Muscle or Fibre, which is either impaired or destroyed."[5] Although neither Lovett nor Wesley possessed a medical degree, both men were reflecting what most people believed when Franklin proceeded to treat a woman suffering from hysteria with electricity, unquestionably the most powerful stimulant of all.

### THE CASE OF C.B.

The young woman who brought Franklin face to face with hysteria might at first have seemed to have epilepsy. But this woman's seizures were not like those of a true epileptic—they appeared to be controllable and related to her emotional state. Franklin worked on this case of hysterical epilepsy with

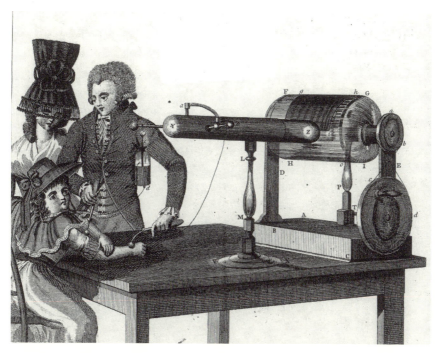

*A young woman undergoing treatment with medical electricity toward the end of the eighteenth century. Although the means of creating, storing, and administering electricity were similar, Franklin would not have had this particular apparatus at mid-century. (From John Birch, "A Letter to Mr. George Adams," in* An Essay on Electricity . . . by George Adams, *4th ed. [London: Hindmarsh, 1792].)*

Cadwallader (sometimes spelled Cadwalader) Evans, who had started in medicine as an apprentice to Thomas Bond in 1736.[6] Six years later, Evans set off to Edinburgh to complete his medical studies. But while on the high seas, a Spanish privateer captured his ship. He then spent some years in Haiti and Jamaica before making his way back to Philadelphia.

In 1752, two years before he set off for Edinburgh again, he and Franklin combined forces to treat the young woman, who might have been Evans's sister.[7] Evans took notes of the case and published a full report of what transpired in *Medical Observations and Inquiries* in 1754; their case of hysterical epilepsy treated by electricity was also summarized in *Gentleman's Magazine*.[8]

Evans tells us that C.B. was about fourteen during the summer of 1742, when she "was seiz'd with convulsions fits, which succeeded each other so fast, she had near 40 in 24 hours after the first attack. She struggled with such violence in the fits, that three strong people cou'd scarcely keep her in bed; but after bleeding, blisters, with the use of anodine and nervous medicine, they now abated in severity, and did not return above one or twice a day."

"Notwithstanding this," he went on, "her disorder continued in one shape or other, or, return'd after an intermission of a month or two, at farthest. Sometimes she was tortur'd almost to madness with a cramp in different parts of the body; then with more general convulsions of the extremities, and a choaking deliquium; and, at times with almost the whole train [of] hysteric symptoms." The hysterical symptoms "continued and harrass'd her alternatively for 10 years, tho' she had the best advice the place afforded, and took a great number of medicines."

In September 1752, C.B. made up her mind to find out whether electricity, which might have been suggested by Evans, would work for her. Evans now quoted directly from one of C.B.'s letters, dated February 1754:

At length my spirits were quite broke and subdued with so many years of affliction, and indeed I was almost grown desperate, and being left without hope of relief. About this time there was a great talk of the wonderful power of electricity; and as a person reduc'd to the last extremity, is glad to catch anything; I happen'd to think it might be useful to me. Altho' I cou'd have no encouragement from any experiment in the like case, I resolv'd to try, let the event be what it might; for death was more desirable than life, on the terms I enjoy'd it. Accordingly I went to Philadelphia, the beginning of September 1752, and apply'd to B. Franklin, who I thought understood it best of any person here.

C.B. further writes that she "receiv'd four strokes morning and evening . . . and indeed they were very severe. On receiving the first shock, I felt the fit very strong, but the second eventually carry'd it off; and thus it was every time I went through the operation." Happily, "the symptoms gradually decreased, till at length they entirely left me. I staid in town but two weeks, and when I went home, B. Franklin was so good as to supply me with a globe and bottle, to electrify myself everyday for three months. The fits were soon carried off, but the cramp continued somewhat longer, tho' it was scarcely troublesome, and very seldom return'd. I now enjoy such a state of health, as I wou'd have given all the world for . . . and I have great reason to hope it will continue."

The final line in Evans's communication informs the reader that the electrical treatments had lasting effects, which would make his diagnosis of hysteria, as opposed to true epilepsy, all the more likely: "I have other letters from the family of later date, which says she continues to enjoy perfect health."

A publication from 1828 confirms C.B.'s full recovery. "The cure was perfect and permanent. Her mind was not affected, as is common, by the disease; she possessed uncommon powers of reasoning, and was distinguished for the sprightness of her wit, and the charms of her conversation. She lived to the age of 79 years."[9]

Neither C.B. nor hysteria is mentioned in Franklin's known letters, so it is impossible to know why he believed electricity was worth trying in her case. Did he assume C.B.'s body would respond to a powerful stimulant? Did he use electricity as a placebo? Or did he approach her case as would an empiric, without any theory in mind, but hearing or feeling that electricity was worth trying in such cases? All three possibilities deserve comment.

First, both Franklin and Evans might have targeted the machinery of C.B.'s body, given the popular theories of the day. The belief was strong that a stimulant was called for, and electricity was touted as the best stimulant for tightening the nerves and increasing blood flow. Christian Kratzenstein, in fact, had specifically called for thinning the sluggish blood of hysterical women. He wrote that "since the blood is made thinner and less viscous through rapid circulation, electrification must be an excellent remedy . . . in women with hysterical conditions."[10]

As for the second possibility, that Franklin was already aware of the power of suggestion, here too a good case can be made. After all, he had long known that gullible people might respond positively to quack remedies.[11] And he had read about the Abbé Nollet's visit to Italy and agreed with him that the miraculous cures associated with medicated electrical tubes were probably due to suggestion.

In addition, suggestion had by this time been used in traditional medicine. John Webster, for example, was convinced that it was a waste of time to try to reason with women who thought themselves bewitched. But, wrote Webster in 1677, "If you indulge their fancy, and seem to concur in opinion with them, and hang any insignificant thing about their necks, assuring them that it is a most efficacious and powerful charm . . . you may cure them. Yet . . . the common people (and sometimes the learned also) do attribute the whole effect unto the charm, when indeed it effecteth nothing at all."[12] Poor Richard was less wordy in 1734, when he chimed in, "As Charms are nonsense, Nonsense is a Charm."[13]

John Locke, whom Franklin admired, studied the association of ideas and concluded that people could be deceived by incorrectly associating cause and effect.[14] From Locke's premise, Franklin might have wanted to create a false belief, albeit one that would "cure" C.B. And his willingness to use suggestion would not have been out of character for him. He spoke about "the hope of success" with his palsy patients (see Chapter 5), and he would use suggestion to treat a despondent Polish noblewoman and to account for the successes that Mesmer and his followers were attributing to animal magnetism (see Chapters 13 and 14).

But what about the third possibility, that Franklin was an empiricist not guided by theory? Empiricism was very much in the air, especially among non-academic practitioners. Consider Patrick Brydone's case report which led Franklin to present his own findings with medical electricity to the Royal Society in 1757.[15] The afflicted individual described in Brydone's letter was a young woman who began to lose movement and sensation, and who showed other signs and symptoms, just a few years after her father had died of a palsy. Brydone found that, after a series of electrical treatments, all of her symptoms had vanished. Brydone did not have a medical degree or an academic appointment, and said nothing about a guiding theory.

Just what was going through Franklin's mind before, during, and after working with C.B. may never be known. We can only wonder whether he was wearing the hat of a physiologist, a psychologist, or an empiric, while he administered electricity to this troubled young lady. For all we know, he might have entertained all three possibilities, perhaps knowing that the same protocol would be called for in each instance anyway. But, Franklin would go on to ask, would electricity also work with a closely related disorder, specifically, melancholia?

## MELANCHOLIA'S DARK PAST

The term "melancholia," which was so popular in Franklin's lifetime, included severe depression, but it also applied to less severe, non-febrile disorders marked by sadness, tiredness, sleeplessness, fear, irritability, uneasiness, loss of appetite, self-loathing, and social isolation. To the eighteenth-century medical mind, melancholia was the opposite of mania and a cousin of hysteria. In humoral theory, melancholia, like hysteria, was usually attributed to an over-abundance of cold and dry black bile that the spleen would normally absorb. In fact, the term "melancholia" is derived from the Greek term for dark bile. By mixing with the blood to the brain or by gumming up other passages and organs, an excess of this gloomy humor was believed to cause mental and physical lethargy.

During the second half of the seventeenth century, Thomas Willis, England's leading physician, dismissed the "melancholick Humour" in favor of a "Distemper of the Brain and Spirits dwelling in it."[16] Willis was an iatrochemist, and he attempted to explain melancholia chemically, without recourse to the supernatural. His approach created a gap between him and Robert Burton, the author of *Anatomy of Melancholy*, whose classic text appeared in 1621 and presented original sin and the devil as causes of the disorder.[17]

By the end of the seventeenth century, in accordance with newer mechanical theories, the most popular explanation for melancholia was that sufferers' nerves were too limp or flaccid. Further paralleling the emerging view of its cousin, hysteria, psychological factors began to be incorporated into theoretical formulations. For a growing number of physicians, amalgams of physical and psychological variables seemed to make the most sense.

The use of stimulants was once again high on the list of almost all physicians, whether they stressed the physical or mental causes of melancholia. After all, stimulants could counteract the dark humors, strengthen the slack nerves, increase the sluggish activity of the brain, sharpen the mind, and induce physical activity. The idea of giving melancholics electrical shocks to the head was, however, slow in coming. One reason for this was that many electrotherapists were simply unwilling to administer shocks to the head, perhaps because they thought they might be dangerous or too psychologically traumatic for their patients to handle. Another was that melancholia tended to be perceived as a moral problem in some circles. For these and other reasons, this sort of therapy might not have been attempted until Jan Ingenhousz and Benjamin Franklin proposed giving severely melancholic patients electrical shocks to the head, and that was not until the mid-1780s.

## ELECTRICAL ACCIDENTS

The successful use of mild electrical shocks to treat hysterical patients added to the general enthusiasm for the electrical cure. But the catalyst for Franklin's use of electricity to treat patients with melancholia was not his success with C.B., the Brydone case of hysteria, or any of the enthusiastic reports about medical electricity in general that he might have been reading in *Gentleman's Magazine*. Instead, it stemmed from his own electrical accidents, which he considered rather embarrassing, knowing they could easily have been prevented.

One of Franklin's mishaps was briefly mentioned in a letter to John Lining of Charleston, South Carolina. Lining was a physician and a man with broad interests like Franklin's: meteorology, health, electricity, and the like.[18] In his letter, which was dated 1755, Franklin first described an electrical demonstration on a column of six men.

I laid one end of my discharging rod upon the head of the first; he laid his hand on the head of the second; the second his hand on the head of the third, and so to the last, who held, in his hand, the chain that was connected to the outside of the jarrs. When they were thus placed, I applied the other end of my rod to the prime-conductor, and they all dropt together. When they got up, they all declared they had not felt any stroke, and wondered how they came to fall; nor did any of them hear the crack, or see the light of it.[19]

After describing how the six men experienced what we would call retrograde amnesia as a result of the electrical charge that surged through their heads, Franklin informed Lining that he had once also endured a jolt of electricity that knocked him down. "You suppose it a dangerous experiment," he wrote, "but I had once suffered the same myself, receiving by accident, an equal stroke though my head, that struck me down, without hurting me."[20]

Next, Franklin told Lining about a young lady under his care, who accidentally experienced a shock directly to her head: "And I had seen a young woman, that was about to the electrified through the feet (for some indisposition) receive a greater charge through the head, by inadvertently stooping forward to look at the placing of her feet, till her forehead (as she was very tall) came too near my prime-conductor. She dropt, but instantly got up again complaining of nothing."

Franklin deduced several things about electricity involving the head from what he had witnessed with the line of six men, his own accident, and the incident involving one of his patients. First, electricity could cause a loss of consciousness. Second, it could produce a memory loss for the event. And third, even moderately severe shocks could be applied to the cranium without risking a loss of life. But Franklin was not yet thinking about trying cranial electricity with melancholic patients. In fact, what Lining and he had been discussing was not healing, but whether electricity might be a more humane way to execute criminals. Lining first raised the idea and Franklin concurred with the words "it would certainly . . . be the easiest of all deaths."[21] Many more years would pass before another development would entice him to think about shocks involving the head in a more positive, therapeutic way.

## JAN INGENHOUSZ

Jan Ingenhousz, the Dutchman who had studied medicine in Louvain, Leiden, Paris, and Edinburgh, first met Franklin in 1765, when they were both in London.[22] The two men knew John Pringle and had many common interests, including smallpox inoculation, medical experimentation, and the improvement of practical medicine.

In 1768, after Empress Maria Theresa of Austria survived her own smallpox but saw family members die from it, she asked the king's physicians in England to recommend a skilled physician to inoculate her remaining children. Pringle felt Ingenhousz was the ideal physician, since he had spent time studying inoculation at the London Foundling Hospital and was enthusiastic about the procedure. So Ingenhousz went off to Austria, where he inoculated successfully and stayed on as a royal physician.

Franklin and Ingenhousz remained the best of correspondents, exchanging more than seventy letters between 1773 and 1788.[23] And Ingenhousz, like Franklin, never tired of reading about or dabbling with electricity. Further, he also had his mishaps. His most significant accident occurred in Vienna in 1783, when he was knocked unconscious by a shock to his head. Once he felt more stable, he picked up his pen and described his mental state to Franklin, who was then in France, and he asked him for more information about his own electrical accidents.[24] In his broken English, poor spelling, scratched out terms, and undecipherable words, Ingenhousz stated:

The flash enter'd the corner of my hat. Then it entred my forehead and passed thro the left hand, in which I held the chaine communicating with the outward Coating of the yarr [jar]. I neither saw, heared nor [sensed?] the explosion by which I was Struck down. I lost all my senses, memory, understanding and even sound judgment. . . . after having answered unadequately to some questio[ns] which were asked me by people in the room, I determined to go home. But I wa[s] surprised that, though the accident happened in a hous in the same street where I lodged, yet I was more than two minutes considering whether, to go hom[e], I must go to the right or to the left hand.

He continued: "Having found my lodgings, and consider[ed?] that my memory was become very weak, I thought it prudent to put down in writing th[e] history of the case. I placed the paper before me, dipt the pen in the ink, but when I applyed it to the paper, I found I had entirely forgotten the art of writing and reading and did not know more what to doe with the pen, than a savage, who never knew there was such an art found out. This struck me with terror, as I feared I should remain for ever an idiot."

Ingenhousz went to bed, and upon awakening several hours later he discovered that his "mental faculties were at that time not only returned, but I felt the most lively joye in finding, as I thought at the time, my judgment infinitely more acute." He added, "I saw much clearer the difficulties of every thing, and what did formerly seem to me difficult to comprehend, was now become of an easy solution. I found moreover a liveliness in my whole frame, which I never had observed before."

### FRANKLIN'S RESPONSE

In effect, Ingenhousz told Franklin that a strong shock to his head, powerful enough to cause unconsciousness, produced better judgment and "a liveliness" in his body unlike anything he had experienced. He now went on to tell his close friend that he had already taken steps to put his discovery to good use: "This experiment, made by accident, and on my self . . . has induced me to advise som[e] of the London mad-Doctors, as Dr Brook, to try a similar experiment o[n] mad men, thinking that, as I found my self, my mental faculties impro[ved] and as the world well knows, that your mental faculties, if not improved [by] the two strooks you received, were certainly not hurt, by them, it might perhaps be[?] a remedie to restore the mental faculties when lost."[25]

Franklin was intrigued, but he did not write back until April 1785, just before he received permission to return home from France. In his reply, he referred to two accidents involving electricity that passed through his head. For the first one, he directed Ingenhousz to the 1774 edition of his pamphlet on electricity, which included a letter to Peter Collinson with a detailed description of his experience. For his second accident, he wrote:

I had a Paralytick Patient in my Chamber, whose Friends brought him to receive some Electric Shocks. I made them join Hands so as to receive the Shock at the same time, and I charg'd two large Jars to give it. By the Number of those People, I was oblig'd to quit my usual Standing, and plac'd myself inadvertently under an Iron Hook which hung from the Ceiling down to within two Inches of my Head, and communicated by a Wire with the outside of the Jars. I attempted to discharge them, and in fact did so; but I did not perceive it, tho' the charge went thro' me, and not through the Persons I entended it for.

I neither saw the Flash, heard the Report, nor felt the Stroke. When my Senses returned, I found myself on the Floor. I got up, not knowing how that had happened.

I then again attempted to discharge the Jars; but one of the Company told me they were already discharg'd, which I could not at first believe, but on Trial found it true. . . . A small swelling rose on the Top of my Head, which continued sore for some Days, but I do not remember any other Effect good or bad.[26]

Franklin suffered retrograde amnesia after this direct shock to the head. But because he did not consider his memory loss very serious, and because there were no other lasting effects of the incident, he brushed it aside and agreed with Ingenhousz that shocks to the head could be tried with mad patients without fearing for their safety. Before he left France, Franklin contacted a French medical electrician, who he thought might act on the idea. He informed Ingenhousz: "I communicated that Part of your Letter to an Operator, encourag'd by the Government here to electrify epileptic and other poor Patients, and advis'd his trying the Practice on Mad People according to your opinion."[27]

Noticeably absent from both Franklin's and Ingenhousz's communications is any speculation about why cranial electrotherapy might improve thinking and enhance one's feeling of well-being. Both men stuck with the facts.

## THE REACTION

Did any clinical trials immediately follow the proposals by Ingenhousz and Franklin to the English and French authorities? Franklin told Ingenhousz in his 1785 letter that he suggested shocking "Mad People" to a French health officer, but that "I have not heard whether he has done it."[28] As for Ingenhousz, he ended his 1783 letter to Franklin by telling him that, despite efforts to get the "mad-Doctors" of London to take the next step, "I could never persuade any one to."[29]

The records show, however, that a few practitioners began to treat melancholic and other mad patients with electrical shocks to the head soon after Ingenhousz and Franklin made the suggestion. One such person was John Birch, a surgeon and the founder of the electrical department at St. Thomas's Hospital in London.[30] He might have been the first electrotherapist to try electricity to the head with melancholics, and he tells us that he successfully treated a despondent porter in 1787 with shocks passed through the brain in different directions, and that he similarly helped a suicidal singer. But it was his third patient who received the strongest shocks of all "from the frontal to the occipital bone, and from one temporal bone to the other." Birch expressed surprise that he "could practice so boldly, without any serious inconvenience to the brain," but, unwilling to go further, he dismissed this patient "in the same unhappy state he had so long suffered."[31]

Giovanni Aldini followed Birch, treating his first mad patient in Bologna in 1801.[32] Aldini tells us he was able to help Louis Lanzarini, a farmer with a "taciturn and dreamlike demeanor," who withdrew from other people, and Charles Bellini, a laborer, "who was restored to society."

In 1803, T. Gale, an obscure American practitioner, published a book on medical electricity that included a section on "Madness."[33] Three cases were described: an obviously depressed woman ("deep dejection of spirits, gloomy and melancholy") and two suicidal men. The first man was given "exceedingly heavy shocks" to the head, and the second a shock "as high as I thought he could bear, and live through."[34] All improved.

Neither Birch nor Aldini nor Gale mentioned Franklin or Ingenhousz when describing how they applied shocks to the head. But citing sources, especially unpublished notes, was not the rule at the time. Given the chronology, Franklin and Ingenhousz, directly or indirectly, might have planted the seeds for what these well-intentioned physicians began to do for melancholic, and, in the case of Aldini, possibly also schizophrenic patients.

The idea of shocking the heads of severely debilitated mental patients would resurface again in the 1930s, and thereafter be widely employed, particularly for patients with severe depression. Its resurrection would begin with Ugo Cerletti, an Italian physician who initially worked with schizophrenics.[35] Cerletti was unaware of what Ingenhousz and Franklin had proposed in the 1780s, and his work was not based on the clinical trials that followed the proposals of these two men, but on the mistaken idea that epileptics are immune to schizophrenia.

Following Cerletti, many people have mistakenly concluded that treating mental patients with controlled electrical shocks to the head is something new. Moreover, even the loss of memory that accompanied the head-shock treatments has been regarded as a twentieth-century discovery. Yet, as we have seen, the use of cranial electricity with severely mentally ill patients has roots that go back to Franklin and Ingenhousz in the 1780s. And further, several excellent descriptions of shock-induced retrograde amnesia can be found in Franklin's writings, including his 1755 letter to Lining and his 1751 letter to Collinson, which were published in the 1774 edition of his pamphlet on electricity. In both the electrical therapy and memory disorder domains, Franklin was a thoughtful and astute observer, and he was well ahead of his time.

# PART II
# MEDICINE IN
# GREAT BRITAIN

CHAPTER 7

# Friends and Medical Connections

Without my having made any application for that honor, they chose
me a member.
—Benjamin Franklin on his election to
the Royal Society of London in 1756

Benjamin Franklin made two extended diplomatic trips to England prior to the American War for Independence. Both occurred because he was active in the Pennsylvania Assembly, which represented the citizens of the colony. In the first mission, from 1757 to 1762, his main goal was to try to convince the two surviving sons of William Penn, Thomas and Richard, to pay taxes on their vast Pennsylvania lands for the security and welfare of their colony. There were other issues as well, such as having to work with an inflexible governor—a man appointed, instructed, and salaried by the Penns.

Faced with their own problems and having different priorities, the Penns were less than cooperative. In fact, after lengthy delays and then some accusations, they told Franklin that they would no longer meet with him, because he was not a person of candor. When Franklin sailed home on the *Carolina* five years after arriving in England, he had little to show for his efforts with the Penns. In addition, the Privy Council had exhibited no interest in turning Pennsylvania from a proprietorship into a Crown colony.

Franklin's second mission on behalf of the Pennsylvania Assembly was even lengthier, beginning in 1764 and ending in 1775. This time his diplomacy was largely concerned with the taxes Parliament was imposing or was planning to impose on the colonies. Britain's need for revenue stemmed from the costs associated with the French and Indian War in North America and the partially overlapping Seven Years War in Europe. These conflicts severely depleted the treasury. Supporters of the taxes contended that, because the colonists were the major beneficiaries of the fighting that started in 1754 and ended in 1763, they must contribute more. But many colonists felt that Parliament had no right to impose these taxes, as the colonies were not represented in that legislative body. Moreover, they contended that they had contributed more than their fair share to the war effort.

The second diplomatic mission also proved unsuccessful. Franklin returned home just as blood was being spilled in New England and each side was mobilizing for war. Franklin's many biographers have emphasized what he attempted to accomplish, the methods he employed, how the aristocracy treated him, and how his feelings about the king, Parliament, and mother country changed as a result of this mission. In contrast, much less has been written about Franklin's extensive medical connections and his medical forays during his two lengthy stays in Britain.

## ELECTRICAL CONNECTIONS

With his inquiring mind and love of nature, Franklin sailed from Philadelphia not just with a diplomatic agenda, but with every hope of discussing new ideas in natural philosophy and medicine with kindred spirits across the Atlantic. In fact, one of the first things he did after arriving in London was to purchase the latest copies of *Gentleman's Magazine* to catch up on the newest developments. He also brought with him or soon constructed the most powerful electric machine ever seen in London.

Much has been made of the celebrity status Franklin enjoyed and the popular cult that surrounded him when he went on to become ambassador to France (see Chapter 12). But it is also clear that he was well known and that there were many people who wanted to meet, share ideas, and dine with him after he arrived in Britain. To some of these people, he was a moral philosopher with interesting ideas about self-betterment. To others, he was a perceptive colonist who seemed to understand the needs and hopes of family members and friends living on the western side of the Atlantic. To yet more people, he was the witty author and savvy printer of *Poor Richard's Almanack*. But more than anything else, Franklin's worldwide fame in 1757 rested on his experiments, understanding, and control of electricity. The lifesaving and property-saving attributes of Franklin's pointed lightning rod were by this time widely known among the common people and the gentry. Moreover, his work showing the "sameness" of electricity from machines and lightning had a tremendous impact on natural philosophers, as did his single-fluid theory of electricity and naturalistic explanations for heavenly events, such as thunder and lightning storms.

Major tributes and honors first came Franklin's way in 1753. That year he received an honorary master of arts degree from Harvard College for his

"Improvements in Philosophical Learning, and particularly with Respect to Electricity." A comparable honor followed from Yale just a few weeks later. And in England, the Royal Society had given him its Copley Gold Medal, "on account of his curious experiments and observations on electricity." Franklin, hoping to create a favorable impression in England, had even written back: "Gentlemen, . . . I know not whether any of your learned Body have attain'd the ancient boasted Art of *multiplying* Gold; but you have certainly found the Art of making it infinitely *more valuable*."[1] Three years later, the Royal Society, having taken further notice of him, elected him a member.

As a natural philosopher, Franklin's stature at the time of his arrival in 1757 might have been second only to that of the late Sir Isaac Newton. William Pitt (Lord Chatham) compared Franklin to Newton, calling him "an Honour not to the English Nation only but to Human Nature."[2] But unlike Newton, Franklin had a self-deprecating personality and a wonderful sense of humor. To the brotherhood of experimental natural philosophers, which included many people directly involved in the practice of medicine or with strong interests in medicine, and to many of the leaders in practical medicine, Franklin was a visitor they had to seek out. And he wanted to meet them every bit as much as they wanted to meet him.

## SETTLING INTO LONDON

Franklin's ship arrived in the English port city of Falmouth during the summer of 1757. After a short rest, he headed overland, spending his first night in the London area at Mill Hill. This was the home of Quaker Peter Collinson, agent for his Library Company, philanthropist, renowned botanist, and member of the Royal Society. Franklin and Collinson had exchanged dozens of letters prior to their first meeting, the most notable of which were Franklin's landmark pieces on the nature of electricity and the utility of the lightning rod.

Now that he had arrived in England, Collinson introduced Franklin to other enlightened philosophers and physicians. One of the first and most important was John Fothergill, who wrote the preface for his celebrated pamphlet, *Experiments and Observations on Electricity*.[3] A graduate of the Edinburgh medical school, Fothergill had one of the most successful medical practices in the country and was well connected politically. To quote Franklin, he "made daily Visits among the Great in the Practice of his Profession, [and] had full Opportunity of being acquainted with their Sentiments . . . upon the Subject of America."[4] Indeed, Fothergill helped arrange

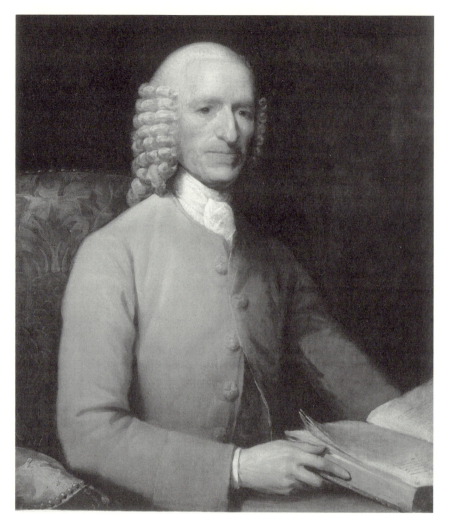

*Painting of Dr. John Fothergill (1712–1780) by Gilbert Stuart.*
*(With permission of the Pennsylvania Academy of Fine Arts.)*

Franklin's first meeting with the Penns at Spring Garden. Moreover, at later dates, he wrote a pamphlet advocating repeal of the Stamp Act and tried to mediate a reasonable compromise. From start to finish, Fothergill provided Franklin with political information, sound advice, and needed support.

Having come down with a recurrent fever soon after arriving, Franklin engaged Fothergill to serve as his physician. Fothergill's other patients included various members of the Penn family, the Earl of Dartmouth, and John Wesley, the cleric who read Franklin's celebrated pamphlet and was extremely interested in therapeutic uses of electricity. Franklin and Fothergill had extensive discussions about preventing and treating diseases while he was sick and afterward. They also discussed hospitals and medical education in the colonies. Years later, Franklin would write: "If we may estimate the goodness of a man by his disposition to do good, and his constant endeavours and success in doing it, I can hardly conceive that a better man ever existed."[5]

John Pringle was another physician in Collinson's illustrious circle.[6] He had studied medicine at Edinburgh and Leyden, and in 1742 was appointed physician to the British Army. Pringle became physician to Queen Charlotte in 1761 and King George III in 1774. With Franklin's influence and support, he also became President of the Royal Society of London. Although highly respected for his thoughts on preventing and treating military and jail diseases, Pringle had broad medical interests, which is why he personally urged Franklin to present his own findings on medical electricity and the palsies to the Royal Society late in 1757. That presentation enhanced Franklin's reputation among physicians even more.

Collinson, Fothergill, and Pringle spent considerable private time with Franklin. Pringle, in fact, became his favorite traveling companion. And although Franklin did not have formal medical training, these men were so impressed with his breadth of knowledge and reasoning powers that they occasionally solicited his medical assistance. A notable example of how they turned to Franklin took place in 1767, when John Pringle asked for more than just his medical opinion.

The case involved Lady Mary Catherine, the twelve-year-old daughter of the Duke of Ancaster. Pringle wanted Franklin to try medical electricity on the girl, who was having convulsions. He knew that Franklin had been successful in treating a convulsive case in the colonies, although C.B.'s convulsions were hysterical and not due to brain damage. And he knew that Franklin had witnessed the successful electrical treatment of a woman who "had for above six weeks lost her speech by convulsive fits," although the brief report in *Gentleman's Magazine* also stated "Mr. *Franklin* of *Philadelphia* . . . expressed his astonishment."[7]

Pringle's urgent note to Franklin read: "I take the liberty to beg that You would come as soon as You can to the Duke of Ancaster's in Berkeley Square, as His Grace and the Duchess are in the greatest distress about their daughter, who has been long in a most Miserable condition with spasms and convulsions . . . the present spasm has shut the Young Lady's jaw and deprived Her both of speech and swallowing. I ventured to name You as the person the most proper for directing the operation, trusting to your friendship to me and humanity towards the distressed."[8]

Franklin's known writings provide us with no more information about this case. But Leonard Labaree, who edited his letters from this time period, states: "It seems probable that after the electric shock treatment (though not necessarily because of it) her condition improved enough for her to be moved from Chelsea to the spa at Clifton, near Bristol." He adds that "she soon suffered a relapse, however, and died on Palm Sunday."[9]

In retrospect, whether treated by Franklin or not, had Lady Mary Catherine been suffering from a malignant brain tumor, as seems likely, she would not have responded to electricity anyway. Yet, if nothing else, Pringle's appeal for Franklin's help tells us a lot about Franklin's stature in Britain's medical community and how highly his thoughts and acumen on some subjects were regarded. It also helps to explain why many exclusive organizations sought out and warmly welcomed Franklin into their ranks.

## FRANKLIN AND THE ROYAL SOCIETY

Historian J. L. Heilbron has written that, "During the Enlightenment natural philosophy was a pursuit of clubbable men, and every natural philosopher of any standing was a member of at least one academy or society. These bodies," he tells us, "tended to restrict ordinary membership to people living nearby, but by bestowing corresponding, associate, honorary, and foreign memberships they at once raised their prestige, flattered the vanity of their colleagues at a distance, and enrolled themselves in a wide cooperative movement. The natural philosopher," Heilbron concluded, "was a social as well as a rational animal."[10]

Franklin, by any standard, was a most "clubbable man." He had started his Junto in 1727 to discuss pertinent issues in philosophy, and presented his plan for an American Philosophical Society in 1743. Now, with his thirst for intellectual stimulation, love of natural philosophy, and interest in medicine growing, he involved himself with a number of British organizations and clubs.

The oldest and most prestigious scientific organization in London was the Royal Society, established in 1660 for the promotion of useful knowledge. Its motto was *Nulius in Verba* (On the Words of No One), signifying its commitment to experiments and careful observation, rather than to authority. The Royal Society had received its charter and mace from King Charles II, and Robert Boyle, Robert Hooke, William Petty, Thomas Willis, and Christopher Wren were among its illustrious early members. Isaac Newton was also active in the society in the seventeenth century, and he directed the organization through most of the first quarter of the eighteenth century.

Peter Collinson had recommended Franklin for membership in the Royal Society on the basis of his electrical contributions, and he was duly elected on April 29, 1756. In his *Autobiography*, Franklin would boast that he never submitted a formal application or was asked to pay a fee, both of which were expected from other candidates. Nevertheless, he was not really "official" until November 24, 1757, when he finally showed up to sign the requisite papers. Franklin would serve the society with distinction under the Earl of Macclesfield, who governed it until 1764. He would then serve under five other presidents: the Earl of Morton (1764–1768), James Burrow (1768–1768), James West (1768–1772), John Pringle (1772–1778), and Joseph Banks (1778–1790). Whenever he could, Franklin attended the formal meetings of the Royal Society at Crane Court, its home since 1710. Sometimes he even brought young American medical students along with him, to inspire them and to introduce them to people who might help them in their careers. He also nominated other enlightened people for membership in the society, many for their work on electricity, but some for other contributions, including medicine.

Franklin made his first nomination in 1759. Edmund Hussey Delaval was a Cambridge-based scientist with a penchant for electricity. Interestingly, his playing of the musical glasses would stimulate Franklin to invent his glass armonica. Delaval was followed by at least thirty-six other nominations, one of whom was a promising young anatomist by the name of William Hewson.[11] Franklin had no reason to suspect at the time of Hewson's nomination, in 1770, that he would literally turn Franklin's London residence into an anatomical museum and school. Yet that is exactly what happened, and it brought Franklin into even greater contact with the British medical community.

Shortly after arriving in London, Franklin began to board at 7 Craven Street.[12] Margaret Stevenson, a widow close to his age, owned the brick dwelling just around the corner from what is now Trafalgar Square and close to Whitehall and Parliament. Her eighteen-year-old daughter "Polly" (Mary) also lived on the premises. Franklin recognized Polly's intellect and her unusual love of knowledge. Hence, he introduced her to Hewson, who had studied medicine at hospitals in London and Edinburgh, midwifery with Colin Mackenzie in London, and anatomy and pathology with the Hunters at their private school in that city.

After John Hunter left in 1760 for a four-year tour of duty with the army,

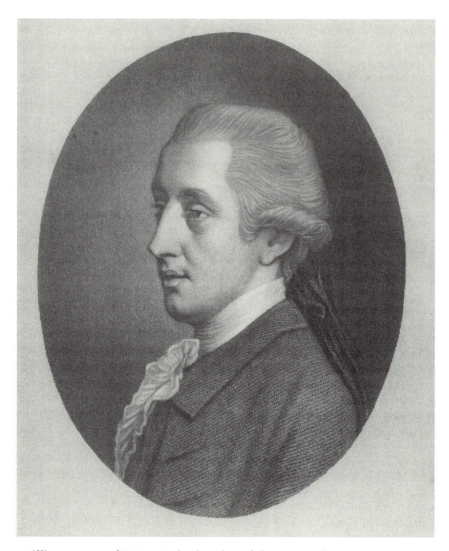

*William Hewson (1739–1774), the talented dissector and anatomy teacher who married Polly Stevenson and lived for some time under the same roof as Franklin.*

his brother William, who ran the school, needed assistance and asked Hewson to help. When Hewson married Polly Stevenson in 1770, he was teaching in the Hunterian Medical School, which had moved to 16 Great Windmill Street two years earlier, and he had become a partner in the enterprise.

Hewson also conducted research, mostly on the lymphatic system and blood corpuscles. His preparations, observations, and theories were consid-

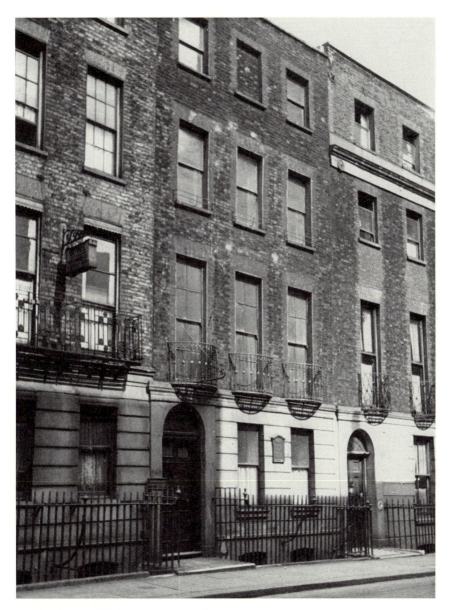

*Benjamin Franklin's Craven Street home.*

ered so good that he was awarded the Copley Prize in 1768 and nominated for membership in the Royal Society two years later. William Hunter and John Pringle joined Franklin in supporting his candidacy.

Unlike Hewson, William Hunter remained a confirmed bachelor.[13] He thought nothing about working through the night at the dissection table and expected Hewson to do the same, even after his marriage to Polly Stevenson. Consequently, he was upset when Hewson began to spend more of his evening hours with his new wife. Soon Hunter was also complaining when Hewson left on short trips; conversely, Hewson did not like the idea that Hunter was claiming ownership of everything he worked on.

Hunter contacted Franklin as a friend of both parties, hoping to resolve the dispute. Franklin did his best to mediate, but Hewson still opted to leave Hunter in 1772. Hunter contacted Franklin again, this time asking if he wanted to collect some of the anatomical preparations Hewson had left behind. Franklin obliged and immediately gave them to Hewson, who had moved with Polly into the house occupied by him and her mother, his landlady.

Not lacking in ambition, Hewson planned to open a new school of anatomy with an anatomical theater at the back of the residence. This led to "prepar'd fetuses" and a buildup of animal and human bones, the latter most likely purchased from "resurrectionists" or grave robbers.[14] Yet as much as Franklin enjoyed discussing medicine with Hewson, he and Margaret Stevenson opted to move to a less crowded house on Craven Street after Polly gave birth to the Hewsons' first child.

Hewson opened his Craven Street school of anatomy during the fall of 1772, and he soon had a sizable number of students. Unfortunately, he cut himself during a dissection and died of septicemia in 1774. Franklin, who would remain close to Polly, took his death as a blow to medical science and as a personal loss. As for the Hunters, Franklin would continue to stay on good terms with them, and, as we shall see, even helped them at the Royal Society.

With his dedication to the Royal Society, reputation as an experimental natural philosopher, and visibility, Franklin was elected to the group's governing council several times. His first appointment was in 1760, and he was reelected again in 1765, 1766, and 1772. In his leadership role, he helped maintain the society's high standards by evaluating submissions for publication in the organization's *Philosophical Transactions*. He was not one to delve into things he knew little about. But when papers from England, the North American colonies, or elsewhere were on subjects that people knew interested him, such as electricity or clean air, they often wound up on his desk. In some cases, the submissions were addressed to, or dedicated to, "Doctor Franklin."

The manuscripts he looked over on electric fish had to be among those he found most intriguing. It was not until the second half of the seventeenth century that Western European natural philosophers began to exam-

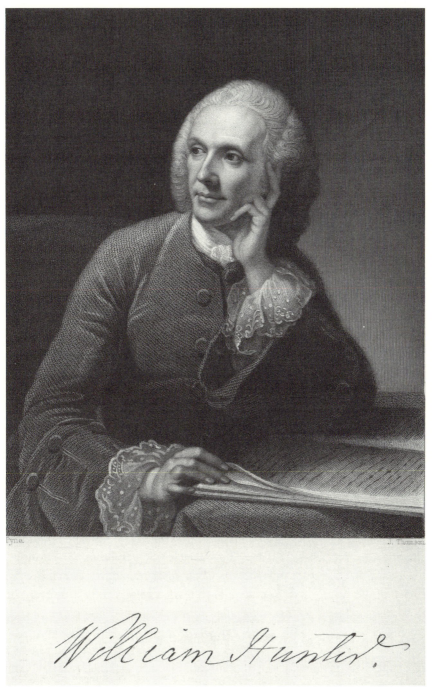

*William Hunter (1718–1783), head of a famous London school of anatomy
and pathology.*

ine these specialized creatures in detail. With electricity now so much on everyone's mind, people wanted to know whether these creatures actually produced electricity. And if they did, what did this mean in the great scheme of things?

Early in the 1770s, John Walsh conducted a clever series of experiments on the electric rays (torpedoes) caught off the coasts of France and England that went a long way toward answering these questions. He sent his material to Franklin with the words, "It is with particular satisfaction I make to you my first communication, that the effect of the Torpedo appears to be absolutely electrical."[15] Walsh then described how an electric ray could discharge fifty or more shocks per minute—shocks that could be transmitted through wires and even people holding hands. What the participants in the experiment felt was indistinguishable from the shocks produced with Leyden jars.

John Hunter did not train in medicine at Edinburgh like his older brother William, but he was even more skilled at dissection. And he became directly involved with these experiments. In 1773, "Mister" Hunter wrote: "I was desired for some time since, by Mr. Walsh, whose experiments at La Rochelle had determined the effect of the Torpedo to be electrical, to dissect and examine the particular organs by which that animal produces so extraordinary an effect. This I have done in several subjects furnished to me by that Gentleman."[16]

John Hunter verbally described and beautifully illustrated the physical structure of the ray's electric organ. In fact, he showed that it appeared to be made up of hundreds of "perpendicular columns," each made up of about 150 horizontal disks separated by "numerous interstices, which appear to contain a fluid." The columns reached "from the upper to the under surface of the body," and the nerves, "having entered the organs, ramify in every direction, between the columns, and send in small branches upon each partition."[17]

The Walsh and Hunter communications, published in the *Philosophical Transactions* between 1773 and 1775, were important because they supported the theory that living creatures can produce electricity and the idea that electricity is the mysterious force coursing through the nerves.[18] As Hunter expressed it: "May we not conclude that they [the nerves to the electric organs] are subservient to the formation, collection, or management of the electric fluid; especially as it appears evident from Mr. Walsh's experiments, that the will of the animal does absolutely controul the electric powers of it's body; which must depend on the energy of the nerves."[19]

John Pringle, who had by this time become the society's nineteenth president, handed Walsh the Copley Medal in 1774. Pleased but not finished with

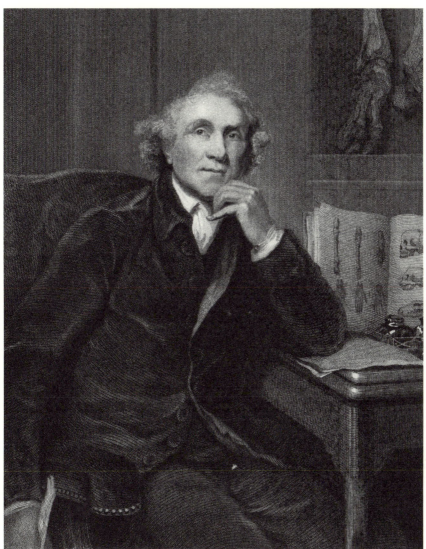

nted by Sir Joshua Reynolds.                    Engraved by G.H.Ad

JOHN HUNTER.

*John Hunter (1728–1793), anatomist, teacher, and brother of William Hunter.*

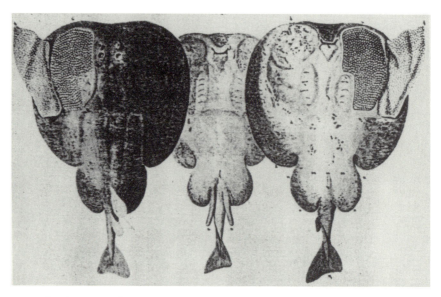

*One of John Hunter's 1773 illustrations of the electric organs of the torpedo, or electric ray. (From John Hunter, "Anatomical Observations on the Torpedo,"* Philosophical Transactions of the Royal Society of London 63 *[1773].)*

his research, Walsh continued to build the case he had made for electricity being generated by these fish. He went on to demonstrate, to the amazement of the skeptics, that the discharge from a healthy ray could actually produce a spark capable of jumping across a cut in a piece of tin foil.[20]

In the larger scheme of things, John Walsh and John Hunter's efforts helped to overthrow the idea that miniscule "spirits" are in some way transmitted through the hollow nerves, an idea that can be traced back to the ancient Greeks and Romans, and one adopted by Descartes and then Leeuwenhoek. Their work also served as the death knell for the theory of watery nerve juices. Before the century would be over, Luigi Galvani and his nephew Giovanni Aldini would expand the idea of electricity in specialized fish to electricity as the nerve force in frogs and then mammals. The jump to humans would no longer be so large.

The new idea, that nonspecialized creatures can produce electricity, a force capable of traveling through the nerves at speeds too fast to be measured, resulted in fundamentally new ways of thinking about how the nervous system functions. And this development, in turn, suggested new ways of looking at diseases of the brain and nerves, including the palsies and seizure disorders that had caught Franklin's attention in the colonies and now in England.

## OTHER CLUBS AND ORGANIZATIONS

Above and beyond listening to or reading formally presented papers, some fellows of the Royal Society liked to gravitate to the Mitre Tavern on Fleet Street to dine and talk more informally about natural philosophy and medicine. Franklin never joined this "Royal Society Club," which was organized in 1743. But during his stay in London he might have been its most frequent dinner guest. Estimates are that he attended at least sixty of the club's discussion-dinners between 1757 and 1775, which allowed him to have face-to-face discussions with many distinguished physicians and experimental natural philosophers with an interest in medicine.

George Baker was one such person. He had become a member of the Royal Society in 1762, and joined the Royal Society Club four years later. In the relaxed atmosphere of the Mitre Tavern, over drinks and dinner, he had time to discuss ideas with Franklin. The discourses of these two men led to a much better understanding of lead poisoning (see Chapter 11).

The Grecian Coffeehouse, close to Craven Street on the Strand, was another place where the learned men of the Royal Society tended to congregate and socialize. Coffeehouses were, in fact, the rage at this time, and London boasted more than five hundred. In general, these establishments were quieter and more genteel than the taverns, particularly the pubs frequented by the local gentry. In an era when practicing physicians did not have offices, some of London's most sought-after physicians, such as Richard Mead, liked to meet apothecaries and dispense advice from reserved tables in their favorite coffeehouses.

Franklin also involved himself in John Ellicot's coterie, which met on Monday nights at the George and Vulture. Ellicot was an instrument maker and had written some essays on electricity that impressed Franklin. But he also had medical interests, and he served as a governor of the London Foundling Hospital and the London Hospital. Knowing Franklin's involvement with Pennsylvania Hospital and his penchant for studying hospital records to evaluate treatments, trends, and even occupational hazards, it is easy to understand why he was drawn to Ellicot, who, in turn, gave him such a warm welcome.

St. Paul's Coffeehouse was yet another of Franklin's drinking and dining establishments. This was the meeting place on alternate Thursdays for a group that he would later refer to as his "Club of Honest Whigs."[21] When the manager of this coffeehouse moved early in 1772 to set up the London Coffeehouse on Ludgate Hill, the club moved with him.

Peter Collinson first brought Franklin into this club, and it was here that he often met his closest medical and political friends, including John Fothergill and John Pringle. Although many members of the Club of Honest Whigs were also active members of the Royal Society, the meetings of the two clubs differed in many significant ways. Among other things, the Club of Honest Whigs was smaller, dominated by Quakers and other dissenters, decidedly pro-American, and open to discussions on a wide range of topics. Medical electricity or the threat of smallpox might be discussed on some nights. On others, this freethinking group might devote its attention to how the colonies were being treated by Parliament and to moral philosophy.

Most of the Honest Whigs lived in or near London, but there were exceptions. Joseph Priestley, for instance, lived quite far away. He first met Franklin in 1765 and later reminisced: "My winter's residence in London was the means of improving my acquaintance with Dr. Franklin. I was seldom many days without seeing him, and being members of the same club, we constantly returned together."[22] Although trained as a minister, Priestley was very interested in writing the history of electricity, including medical electricity. He also studied the chemistry of gasses and shared Franklin's interest in fresh air and health. He made experimental discoveries with plants, and Franklin helped Priestley through his career, including when his protégé came to realize that plants could purify the air (see Chapter 10).

Peter Collinson died in 1768, but Priestley, Fothergill, and Pringle remained close to Franklin throughout his two stays. Priestley, in fact, was with Franklin on his last day in England. "He dreaded the war," he wrote about that somber day, "and often said that, if the difference should come to an open rupture, it would be a war of *ten years,* and he should not live to see the end of it. . . . That the issue would be favourable to America, he never doubted. The English, he used to say, may take all our great towns, but that will not give them possession of the country. The last day that he spent in England, having given out that he should leave London the day before, we passed together, without any other company; and much of the time was employed in reading American newspapers . . . the tears trickled down his cheek."[23]

The verbal picture that Priestley painted of Franklin in 1775 was one of a frustrated, abused, and beaten diplomat. But when Franklin had been able to lay his diplomatic chores aside to discuss science and medicine, he could not have been happier. For example, his frame of mind was bright when he traveled to Scotland in 1759 on a trip that brought him in contact with a number of illustrious physicians, and that had important ramifications for the future of American medical education.

CHAPTER 8

# Scotland and the First American Medical School

[I] am pleas'd to see our College begin to make some Figure as a School of Physic, and have no doubt but in a few Years . . . it may acquire a Reputation similar and equal to that in Edinburgh.
—Benjamin Franklin to John Morgan, 1772

When time permitted, Franklin left London for two reasons. One, as we have seen, was to get the exercise associated with traveling, which he believed was beneficial to body and mind. The other was to meet and exchange ideas with some of the most learned men of the Enlightenment outside London.

He visited the Birmingham region in the English Midlands several times to meet with Erasmus Darwin, a graduate of the Edinburgh Medical School and one of the most distinguished natural philosophers and medical scholars of the century. He also traveled south from London on several occasions to visit Jonathan Shipley, an Honest Whig who lived in Twyford. It was here, with Shipley, his wife, and his five daughters in attendance, that Franklin started to write and read aloud his *Autobiography* in 1771, when he was sixty-five.

Franklin also made several trips to Continental Europe, beginning with a visit to the Lowlands with his son William in 1761. The highlight of this trip was a stop in Leyden, where he met Pieter Van Musschenbroek, the Dutchman who invented the Leyden jar. He also visited France, but not until hostilities with Britain ended. In 1767, he traveled to Paris with John Pringle, who had accompanied him to Germany and the Netherlands the previous summer. Louis XV and his wife Queen Marie invited the distinguished foreigners to Versailles for a grand *couvert* (public supper) and, in Franklin's words, the French monarch spoke to them "very graciously and very cheerfully." Franklin enjoyed his visit to France so much that he returned two years later.

Yet of all the countries he visited, Franklin repeatedly said that he enjoyed

Scotland the most. In Scotland Franklin received his first doctorate, and although the diploma was not in medicine but in law, it enhanced the misperception of him as a man trained in medicine. In addition, what he saw and the contacts he made helped change the course of American medical education.

## DOCTOR FRANKLIN

Franklin made his first trip to Scotland in 1759, accompanied by his son William, then almost thirty.[1] He left London late in the summer and arrived on Scottish soil on September 2. His ledger at Craven Street shows no new entries until November 2, 1759.

He now visited St. Andrews University, which had honored him for his work on electricity by mailing him an honorary doctor of laws degree earlier in the year.[2] Prior to this time he possessed only honorary master's degrees from Harvard, Yale, and William and Mary in the colonies.

With his doctorate, Benjamin Franklin's image underwent a further transformation. Earlier, he had cultivated the image of a hard-working printer. Later, at the time of his electrical experiments, he worked hard to portray himself as a gentleman-philosopher. But now, for the first time, people began to address him as "Doctor" Franklin, and he was both honored and thrilled. Of course, the Scots who honored Franklin as "the most Worthy Doctor" knew that he had never attended medical school, nor had he been apprenticed to a physician. So did his close friends and associates, many of whom also began to use the title "Doctor" when referring to him or addressing him in public. But, as he continued to involve himself in medicine, and as his reputation as a great man of the Enlightenment grew, others seemed less sure. Some portraits of Franklin even began to include "Doctor of Medicine" or its equivalent in another language under the image.

While Franklin was at St. Andrews for his academic investiture in October, an event took place that could only have added to the subsequent confusion about Franklin's medical education.[3] It involved a feverish student, David Steuart Erskine (Lord Cardross, later the Earl of Buchan). Franklin was asked to look at him and venture an opinion about whether he should undergo painful blistering, as recommended by one physician. Franklin was cautious, if not skeptical, and ultimately advised against the unpleasant procedure, which was thought to act as a strong stimulant.[4] Franklin's conservative approach was heeded and the boy slowly recovered from his illness. The young Lord, who would garner a reputation for being eccentric, thereafter claimed that Doctor Franklin "gave a turn to the career of a disorder which

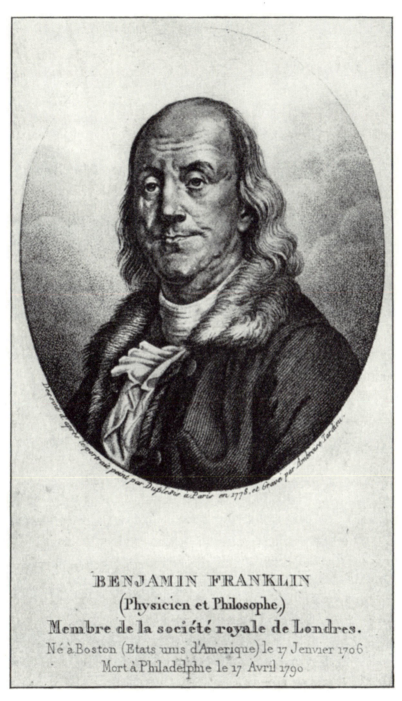

BENJAMIN FRANKLIN
(Physicien et Philosophe,)
Membre de la société royale de Londres.
Né à Boston (Etats unis d'Amerique) le 17 Janvier 1706
Mort à Philadelphie le 17 Avril 1790

*An engraving from Franklin's lifetime in which he is referred to as a doctor of medicine.*

then threatened my life."[5] With the help of people like Lord Cardross, the myth that Franklin had been trained in medicine continued to grow.

## EDINBURGH

Franklin also visited Edinburgh during this visit to Scotland. He first stepped foot in the burgeoning city of 50,000 people on September 6, 1759. Sir George Drummond, Lord Provost and the father of modern Edinburgh, warmly welcomed him. Drummond was in many ways the man behind Edinburgh's successful medical school. He saw its creation in the 1720s as a way to reverse the city's declining status, and he wisely modeled the school after Hermann Boerhaave's medical institution at Leyden.[6] Moreover, Drummond supported clinical lecturing and helped make it a reality in Edinburgh.

After lodging for a few nights in a building in the city's Milne Square, Franklin was invited to spend a full week with Sir Alexander Dick and his family at Prestonfield House on the slopes of Arthur's Seat, two miles from the center of the city. Sir Alexander had received his medical degree from Leyden and was president of the Royal College of Physicians of Edinburgh.

Knowing Franklin's interest in medicine, and eager to show off some of the crown jewels of the city, Dick and Drummond took Franklin to see the medical school. They also showed him the hundred-bed infirmary that had served as a model for Franklin's Pennsylvania Hospital. At the time of Franklin's visit, it had a special ward with about thirty beds for clinical instruction.

Franklin's two hosts also made sure he was introduced to some of the greatest Scottish medical minds of the time. At the end of a letter dated December 11, 1763, to Sir Alexander Dick, Franklin wrote: "Be pleased to present my Respects to our Friends the Russels, when you see them; to the two Doctors Monro, Dr. Cullen, Dr. Clark, Mr. M'Gawen, and any other who may do me the Honour to enquire after me."[7]

James Russel was a leading surgeon-apothecary, the man who was about to become the university's professor of natural philosophy. The elder Alexander Monro had been a surgeon and received the first professorship at the Edinburgh medical school, where he was granted life tenure in 1722 and taught an annual course in anatomy. His son of the same name was an even more talented anatomist and the discoverer of the foramen of Monro, a canal that connects the cerebrospinal fluid-filled ventricles of the brain. As for William Cullen, he was a professor of chemistry and medicine at the university, and a lecturer at the Royal Infirmary.[8] He would later become president of the Royal College of Physicians of Edinburgh. Franklin also met William Robertson on this trip, the historian soon to be appointed principal of the University of Edinburgh.

Franklin spent more than two weeks in Edinburgh before circling west to Glasgow, which also boasted a medical school. He then went back east to St. Andrews to receive his degree, and then south once again to Edinburgh, further down the coast. On his return visit he stayed with philosopher David Hume, saw Cullen's patron Lord Kames (Henry Home), and spent

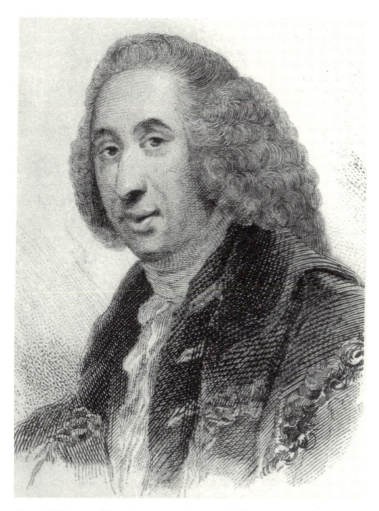

*Dr. William Cullen (1710–1790), one of the most popular teachers on the Edinburgh faculty.*

additional time with some of his new physician friends at the university and infirmary.

Franklin felt very comfortable in Scotland, in part because he was treated with so much respect, but also because the Scots were less concerned with inherited titles and family money than were many Englishmen. The Scots he met seemed to value significant achievements and good deeds more than anything else. Recognizing this, and having similar ideals, Franklin was not in the least bashful about asking several members of Edinburgh's medical community to help with a good cause. He wanted deserving medical students from the colonies to get the best training possible, and the British North American colonies still did not have a medical school in 1759.

## STUDENTS ABROAD

In his essay on medical training in Philadelphia, medical historian Francis Packard asked: "Why did the majority [of Philadelphia's Colonial-Era physicians] go to Edinburgh?" Packard provided a three-part answer to his rhetorical question. "In the first place," he wrote, "they naturally went to a British rather than a continental university because Great Britain was their mother country. Secondly, Edinburgh was at the height of its fame as a medical center. Robert Whytt, the Monros, William Cullen, Joseph Black and other members of its faculty were unsurpassed as teachers in their various fields. Lastly, young Philadelphians had a special reason for going to Edinburgh. It was the Alma Mater of John Fothergill, the great Quaker physician of London, friend of Benjamin Franklin, and benefactor of the Pennsylvania Hospital."[9]

All this is true. But Packard could also have given direct credit to Franklin, who served as an important intermediary between a number of aspiring colonial medical students and the Edinburgh faculty that helped to train them. The records show that, within a year after visiting Scotland and making many friends there, Franklin began to recommend training in Edinburgh to Philadelphia's brightest medical students, and to write personal letters of recommendation on their behalf.

Consider a letter dated September 17, 1760, to Sir Alexander Dick on behalf of William ("Billy") Shippen, Jr., who would drop the "Jr." from his name while in London and later play a prominent role in the founding of the first American medical school. "Mr. Shippen," Franklin began, is "an ingenious worthy young Man, and the Son of my Friend. He goes to Edinburg to improve himself in Physic and Surgery, and hopes to obtain there the Sanc-

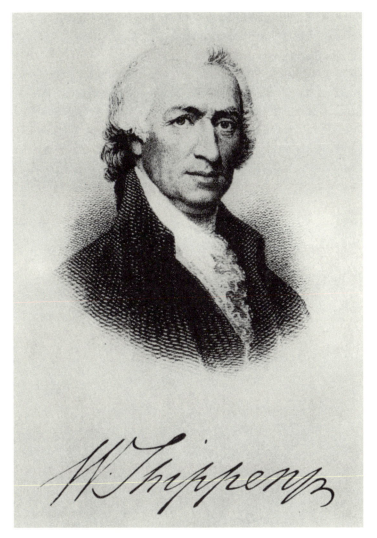

*Dr. William Shippen, Jr. (1736–1801) of Philadelphia.*

tion of a Degree, if found to merit it. Your friendly Advice with regard to his Studies, and kind Influence and Interest in facilitating his Affair, will, I am persuaded, be a Favour conferr'd not improperly."[10]

A second letter of recommendation on behalf of Shippen was sent the same day to William Cullen, the professor who oversaw bedside instruction at the Edinburgh Infirmary and managed the twenty-bed teaching ward. In this letter, Franklin described Shippen as an "ingenious sober and discreet young Man" worthy of Cullen's consideration.[11]

A year later, Cullen received a letter from Franklin on behalf of John Morgan, who would also play a role in establishing the first medical school in the colonies. Morgan, the son of Franklin's friend Evan Morgan, had been undecided about whether to go to Edinburgh or Leyden. Franklin persuaded Morgan to head to Scotland. His letter of recommendation reads: "Mr. Morgan, who purposes to reside some time in Edinburgh for the completion of his studies in Physic, is a young gentleman of Philadelphia whom I have long known and greatly esteem. And as I interest myself in what relates to him, I cannot but wish him the advantage of your conversation and instructions. I wish it also for the sake of my country, where he is to reside, and where I am

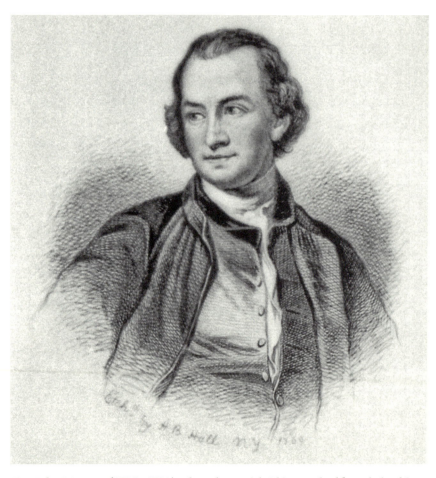

*Dr. John Morgan (1735–1789) who, along with Shippen, had been helped in his medical education by Franklin. (Image courtesy of the National Library of Medicine.)*

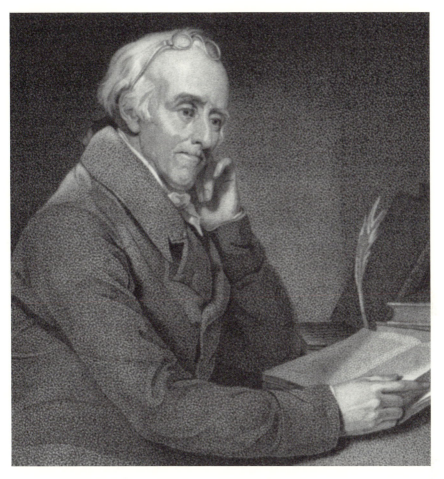

*Dr. Benjamin Rush (1746–1813), who had also been helped early in his career by Franklin.*

persuaded he will be not a little useful."[12] As was the case for Shippen, Franklin sent more than one letter on the behalf of Morgan.[13]

Franklin also sent a number of letters on behalf of Benjamin Rush, who would return to join the new medical school faculty and become the most influential American physician of the post–Revolutionary War era. Charles Thomson had originally asked Franklin to help Rush, writing: "As his design in going abroad is for the sake of acquiring medical knowledge, he is Ambitious of being under your patronage, and should think himself extremely happy if by a line from you he could be introduced to the Notice of Men of Letters especially such as are eminent in Physick."[14] Rush also sent letters to Franklin, explaining that he regretted having to ask him for help without first stopping to see him in London. He added, "[I] beg of you to write to such of your Friends in Edinburgh in behalf of my good Friend Mr. Potts and myself as you think will be most useful to us in the prosecution of our Studies."[15]

Franklin provided the requested letters for Rush and Potts in 1766,[16] but he also warned the two young men that their destiny would ultimately depend on them, not him. "Letters of Recommendation may serve a Stranger for a Day or two," he explained, "but where he is to reside for Years, he must depend on his own Conduct, which will either increase or totally destroy the Effect of such Letters."[17] He added: "You have great Advantages in going to study at Edinburgh at this Time, where there happens to be collected a Set of as truly great Men, Professors of the several Branches of Knowledge, as have ever appeared in any Age or Country. I recommend one thing particularly to you, that besides the Study of Medicine, you endeavour to obtain a thorough Knowledge of Natural Philosophy in general. You will from thence draw great Aids in judging well both of Diseases and Remedies; and avoid many Errors. I mention this, because I have observed that a number of Physicians, here as well as in America, are miserably deficient in it."[18]

Franklin actually advised colonial medical students to do three things while abroad. One was to go to Edinburgh to study principles, systems, theories, and philosophy of medicine—and to obtain their medical degrees there. Second, he encouraged them to get a broad education and especially to learn natural philosophy, in order to enhance perspective and develop a solid, scientific approach to medicine. And third, he advised them to spend ample time in London, where they could watch attending physicians treat patients in a large city hospital and receive training in pathological anatomy and surgery from the Hunters and from William Hewson, at their private school.

The significance of separate training in pathological or morbid anatomy in London lay in the fact that the voluntary hospitals, such as the Edinburgh Infirmary, depended on charitable donations. Fearing the bad publicity that would result from doing autopsies, the managers of these institutions passed regulations that made postmortems very difficult to perform. In addition, the voluntary hospitals were largely concerned with curable patients, not those with life-threatening diseases. In contrast, the private school of anatomy run by the Hunters was tuition driven, nor pinned down by frightened, cash-strapped managers. In addition, they were located where unwanted corpses of executed felons could be obtained almost at will.[19]

William Shippen, John Morgan, and Benjamin Rush did everything that Franklin could have asked of them before heading home.[20] And when these young men returned with their academic knowledge and practical training, they worked hard to establish the first medical school in the colonies. Shippen and Morgan would take the lead, and Rush and others would follow, but feathers would be ruffled in the process.

## WILLIAM SHIPPEN

The younger William Shippen was born in 1736 to an old line Philadelphia family.[21] Valedictorian of the College of New Jersey in 1754. He then apprenticed for three years with his physician-father, who was well known to Franklin, having been a member of his American Philosophical Society, a founding member of his Academy of Philadelphia, and on the board of Pennsylvania Hospital. By 1757, the elder Shippen was "casting about to raise a sum of money for Billey's improvement abroad."[22] The money was eventually obtained and young Shippen left for London in the fall of 1758. Unfortunately, severe storms wrecked his ship and left him stranded in Belfast, Ireland. Upon learning of his dilemma, Franklin sent Shippen the funds he needed to make his way to London, and he probably arrived there in November of that year.

Franklin introduced Shippen to John Fothergill, hoping he would give him some helpful advice about his medical education, much as he had done for Thomas Bond, who had visited London two decades earlier. Fothergill now had so many responsibilities that he preferred to meet with visiting students over breakfast at his home.[23] Shippen managed to meet with him several times, although details of their discussions were not recorded. Shippen's diary for August 27, 1759, reads: "Rose at 7 breakfasted with Dr. Fothergil [*sic*] who was very familiar and social."[24] Entries also show that he met and dined on several occasions with Franklin, who even took him to at least one meeting of the Royal Society.[25]

Both Fothergill and Franklin were very impressed by the young man who was determined to make good use of his time abroad. Indeed, Shippen spent his days in London "walking the wards" of several large hospitals, including St. Thomas's, Guy's, and St. George's. Walking the wards permitted paying students to examine individual patients and to follow the clerks, physicians, and surgeons from bed to bed as they made their rounds. It also allowed them to observe and sometimes help with emergency admissions and surgeries. Because this was well before the advent of anesthetics and antisepsis, few operations were on the deep internal body parts; most were for partial limb amputations to prevent the spread of gangrene, to remove superficial tumors, or to drain abscesses.

Shippen also helped Dr. Colin Mackenzie deliver babies at his small "lying-in" charity hospital on Crucifix Lane. Midwifery was still dominated by women who had learned their craft by observing and assisting. But an increasing number of men were now getting trained in what we would now call surgical obstetrics, and Shippen, like Hewson before him, wanted to learn with Mackenzie, a pioneer in the field.

While in London, Shippen became a house-pupil of John Hunter and worked long hours with him on human and animal cadavers, with breaks only to attend William Hunter's lectures. In addition to his time with the Hunters, Shippen was also able to interact with William Hewson, who was then at their school of anatomy and pathology.

When Shippen headed up to Edinburgh in 1760, he was knowledgeable about surgery, pathology, and midwifery. He also had letters of recommendation from Franklin and the idea of an American medical school firmly planted in his head. He received his medical degree with honors after just one year at Edinburgh, and he gave a presentation copy of his thesis to Franklin. It dealt with the separate blood supplies of the fetus and the mother, a subject that the Hunters and Mackenzie had directed him to while he was in London. With the hope of learning even more, Shippen then packed his bags and left to visit some of the major hospitals in France.

Upon returning to Philadelphia in 1762, Shippen opened a school of surgical anatomy modeled on the Hunters' school. In his introductory lecture, he presented his vision of how American physicians and surgeons should be trained in the future. He then turned to anatomy. In subsequent lectures, he used a skeleton given to Pennsylvania Hospital by Deborah Morris in 1757, and various materials recently donated by John Fothergill as teaching aids.

The philanthropic Fothergill had, in fact, gifted eighteen framed crayon drawings of the different parts of the human body by Dutch artist Jan van Riemsdyck, who had been doing illustrations for the Hunters. He also sent three cases of anatomical castings, a skeleton, a fetus, £350 sterling, and a copy of *An Experimental History of the Materia Medica* by William Lewis. These items were intended for student use, with the hope that Philadelphia might soon have its own "School of Physic."[26]

## JOHN MORGAN

John Morgan returned to Philadelphia in 1765, while Shippen was giving his fourth private course in anatomy and beginning a new one on midwifery. Morgan had stronger credentials than Shippen, even before leaving

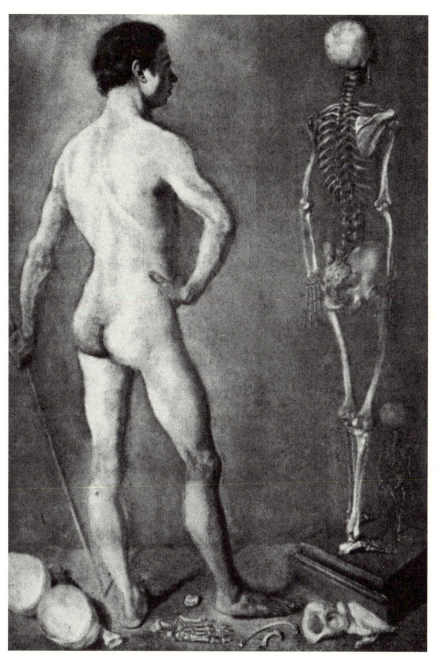

*One of the medical drawings by Jan van Riemsdyck that was sent to
Philadelphia by John Fothergill. (Courtesy of the Pennsylvania Hospital
Historic Collections, Philadelphia.)*

Philadelphia for Europe.[27] He had completed a six-year medical apprenticeship with Dr. John Redman, served a year as resident apothecary of Pennsylvania Hospital, and was in the first graduating class of the College of Philadelphia. Additionally, he had served as a regimental surgeon and line officer in the French and Indian War.

Morgan sailed to Europe in 1760, carrying letters for Franklin and Shippen. While in London, like Shippen, he walked the wards of St. Thomas' and other hospitals and studied anatomy at the Hunters' private school. He did not, however, involve himself with midwifery and surgery, which he did not view as suitable professions for a proper gentleman.

With Franklin's help, Morgan was introduced to John Fothergill, who also graciously helped him plan his course of studies. Shippen had not yet left for Edinburgh when Morgan arrived in London. This overlap allowed Shippen, Morgan, Fothergill, and Franklin to exchange ideas about the future of American medical education. These four individuals were also able to get together during the autumn of 1761, just after Shippen had completed his courses at Edinburgh and had come back to London.

With his coveted letters from Franklin, Morgan was treated well when he arrived in Edinburgh later in 1761. After attending lectures by Cullen, the Monros, Whytt, and others, he even received a personal note from London dated October 1762. Franklin wished him "a prosperous Completion of your Studies, and in due time a happy Return to your Native Country, where if I can be of the least Service to you, I shall be glad of the Occasion."[28]

In 1763, having become the tenth American to receive an Edinburgh M.D. degree, Morgan began a grand tour of Britain, the Lowlands, France, and Italy. He met Pope Clement, Voltaire, and Giovanni Battista Morgagni, the father of modern pathological anatomy. He was also invited to join numerous foreign scientific and medical societies, including the Royal College of Physicians of London, the Royal College of Physicians of Edinburgh, and the Académie Royale de Chirurgie de Paris.

In addition to these honors, Franklin, Fothergill, and Pringle personally nominated Morgan for membership in the Royal Society of London. Since Morgan was already sailing back to Philadelphia when admitted, Franklin covered Morgan's initiation fee.

## ESTABLISHING THE FIRST AMERICAN MEDICAL SCHOOL

Morgan worked out a detailed plan for the first American medical school before he even returned to Philadelphia. He felt it wise to follow the Edin-

burgh example of placing the medical school under the auspices of an institution of higher learning, in this case the College of Philadelphia, rather
than using the London model of a hospital-based school without a university
affiliation. He also wanted to base the new curriculum on Edinburgh's, which
was, in his estimation, the best in Europe.[29]

Morgan discussed his ideas with John Fothergill, William Hunter,
William Cullen, William Watson, and trustees of the College of Philadelphia who happened to be abroad. He also solicited advice through the mails
from elderly physician John Redman, who had gone to Edinburgh in 1746
and was still influential in Philadelphia. To top things off, he managed to
secure a letter from Thomas Penn to the Trustees of the College of Philadelphia that virtually mandated immediate action.

Morgan wasted little time after his return before approaching the Trustees
of the College of Philadelphia with his elaborate plan. The group included
physicians Thomas Bond, Phineas Bond, Thomas Cadwalader, and John
Redman. The elder Shippen was also a trustee, but he was notably absent
from the meeting. Those present responded favorably to most of what Morgan was proposing, and he was invited to present his proposals at the college's commencement in 1765.

Morgan took the occasion to assail the old apprenticeship system and to
enumerate the advantages of having a medical school in Philadelphia. He
pointed to the number of practicing physicians in the area, the central location
of the city, its fine hospital, the growth of the college, and the needs of the
rapidly growing community. He then discussed the importance of having a
liberal education before starting formal medical training. Proper training in
medicine, he told his audience, should include lectures, bedside training, and
an apprenticeship at Pennsylvania Hospital.

Franklin was aware of what Morgan was proposing. He sent Morgan a
letter in July that began, "It rejoices me to hear that you got well home, and
that you are like[ly] to succeed in your Scheme of establishing a Medical
School in Philadelphia."[30] To Morgan's delight, the trustees voted to go
along with his proposal on everything but his contention that the gentle-
manly practice of physick, the manual craft of surgery, and the dispensing of
medicines should be taught as distinct and separate professions. Although
this tripartite division was in effect in Britain, the trustees felt that the
colonies, having few large cities and endless frontiers, would be better served
by generalists.

The trustees appointed Morgan "Professor of the Theory and Practice of
Physic"—the first medical professorship in colonial America. Soon after

receiving the honor, Morgan wrote to Franklin: "I am under so many Oblig-ations to You that I fear I shall never have it in my power to make you any due acknowledgement."[31]

Shippen, who did not mind getting his hands bloodied and apron stained, was appointed professor of anatomy and surgery. But he was very upset. In his acceptance letter, he explained: "I should long since have sought the patronage of the Trustees of the College, but waited to be joined by Dr. Mor-gan, to whom I first communicated my plan in England, and who promised to unite with me in every scheme we might think necessary for the execution of so important a point."[32] He did not indicate where the idea that led him to his plan emerged, but he spoke about it being on his mind for seven years.

Morgan's preemptive actions also enraged Shippen's father and the fam-ily's close medical friends. Even John Fothergill, who had expected Morgan and Shippen to approach the trustees together, was disturbed. He had writ-ten to James Pemberton of Philadelphia to tell him that he had advised Ship-pen give a course of anatomical lectures, while waiting for Morgan to return. He stated that Shippen "will soon be followed by an able assistant, Dr. Mor-gan, both of whom I apprehend will not only be useful to the Province in their employments, but if suitably countenanced by the Legislature will be able to erect a School of Physick amongst you."[33]

Hence, a deep schism developed between Shippen and Morgan, one that also involved others.[34] Moreover, this was not the first time Morgan had exhibited questionable ethics. John Hunter believed that Morgan had used his ideas in his dissertation without proper acknowledgement, and William Hunter and William Hewson were angry with him for taking credit for a technique that was not his. Even James Boswell, who had stud-ied law at Edinburgh and traveled with Morgan through Holland, was put off. He parted company with him saying that he was a conceited fool—"*un fat bonhomme.*"

Despite the problems caused by Morgan's aggressive, self-centered actions, the first medical school in British North America opened its doors in 1765 with both Morgan and Shippen on its faculty. It antedated the medical schools in Manchester, Liverpool, and Leeds by more than fifty years. Ship-pen opened the semester with the first of his anatomical lectures and four days later Morgan began his course on the theory and practice of physic.

Two years later, the curricula leading to the bachelor's and the doctorate degrees in medicine were formalized. The school of almost forty students graduated its first class a year later. Jonathan Potts gave the valedictory address in 1768, which was on the advantages that can be gained from a liberal education that included natural philosophy. Had Franklin been there, Potts's talk would have made him smile, since he had been the one to advise Potts and Rush to "obtain a thorough Knowledge of Natural Philosophy in general," when he provided them with letters of introduction for Edinburgh.

The faculty of the medical school quickly grew. Adam Kuhn, who had studied botany under Linnaeus in Sweden before Franklin sponsored his medical training in Edinburgh, obtained an appointment. He joined Morgan, Shippen, and William Smith, who owed his original appointment at the college to Franklin and now lectured on natural and experimental philosophy. Benjamin Rush next came on board as professor of chemistry. As for Thomas Bond, although he did not receive an official faculty appointment, he proposed a formal course of clinical lectures at the hospital each year, which the board made into a requirement for the M.D. degree.[35]

But just how good was the teaching by Morgan, Shippen, Rush, and the others at the new medical school? Medical historian John Duffy assessed the overall quality of the lecturing as "probably not too high" and not comparable to Edinburgh. Duffy continued: "For example, the first chemistry course at the College consisted of the instructor reading back the notes, which he had taken in Cullen's classes at the University of Edinburgh."[36] Using detailed notes from Cullen, Whytt, or another Edinburgh professor was, in fact, the norm for teaching when the school opened.[37] Although this approach to lecturing would be discouraged today, Duffy reminds us that note reading was common in most teaching institutions during the eighteenth century.

Still, the new professors were innovative in some areas. They did their best to emphasize New World diseases, America's unique environmental conditions, and the local botanicals. Hence, some historians disagree with Duffy, and Carl and Jessica Bridenbaugh go so far as to write: "Philadelphia on the eve of the Revolution enjoyed the services of a medical faculty perhaps unequaled outside London and Edinburgh."[38]

Franklin's own assessment is noteworthy, because it falls midway between the extremes. In 1772, he wrote that he was "pleas'd to see our College begin to make some Figure as a School of Physic, and have no doubt but in a few Years, with good Management, it may acquire a Reputation similar and equal to that in Edinburgh."[39] He mailed this optimistic thought to John Morgan, who was continuing to inform him about the gains being made at the institution that was largely staffed by physicians he had personally helped from his base in London.

EPILOGUE

We may never know who first proposed an American medical school, particularly if the idea emerged during a casual conversation over a breakfast table. Although Morgan and Shippen are usually considered the school's fathers, given what they did upon returning to Philadelphia, it would be a mistake to overlook the roles played by two of the greatest names of the Enlightenment, Fothergill and Franklin. These two "doctors," albeit with different backgrounds and degrees, preferred to work behind the scenes rather than in the spotlight.

In retrospect, Benjamin Franklin might well have been in the best position of all to see the opportunity and need for a medical school in America. He had been instrumental in founding and governing Pennsylvania Hospital, which had been used from the start for teaching purposes. And he was also a founder of the Academy of Philadelphia, which developed into the College of Philadelphia, the educational institution with which the medical school would affiliate. Moreover, after seeing Edinburgh, he would have recognized what the colonies sorely needed. And he had ample opportunity to discuss his vision for American education with Fothergill and the colonial medical students who braved the dangerous ocean voyage to study abroad.

Of course, it is entirely possible that Franklin merely recognized a good idea that was not his own and then endorsed and encouraged its development. But, even if this were the case, it is clear that what he did after he visited Edinburgh in 1759 had a major influence on the future of American medical education. He returned to London enthused by how the Scots organized their medical school, selected their faculty, and ran their infirmary. He then wrote letters and used his formidable influence to make sure that America's most promising medical students obtained excellent practical and theoretical training abroad. He also instilled in their minds his own firm belief that medicine must be solidly grounded in experimental natural philosophy, not in speculative theories that could not be proven or sustained.

Franklin obviously cared deeply about medical care, which in turn required good training. And he wanted to see the colonial medical school idea developed into a reality. Shippen, Morgan, and Rush knew this and, with the help of Franklin and his friends, they received exceptional training and then directed colonial medical education on a formal, new institutional course, one that no longer required crossing the perilous Atlantic for a degree.

# CHAPTER 9

# Colds, the Weather, and the Invisible World

From many Years Observations on my self and others, I am persuaded we are on a wrong Scent in supposing Moist, or cold Air, the
Causes of that Disorder we call a Cold.

—Benjamin Franklin, 1773

Benjamin Franklin enjoyed reasonably good health for a heavyset male living in the eighteenth century, at least until fairly late in life. Yet, like everyone else, he did catch colds, flus, and other illnesses. During the fall of 1757,
soon after he arrived in London, he was plagued by a disorder for several
months, and it was not until late in November that he was finally able to
inform Debby "that my intermitting fever which had continued to harass
me, by frequent relapses," finally seemed over. "My doctor, Fothergill, who
had forbid me the use of pen and ink, now permits me to write as much as I
can without over fatiguing myself." He then told her about his ordeal and
how he was treated.

The second of September I wrote to you that I had had a violent cold and something of a fever, but that it was almost gone. However, it was not long before I had
another severe cold, which continued longer than the first, attended by great pain in
my head, the top of which was very hot, and when the pain went off, very sore and
tender. These fits of pain continued sometimes longer than at others; seldom less
than 12 hours, and once 36 hours. I was now and then a little delirious.

They cupped me on the back of the head, which seemed to ease me for the present; I took a great deal of bark, both in substance and infusion, and too soon thinking myself well, I ventured out twice, to do a little business . . . and both times got
[a] fresh cold and fell down again; my good Doctor grew very angry with me. . . .

I took so much bark in various ways that I began to abhor it; . . . at last I was
seized one morning with a vomiting and purging, the latter of which continued
the greater part of the day, and I believe was a kind of crisis to the distemper,

carrying it clear off; for ever since I feel quite lightsome, and am every day gath-
ering strength; so I hope my seasoning is over, and that I shall enjoy better health
during the rest of my stay in England.

It is now twelve days since I began to write this letter, and I still continue well,
but have not yet recovered my strength, flesh, or spirits. I every day drink a glass of
infusion of bark in wine, by way of Prevention, and hope my fever will no more
return; on fair Days, which are but few, I venture out about noon.[1]

Franklin's allusions to "my intermitting fever, "the bark," "a kind of crisis," and "my seasoning" reflect important beliefs at this moment in time, and
each deserves comment.

Intermitting fever, as previously noted, was a term often used for malaria,
a disorder characterized by wide fluctuations in body temperature. But
Franklin might have been using the term in a more generic way. He went on
to describe what he had as a cold that seemed to linger only to be followed by
another, more severe cold. And he alluded to "something of a fever," which
would not be how the fever associated with malaria would typically be
described. His language would suggest that he might have had only a nagging cold or a miserable flu that just would not go away.

But what about "the bark"? Powdered bark from evergreen trees that
grew on the western slopes of the Andes was found to be effective in treating malaria in the previous century. This bark was given a number of names,
including "Jesuit's bark," "Peruvian bark," and "cinchona bark," and its
active ingredient would later be found to be quinine. Thomas Sydenham
confirmed that the new cure worked well for intermitting fever, and he was
among the physicians who also began to administer it for colds, flus, smallpox, and other febrile diseases. It took a while before some practitioners
began to realize that the bark was not a cure for all fevers. But Franklin's illness did seem episodic, which might have been one of the reasons why John
Fothergill, who was well read, decided to administer it to him.

Franklin's own thoughts about the bark seemed to be favorable. In 1749
he included a lengthy discourse on the history of the bark's use "for the cure
of intermitting fevers, agues, &c." in *Poor Richard's Almanack*. Readers were
told that, "after it had been introduced into Europe with great applause," it
fell into disrepute and then became esteemed again.[2] Seven years later, Poor
Richard was still touting it for "Ague or Intermitting Fever," and in his 1758
almanac, which went to press soon after Franklin recovered, it was again recommended for these fevers.[3] Years later, he would tell Debby that "three or
four Doses of Bark taken on the first Symptoms of a Cold, will generally put

it by," suggesting that he and the medical people he consulted did not view it as a specific treatment for malaria.[4]

The major problem with Peruvian bark was that it had to be imported, making it expensive. Recognizing this drawback, British clergyman Edward Stone set out to find a cheaper substitute. He noticed that willow bark tasted just as bitter, and by testing it on rheumatic fever patients discovered that it was a good pain reliever and fever fighter. But this was six years after the illness that affected Franklin in 1757. Hence, when he fell ill soon after settling in London, Fothergill would not have given him this alternative bark, which we now know has salicylic acid, the key ingredient in aspirin.

Franklin's belief that he would get better after having gone through some sort of a "crisis" has roots that go back to Greek medicine. The basic idea was that some signs and symptoms must first peak before they can undergo remission. To Franklin, an intense headache with a very high fever followed by profuse sweating and dramatic pain relief suggested that he had endured a successful crisis, and it gave him reason to be cautiously optimistic about the worst being behind him.

"Seasoning" referred to acclimating to a new environment. Franklin and his contemporaries believed that it involved not just adjusting to new climates, waters, and foods, but managing to survive the diseases common to the new region. Having undergone two months of intense seasoning that left him weak, Franklin now had another reason to expect better health in London.

Of course, Franklin knew that his seasoning would not provide him with complete immunity against new colds, the flu, or even intermitting fever. In fact, he suffered what he called another "Epidemical Cold" in 1760, characterized by headaches and dizziness. John Fothergill again served as his physician, and he drew eight ounces of blood from the back of his head on one occasion and sixteen ounces on another.[5] In addition, his learned physician-friend subjected him to a plethora of other "heroic" treatments. In Franklin's own words: "I have been cupp'd, blooded, physick'd and at last blister'd for it."[6] He griped that these treatments weakened him, but joked that they had one positive effect—they helped him lose weight.[7]

During his prolonged, physician-ordered confinements, Franklin had ample time to ponder the nature of colds. And in John Fothergill and John Pringle, he had two exceptional men of medicine for discussing the ideas about colds that were fermenting in his mind. Franklin would soon tie a number of notions together, including minute living organisms as the cause of colds, the belief that a poorly regimented body would be most susceptible to colds, and the seminal thought that people can act as vectors. He would also contend that wet or cold weather cannot by itself be regarded as a causal agent, an idea that ran contrary to popular opinion.

## ANCIENT THEORIES, NEW NEEDS

The Hippocratic physicians of the Golden Age of Greece were very interested in epidemics and how they might be triggered by the weather and other environmental factors.[8] Their treatises, written approximately 450 to 350 years before the current era—especially one appropriately titled *Air, Waters, and Places*—are filled with details about seasonal changes, prevailing winds, humidity, topography, and illnesses.[9] These Greek healers sought naturalistic as opposed to religious explanations for diseases, and they believed climatic factors ("atmospheric constitutions"), such as hot or cold and wet or dry, could trigger imbalances among the four bodily humors. The physician's job was to keep the blood, phlegm, black bile, and yellow bile in balance, and to return the body to its proper equilibrium if an imbalance occurred.

The Hippocratic emphasis on the role played by the environment was incorporated into Roman medicine, with modifications. The most important medical writer in the Roman era was Galen, who lived in the second century. He asked why certain people and not others might become ill in the same environment. A "plethoric" body corrupted by overeating and excessive drinking, he opined, was more prone to illness than one in good physical condition.[10] Maintaining a proper balance between sleeping and waking, exercising, controlling the evacuations, properly managing one's passions, and breathing good air were also important. These factors, all of which could be controlled by free men of means, were called the *res nonnaturales* or "non-naturals."[11]

Galen, like just about every other Roman physician, warned that people should stay clear of marshes, swamps, and sewers on sticky, sweltering days, and that the stench of rotting corpses and decaying vegetation must also be avoided. In several places he even theorized that "pestilential seeds" *(loimou spermata)* of illness might be carried in the air from these sites or even from person to person.[12] These seeds of contagion, he speculated, could cause havoc, especially in plethoric, poorly regimented bodies.

The idea of virulent seeds was itself in the air when Galen expressed these thoughts. Lucretius and Varro, two writers from the previous century, used comparable terminology and the latter even raised the possibility of tiny, invisible animals poisoning the atmosphere.[13] Thus, even among the ancients there were two basic notions about illnesses and the air, ideas that were sometimes blended. One was that extreme temperatures, certain wind directions, and wetness are to blame for colds. And the other was that pestilent seeds carried by the air posed the real danger. The concept of pestilent seeds, however, attracted very little attention before Girolamo Fracastoro and his followers revived it in the sixteenth century. And even after its resurgence, more stress tended to be placed on basic air qualities, such as cold and wet.

Thomas Sydenham, who strove to be empirical, took the next significant step. Bothered by the fact that much of what was being said about epidemics was not backed by systematic observations, and urged on by his neighbor Robert Boyle, he set forth to determine whether epidemic diseases could be associated with different seasons and weather patterns.

Sydenham's first publication on the subject appeared in 1666. Ten years later, writing about five epidemics in his *Medical Observations,* he discovered that fairly similar atmospheric conditions were associated with different acute diseases over the years, and that some acute diseases returned under quite different conditions.[14] His findings led him to reject the usual weather qualities as direct causes of epidemics, hypothesizing instead that acute fevers are more likely to result from "unknown particles in the atmosphere." He even used terms such as "morbific particles" and "peccant matter." Further, he stated that "it is a truth that at particular times the air is stuffed full of particles which are hostile to the economy of the human body."[15]

Robert Boyle, who had been maintaining that epidemics might be caused by minute particulate matter from within the earth, had a strong influence on Sydenham. Since 1660, Boyle had been writing about "secret and hidden alterations taking place within the bowels of the earth," "subterraneal effluvia," and "pestiferous or other morbific corpuscles," minute enough to ascend into the atmosphere and "insinuate themselves . . . in human bodies."[16] Sydenham, however, went beyond the earthly emanation idea that has roots in the writings of Seneca and drew Boyle's attention. He postulated that "exhalations from those who have sickened" could also pollute the atmosphere and cause acute illnesses.

Sydenham's clarion call for more and better data was heeded by a number of people whose writings were also read by Franklin. John Locke, for example, read Sydenham's books, visited the sick with him (as did Boyle), and began keeping a daily weather log nine years before getting his medical degree from Oxford in 1675. Locke published his records from 1666 to 1683 in 1692, and he even tried to start a worldwide clearinghouse of information.[17]

By Franklin's time, what we would now call medical meteorology was advancing rapidly. There were new thermometers, barometers, hygroscopes, rain gauges, and wind recorders, at least for those who could afford them.[18] In addition, more informative data began to be compiled about environmental conditions surrounding illnesses and deaths. And stimulated by what was being published about the weather and diseases in London, correspondents around the world, including in the British North American colonies, began to make their own contributions.[19]

In 1732, while Philadelphia was undergoing an epidemic of colds, Franklin published a piece in his *Pennsylvania Gazette* with the simple title "On Colds."[20] "From all Parts of this Province, and even from Maryland," he began, "People complain of Colds, which are become more general than can be remember'd in these Parts before. Some ascribe this Distemper to the sudden Change of Weather into hard Frost, which we had about the middle of November; but others believe it is contagious, and think 'tis communicated by infected Air, after somewhat the same manner as Smallpox or Pestilence."

Franklin noted that "this Cold was first heard of in the eastermost Parts of New-England . . . from whence it has gradually made its Progress thro' all the English Settlements." He then quoted Thomas Molyneux, an Irish physician and a friend of John Locke, on a comparable epidemic of colds that spread from Britain to Ireland and then on to the Continent in 1793.[21] He wrote that Molyneux's study "seems . . . to favour both opinions" (a sudden change in the weather and contagion). But unsure of himself, Franklin was not yet ready to take a stand of his own.

Franklin's interest in the weather was enhanced by John Lining's research in Charleston, South Carolina.[22] Praised even by the usually critical William Douglass, Lining began making meteorological observations with quality instruments in 1737, and he continued his work for almost two decades, publishing many of his findings about weather and diseases in the *Philosophical Transactions*.[23] Among his many achievements is the first good description of the "American Yellow Fever," which he was unable to link to "any particular constitution of the weather."[24]

Lining and Franklin exchanged many letters. Nevertheless, it was only after he was treated for his own illness in 1757 by John Fothergill, who had recently published a series of monthly "Essays on the Weather and Diseases of London," that Franklin seemed to have fully embraced the idea that tiny animals lurk behind the colds that plague humankind. Significantly, he was also meeting with John Pringle at the time.

## THE INVISIBLE WORLD

John Pringle had a professional interest in the spread of diseases.[25] In 1750, he published his *Observations on the Nature and Cure of Hospital and Jayl-Fevers*, and two years later came out with his lengthier *Observations on the Diseases of the Army*.[26] Pringle argued that poisonous emanations from the sick, which might be inhaled or swallowed, were to blame for a slow type of fever he called "typhus," in which internal body parts putrefy. In later editions of his *Observations*, such as the fourth edition of 1764, he would again suggest that some of the dangerous emanations might involve tiny living organisms.[27]

Eighteenth-century interest in the idea that foreign agents could enter the body stemmed from the work of Anton van Leeuwenhoek, who opened up the previously invisible world with his microscopes in the second half of the seventeenth century. After observing swarms of minute, living animals or "insects" in the bodies of animals and on plants, he raised the possibility that these tiny life forms could enter the body in food and drink, by touch, and even in the air we breathe.[28] In a sense, he gave new life, if not life itself, to the ancient idea of seeds of contagion.

Boyle and Sydenham did not respond to the observations that van Leeuwenhoek sent to the Royal Society from 1676 onward, perhaps viewing the microscope as unreliable and his thoughts too speculative. Benjamin Marten, however, contended that some species of "Animalculae," because of their peculiar shapes or "disagreeable Parts," may be disruptive to humans.[29] Capable of sustaining themselves in the fluids and vessels of the body, these tiny animals or their "Seed" could cause illnesses, which could then spread from person to person. Marten presented these intriguing thoughts in 1720, three years before van Leeuwenhoek died, and he gave the example of a tubercular person who might make a healthy person sick by lying in the same bed, sharing the same food, or by breathing on him or her.

Cotton Mather adopted this concept in 1721, at the same time that he was advocating inoculation as the best way to deal with smallpox. In a letter to physician John Woodward of the Royal Society, he wrote that he "suspected that the Small-Pox may be more of an animalculated Business" than was thought, and he made a similar statement in his 1722 pamphlet on the disease. He stopped short, however, of saying that smallpox inoculation involved the transmission of his "invisible worms."[30]

Mather took the concept of tiny life forms further in *The Angel of Bethesda*.[31] Although this substantive work from 1724 was not published in his lifetime, he theorized that tiny animals, of which we may only be seeing the largest, even with our best lenses, could "multiply prodigiously" in the body and affect the blood. Moreover, "one Species of these Animals may offend in one Way, and another in another, and the various Parts may be variously offended: from whence may flow a Variety of Diseases." By affecting travelers, the food, or even the air, "vast Numbers of these Animals keeping together, may at once make such Invasions, as to render Diseases epidemical."[32]

Before he even left for England in 1757, Franklin had been intrigued by what was being seen under the microscope. Poor Richard even included pieces on how the invisible world was now becoming visible. An entry from 1748 is particularly interesting: "*Muschitoes* or *Musketoes*, a little venomous fly, so light, that perhaps 50 of them, before they've filled their bellies, scarce weigh a grain, yet each has all the parts necessary to life, motion, digestion, generation, &c. as veins, arteries, muscles, &c. each has in his little body room for the five senses of seeing, hearing, feeling, smelling, tasting: How inconceivably small must their organs be! How inexpressedly fine the workmanship! And yet there are little animals discovered by the microscope, to whom a *Musketo* is an Elephant!"[33]

Three years later, we can find a longer entry on the microscope in *Poor Richard's Almanack*.[34] Twelve things that can now be observed in greater detail, from thin pieces of brain to "Globules of the Blood," are presented. Entry 7 is particularly deserving of attention:

By the Help of a Microscope the innumerable and inconceivably minute Animalcules in various Fluids are discovered, of the Existence of which we have no Reason to suppose any Mortal had the least Suspicion, till the last Century. . . . Of Animalcules, some Species resemble Tadpoles, Serpents or Eels, others are of a roundish or oval Form, others of very curiously turned and various Shapes; but in general they are very vigorous and lively, and almost constantly in Motion. Animalcules are to be found . . . in our Skins when affected with certain Diseases. . . . By this Instrument it is found that what we call Mouldiness upon Flesh . . . is no other than a great number of extremely small, but perfect Plants.[35]

Hence, even before Franklin met Fothergill and Pringle, he was aware of what the microscope was showing and familiar with the theory that some diseases could result from tiny life forms entering the body. Historically, this was more than a century before Louis Pasteur would receive the lion's share of the credit for "his" germ theory of diseases.

## FRANKLIN'S THEORY

By 1771, if not earlier, Franklin was thinking about writing a major essay on colds. "It concerns the publick Interest that your Treatise on Colds should not be deferr'd too long," wrote his good friend and Honest Whig, Jonathan Shipley, that year.[36] But Franklin was still trying to gather information when he received Shipley's not so gentle push. He wrote back: "I own that I do flatter my self that my Pamphlet upon Colds may be of some Use. If I can persuade People not to be afraid of their real Friend *Fresh Air,* and can put them more upon their guard against those insidious enemies, *full Living* and *Indolence,* I imagine they may be somewhat happier and more healthy."[37]

Franklin had, in fact, just written to William Small in Birmingham, England, to try to get a better feel for what the ancients had written about the subject. Small had previously been a professor at the College of William and Mary, and the teacher of Thomas Jefferson, who considered him "a man profound in most of the useful branches of science."[38] In response to Franklin's inquiry, Small wrote back that "the prevailing opinion of their time seems to have been that what we now commonly call colds and catarrhs arose solely from excess and indolence."[39]

Franklin incorporated Galen's idea that excesses made the body more prone to diseases into his theory of colds. It fit well with his personal philosophy that people should not overeat, drink to oblivion, or fail to exercise. But the more he read and thought, the more he felt that colds are probably spread by contaminated air to susceptible bodies. Rain, freezing cold, and other changes in the weather were not, in and of themselves, direct causes of colds; nor should wet clothes be to blame.

By 1773, Franklin was ready to present his ideas to several highly influential men of medicine in Europe and North America. Some of his letters went to Jacques Barbeu-Dubourg, the physician and natural philosopher who had translated some of his writings on electricity into French. "I do not attempt to explain why damp Cloaths cause Colds, because I now doubt the Fact," he wrote. "I think Colds (the Disease so called) proceed from other Causes, and have no Relation to Wet or Cold."[40]

Three months later, he wrote again to Barbeu-Dubourg, this time asking him to do a survey for him. "I do not have time now to write what I intend upon the Cause of Colds, or Rheums, and my Opinions on that Head are so singular here, that I am almost afraid to hazard them abroad," he explained. "In the mean time, be so kind as to tell me, at your leisure, whether in France, you have a general Belief that moist Air, and cold Air, and damp Shirts or Sheets, and wet Floors, ... and wearing leaky Shoes, and sitting near an open Window or Door ... are all or any of them capable of giving the Distemper we call *a Cold*, and you a *Rheum* or *Catarrh?*"[41]

Another of his correspondents was Benjamin Rush, who was now teaching at the new medical school in Philadelphia. Rush had expressed some of his own opinions on colds to Franklin. He also informed Franklin that William Cullen, his teacher at Edinburgh and a man Franklin had corresponded with, "speaks of a great many Catarrhs or Colds from Contagion, but includes with these One Species *a frigore*," meaning caused by cold weather itself.[42]

In his letter back to Rush in July 1773, Franklin wrote: "I shall communicate your judicious Remark relating to Air transpir'd by Patients in putrid Diseases to my Friend Dr. Priestly. I hope that after having discover'd the Benefit of fresh and cool Air apply'd to the *Sick*, People will begin to suspect that possibly it may do no Harm to the *Well*." He continued:

I have not seen Dr. Cullen's book: But am glad to hear that he speaks of Catarrhs or Colds by *Contagion*. I have long been satisfy'd from Observation, that besides the general Colds now termed *Influenza's*, which may possibly spread by Contagion as well as by a particular Quality of the Air, People catch Cold from one another when shut up together in small close Rooms, Coaches, &c. and when sitting near and conversing. . . . I think too that it is the frowzy corrupt Air from animal Substances, and the perspired Matter from our Bodies, . . . which infects us. . . . From these Causes, but more from *too full Living* with too *little Exercise*, proceed in my Opinion most of the Disorders which for 100 Years past the English have called *Colds*.

As for Dr. Cullen's Cold or Catarrh *à frigore*, I question whether such an one ever existed. Traveling in our severe Winters, I have suffered Cold sometimes to an Extremity only short of Freezing, but this did not make me *catch Cold*. And, for Moisture, I have been in the River every Evening two or three Hours for a Fortnight together, when one would suppose I might imbibe enough of it to *take Cold* if Humidity would give it; but no such Effect followed: Boys never get Cold by Swimming. Nor are People at Sea, or who live at Bermuda, or St. Helena, where the Air must be ever moist, from the Dashing and Breaking of Waves against their Rocks on all sides, more subject to Colds than those who inhabit Parts of a Continent where the Air is driest. Dampness may indeed assist in producing Putridity, and those Miasms which infect us with the Disorder we call a Cold, but of itself can never by a little Addition of Moisture hurt a Body filled with watery Fluids from Head to foot.[43]

In a follow-up letter in September 1773, Rush told Franklin that he agreed with him that cold and moisture do not *cause* colds. More likely than not, they only predispose bodies to those effluvia that can cause acute illnesses.[44]

Another of Franklin's correspondents from 1773 was Thomas Percival, who studied medicine in Edinburgh and Leyden. Now practicing in Manchester, England, Percival was active in the Royal Society and had just published two pamphlets on subjects dear to Franklin's heart: *Internal Regulation of Hospitals* (1771) and *A Scheme of Professional Conduct Relative to Hospitals and Other Medical Charities* (1772). In his letter to Percival, Franklin again made the point that people who live in moist environments are no more likely to catch colds than those who live elsewhere, provided the air is not putrid like that found in marshes. "It seems strange that a Man whose Body is composed in great Part of Moist Fluids, whose Blood and Juices are so watery, who can swallow Quantities of Water and Small Beer daily without Inconvenience, should fancy that a little more or less Moisture in the Air should be of such Importance. But," he added, "we abound in Absurdity and Inconsistency. From many Years Observations on my self and others, I am persuaded we are on a wrong Scent in supposing Moist, or cold Air, the Causes of that Disorder we call a Cold."[45]

To the chagrin of his medical friends, Franklin never completed his treatise on colds, which would have put his thoughts on regimen, contagion, the invisible world, and weather conditions into a single package. He might have felt that he had already shared his thoughts with some of the best minds and most influential physicians in England, France, and America. These individuals were sure to mull over his ideas and give them proper exposure.

Hence, aside from his various letters, Franklin left us only with notes scribbled on loose sheets of paper for his proposed treatise. These notes were probably written at different times and the collection is anything but systematic. But in certain places we can almost imagine Franklin, with his glasses slipping down his nose and his chin on his hand, thinking about how to organize what he had in front of him. A sheet of paper with the words "Hints Concerning what is Called Catching of Cold" might have been the intended title for his treatise.[46] One section lists a number of theories, those that made sense to him intermingled with those that did not. Additionally, there is a section on how colds might be prevented, again including both thought-provoking ideas and those that he believed had little substance.

The major ideas expressed in Franklin's letters to Shipley, Barbeu-Dubourg, Percival, Rush and others appear again and again in these notes: "Scarce any Air abroad is so unwholesome as Air in a c[lose] Room often breath'd"; "Exercise and fitness can help prevent colds; those interested in preserving health should also watch what they eat and drink"; and "People often don't get Cold where they think they do, but do where they think they do not."[47]

## A THEORY WORTH KEEPING

Franklin continued to promote his beliefs about fresh air and colds to anyone who would listen, not just in England, but after he briefly returned to America before turning around and sailing off to France. In 1776, he presented his thoughts to John Adams, the stodgy New Englander who would later join him in France and then become the second President of the United States.

Franklin and Adams got together shortly after the British had soundly beaten George Washington's forces on Long Island. Lord Howe, the British commander who still hoped for a peace accord, had asked Congress to send a few American representatives to Staten Island to discuss ways of quickly ending the war. Franklin, who had enjoyed Howe's company in England, was one of the chosen men. John Adams and Edward Rutledge joined him on the peace mission that really had no chance of succeeding.

Franklin and Rutledge traveled together to an inn at nearby New Brunswick, New Jersey, where they met up with Adams, who had come on horseback. But there were so many American troops and officers in New Brunswick that it was not easy for the three men to find lodging. Adams described what happened next:

At Brunswick, but one bed could be procured for Dr. Franklin and me, in a chamber little larger than the bed, without a chimney, and with only one small window. The window was open, and I, who was an invalid and afraid of the air of the night, shut it close. "Oh!" says Franklin, "don't shut the window, we shall be suffocated." I answered I was afraid of the evening air. Dr. Franklin replied, "The air within this chamber will soon be, and indeed is now, worse than that without doors. Come, open the window and come to bed, and I will convince you. I believe you are not acquainted with my theory of colds."

Opening the window, and leaping into bed, I said I had read his letters to Dr. Cooper, in which he had advanced, that nobody ever got cold by going into a cold church or any other cold air, but the theory was so little consistent with my experience, that I thought it a paradox. However, I had so much curiosity to hear his reasons that I would run the risk of a cold. The Doctor then began a harangue upon air and cold, and respiration and perspiration, with which I was so much amused that I soon fell asleep. . . .

I remember little of the lecture, except that the human body, by respiration and perspiration, destroys a gallon of air in a minute; that two such persons as were now in that chamber, would consume all the air in it in an hour or two; that by breathing over and over again the matter thrown off by the lungs and the skin, we should imbibe the real cause of colds, not from abroad, but from within. I am not inclined to introduce here a dissertation on this subject. There is much truth, I believe, in some things he advanced, but they warrant not the assertion that a cold is never taken from cold air.[48]

Franklin was not bothered by the fact that Adams was not a believer in all parts of his theory. Adams was hardly an expert in medicine and, as far as Franklin was concerned, his theory needed no modification. Even on his voyage home from France in 1784, he would stand by the sharp distinction he had made a decade earlier between moist air and air corrupted by animal matter. In fact, he even noted that he was sailing across the Atlantic in extremely moist air, but that the crew and passengers were just as healthy as were the people of landlocked, mountainous Switzerland.

At the same time, he reasoned that the good health of sailors and people living on small islands has everything to do with, in his words,

the Moisture being pure, unmix'd with the poisonous Vapours arising from putrid Marshes and stagnant Pools, in which many Insects die and corrupt the Water. These Places only afford unwholesome Air: and that is not the mere Water contained in damp Air, but the volatile Particles of corrupted animal Matter mix'd with that Water, which renders such Air pernicious to those who breathe it. And I imagine it a Cause of the same kind that renders the Air in close[d] Rooms, where the perspirable Matter is breath'd over and over again by a number of assembled People, so hurtful to Health. After being in such a Situation, many find themselves affected by that *Febricula*, which the English alone call *a Cold*, and, perhaps from the Name, imagine that they caught the malady by *going out* of the Room, when it was in fact by being in it.[49]

Today we realize just how right Franklin was in his well-reasoned conclusions about common colds and flus. Colds and influenza are contagious; they involve matter that cannot be seen with the naked eye; bad weather or moist clothes do not cause them; and they are most likely to affect badly abused and weakened bodies. In retrospect, no part of Franklin's theory is really original. Still, he did four things for which he deserves more recognition. First, he put a number of salient ideas together into a coherent whole that made sense, one that included minute living matter and the state of the body. Second, his letters forced enlightened physicians to think much harder about colds, their real causes, and long-held false impressions. And third, after concluding that corrupt air plays a causal role, he alerted people to the need for fresh air. Just how Franklin used his many skills to find ways to purify the air of foul matter is the subject of the next chapter.

# CHAPTER 10

# Fresh Air and Good Health

> I rise early almost every morning, and sit in my chamber, without
> any clothes whatever, half an hour or an hour, according to the sea-
> son, either reading or writing.
> —Benjamin Franklin, 1768

Franklin's theory of colds emphasized the transmission of foul matter to susceptible, unregimented bodies. In his estimation, minute particles, most likely of animal matter, bore the responsibility for colds, flus, and related diseases. One ramification of his theory was that he became even more upset at the thought of being forced to breathe the miserable, polluted air of the big cities.[1] In this context, he campaigned even harder for better sanitation. He was also taken back by how people closed themselves up in poorly ventilated homes, shops, offices, and hospitals. This led him to think about ways to purify the air, or at least to remove foul air—to ponder how he might use science and technology to modify dangerous environments, and whether Nature might also have some solutions.

Franklin would go well beyond just looking at air loaded with microscopic insects and animal waste as negative, and at noncorrupted air as neutral. He would argue that fresh air can be a healthy stimulant that can preserve and restore physical and mental health—even if cold, even if damp.

## THE FOUL AIR OF EVERYDAY LIFE

Franklin was notably upset with the putrid, irritating, and smelly air he was forced to breathe from the start of his stay in London. In a 1758 letter to his wife, Debby, he wrote, "The whole Town is one great smoky House, and every Street a Chimney, the Air full of floating Sea Coal Soot, and you never get a sweet Breath of what is pure, without riding some Miles for it into the Country."[2]

Indeed, the great city in which he was now residing had air that was polluted by soot and residue from fireplaces, furnaces, and factories. The liquid and solid waste coming from the thousands of horses on the muddy streets made breathing the street air even worse. And into this noxious cauldron there was the nonstop breathing of healthy and not so healthy people; the mass of London citizens who sold goods, shopped, ran errands, and went outdoors to socialize and meet friends.

By 1773, the year in which Franklin was telling a number of correspondents about his theory of colds, he was clearly stunned by how well-to-do Londoners, including many people he knew personally, were defining "taking the air." In a letter to physician Thomas Percival, he lamented: "Tho' it is generally agreed that *taking the Air* is a good Thing, yet what Caution against Air, what stopping of Crevices, what wrapping-up in warm Clothes, what Shutting of Doors and Windows! Even in the midst of Summer! Many London Families go out once a Day to take the Air; three or four Persons in a Coach, one perhaps Sick; these go three or four Miles, or as many Turns in Hyde Park, with the Glasses both up close, all breathing over and over again the same Air they brought out of Town with them in the Coach with the least change possible, and render'd worse and worse every moment. And this they call taking the Air?"[3]

## THE "UNIVERSAL SMOKE DOCTOR"

Franklin's obsession with air quality, and his desire to improve it, can be traced back to his Junto days in Philadelphia. He not only wanted to pave and clean streets, but asked, "How may a smoky chimney be best cured?" Putting on his experimental philosopher's hat and studying air currents, he soon had one solution. His "open stoves" or "Pennsylvania Fire-Places" (what others called Franklin stoves) stemmed from the observation that standard fireplaces lost most of the heat they produced up the chimney. Narrowing the escape passage to curtail the heat loss made the rooms warmer, which was good, but smokier, which was bad. Franklin's ingenious solution was to construct a free-standing iron fireplace with two separate components, one for heating the room and the other for discharging the dense, choking smoke.

The heating component had an opening below the floor of the fireplace for cool air to enter a separate "air box," which was located right behind the fire, where it could be heated. The hot air was forced back into the room through an opening at the top of the air box; the air current being maintained by the hot air escaping above and the cooler air being sucked in below. As for the soot and smoke from the fire itself, it was forced out a

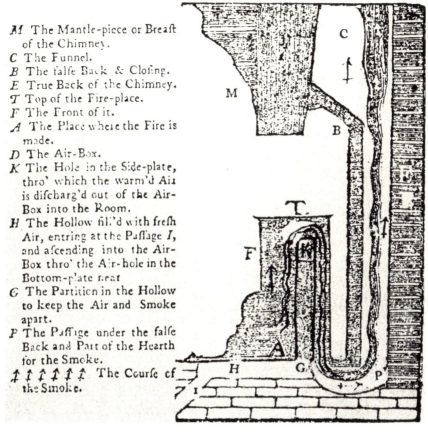

*M* The Mantle-piece or Breaſt of the Chimney.
*C* The Funnel.
*B* The falſe Back & Cloſing.
*E* True Back of the Chimney.
*T* Top of the Fire-place.
*F* The Front of it.
*A* The Place where the Fire is made.
*D* The Air-Box.
*K* The Hole in the Side-plate, thro' which the warm'd Air is diſcharg'd out of the Air-Box into the Room.
*H* The Hollow fill'd with freſh Air, entring at the Paſſage *I*, and aſcending into the Air-Box thro' the Air-hole in the Bottom-plate near
*G* The Partition in the Hollow to keep the Air and Smoke apart.
*P* The Paſſage under the falſe Back and Part of the Hearth for the Smoke.
↑↑↑↑↑↑ The Courſe of the Smoke.

*The Pennsylvania fireplace, 1744. (See Franklin's* Papers *2; 419–446.)*

chimney via a well-designed passage that also prevented the fire from burning too quickly.

Franklin advertised his new fireplaces in his *Pennsylvania Gazette* in 1741. He wrote: "To be SOLD at the Post-Office Philadelphia, The New Invented Iron Fire-Places, Where any Person may see some of them that are now in Use, and have the Nature and Advantages of them explain'd."[4] The master ironworker who was instrumental in putting the new device into production was Robert Grace, a Junto member who also helped Franklin sell them. In an issue of the *Gazette* from 1742, we read: "NEW IRON FIRE-PLACES, large and small, to be sold by Robert Grace at the Upper End of Market Street, and by the Printer hereof."[5]

In 1744, Franklin published a pamphlet to illustrate and promote his new invention. *An Account of the New-Invented Pennsylvania Fire-Places* explained that his fireplaces were less costly to operate and that they kept more warm air in the house.[6] And with an eye on health, he added that they reduced coughing, respiratory problems, and irritated eyes.

The "Pennsylvania Fire-Place" was Franklin's first significant practical invention. He made a little money from it and could have lined his pockets with much more. But because it would help people, he never sought to patent his technology, even though encouraged to do so by others, including the governor of Pennsylvania. "I declin'd it from a principle which has ever weighed with me on such occasions," wrote Franklin. "That, as we enjoy great advantage from the inventions of others, we should be glad of an opportunity to serve others by any invention of ours; and this we should do freely and generously."[7]

After devising his first fireplaces, Franklin continued to work hard to find out everything he could about air currents and chimneys. And as he learned and experimented, he continued to improve his fireplaces. Consequently, well before he arrived in England in 1757, he was the recognized authority on channeling air currents to clean the air and make breathing easier.

In 1758, while Franklin was visiting Scotland, Lord Kames asked him for some advice about ventilating his new home. Kames explained: "I have bought a house in this Town which luckily is absolutely free of smoke except what is commonly called neighbourhood smoke; that is the smoke issuing from one vent sometimes goes down a neighbouring vent and issues into the Room when there is no fire in it. I apply to you for a remedy as to an universal Smoke Doctor."[8]

The affable "universal Smoke Doctor" from the New World gave Kames some helpful suggestions. But Franklin soon faced an even more daunting task—improving the air in the House of Commons in London, which tended to become very stuffy when it was crowded. In response to this unexpected request, Franklin replied that outlets could be made in the perpendicular parts of the seats, by which the stale air could be carried off by ventilators. He also suggested some escapes close to the ceilings. And he added that some of the vents could be associated with flues heated by existing fireplaces. The warming of these vents, he explained, would quicken the expulsion of the hot, stale air.

Even after he went to France, Franklin was still regarded as the most knowledgeable smoke doctor in the world. He fixed the chimneys on the estate of Monsieur Chaumont, on whose property he lived, so there would no longer be an "intolerable malady of smoke." But it was not until he had left France and was sailing back to the new United States at age seventy-eight that he put all of his technological ideas on paper for broader dissemination.

His essay on the causes and cures of smoky chimneys was composed as a letter to Jan Ingenhousz, who had been begging him to spell out his thoughts on this matter, as well as on other subjects, because he knew Franklin was old and sickly and would not live much longer. As Ingenhousz so bluntly put it, "it would be a pity [if] your ideas should sink with you into the grave."[9] Knowing Ingenhousz was right, Franklin picked up his pen and composed a suitable manuscript based on decades of experience, while his ship slowly sailed west. It was published in *Transactions of the American Philosophical Society* in 1786.

In his piece, Franklin listed nine causes of smoky chimneys and, after each cause, suggested a way or various ways to remedy the situation, in order to improve air quality and, of course, preserve heath. Consider this example: "Another cause of smoky Chimneys is too short a Funnel. This happens necessarily in some Cases, as where a Chimney is required in a low Building. Remedies. Contract the Opening of the Chimney."[10] Franklin also suggested a higher funnel, provided it could be properly supported. To those with limited means, some of Franklin's suggestions might have seemed more like ideals. But remembering his own humble roots, he also did his best to come forth with alternatives that would not be terribly expensive.

## THE FRESH AIR TONIC

In his essay on how to make better chimneys, Franklin also took the occasion to try to overcome the irrational fears most people still seemed to have of opening the windows and letting in some fresh air. He explained:

Some are as much afraid of fresh Air as persons in the Hydrophobia [rabies] are of fresh Water. I myself formerly had this Prejudice, this Aërophobia, as I now account it; and . . . clos'd with extreme care every Crevice in the Rooms I inhabited.

Experience has convinced me of my Error. I now look upon fresh Air as a Friend; I even sleep with an open Window. I am persuaded, that no common Air from without is so unwholesome, as the Air within a close[d] Room, that has been often breath'd and not changed. Moist Air, too, which formerly I thought pernicious, gives me now no Apprehensions; for, considering that no Dampness of Air apply'd to the Outside of my Skin can be equal to what is apply'd to and touches it within, my whole Body being full of Moisture, and finding that I can lie two hours in a Bath twice a Week, cover'd with Water, which certainly is much damper than any Air can be, and this for Years together, without catching Cold, or being in any other manner disorder'd by it, I no longer dread mere Moisture, either in Air or in Sheets or Shirts.[11]

Franklin did not always follow what Pool Richard wrote when it came to his diet. But no one could ever say that Franklin did not practice what he preached about fresh air. We need only turn to a letter he had written to French physician Jacques Barbeu-Dubourg from London on July 28, 1768. To put this epistle in context, it must be noted that one of the popular theories at the time held that bathing in cold water was a healthy practice. Among other things, it was thought to stimulate the body's fibers. Franklin accepted this. But why, he asked, should "bathing" in cool air be different from bathing in cool water? Why would an air bath not be just as stimulating and just as healthy?

You know the cold bath has long been in vogue here as a tonic. . . . But the shock of the cold water has always appeared to me, generally speaking, as too violent: and I have found it much more agreeable to my constitution, to bathe in another element, I mean cold air. With this view I rise early almost every morning, and sit in my chamber, without any clothes whatever, half an hour or an hour, according to the season, either reading or writing. This practice is not in the least painful, but on the contrary, agreeable; and if I return to bed afterwards, before I dress myself, as sometimes happens, I make a supplement to my night's rest, of one or two hours of the most pleasing sleep that can be imagined. I find no ill consequences whatever resulting from it, and that at least it does not injure my health, if it does not in fact contribute much to its preservation. I shall therefore call it for the future a bracing or tonic bath.[12]

There may be hundreds of paintings, engravings, and casts of Franklin showing him holding a pen at a desk or with a book in his hand. But to the best of this author's knowledge, none of these working scenes has ever shown Franklin working in the nude, fully enjoying the fresh air on every part of his body. But even if artists missed the opportunity to capture him taking one of his famous air baths, it is hard to deny that the American philosopher of good health was in a class of his own. Although few people seemed to follow the extreme example he provided, his more general message did get though, at least to some highly educated men.

## FRESH AIR FOR SCHOOLS AND HOSPITALS

One of Franklin's most influential friends in England, and a physician who helped him to open more windows, was Erasmus Darwin.[13] At about the same time as Franklin was praising the air bath, Darwin, then in his thirties, jumped off a boat, swam ashore, and hiked, still sopping wet, to a nearby marketplace. He then climbed onto a stand and lectured to a crowd on the benefits of fresh air and leaving bedroom windows at least partly open at night.[14]

Late in his life, Darwin published *A Plan for the Conduct of Female Education in Boarding Schools,* which would have brought a smile to Franklin's face had he still been living.[15] Darwin advised schools to improve the purity of the air in their classrooms. One of his recommendations was to saw an inch of wood off the top of every door and to insert a tin plate at a forty-five-degree angle there. He also recommended opening the windows a few inches, when weather permitted. These suggestions, and others like them for the home, could well have come from earlier conversations with Franklin, who visited him at his Litchfield home near Birmingham, and for whom Darwin professed great admiration.

Franklin was also interested in improving the air quality in both civilian and military hospitals. Hospitals were notorious for housing large numbers of people together in tight quarters with little or no air circulation. In this domain, John Pringle, who spent considerable time with him at the Royal Society, in the Club of Honest Whigs, and as his traveling companion, was a good source of information. In his 1752 book, *Observations on the Diseases of the Army,* which went through many editions, Pringle pressed hard for better ventilation in the British infirmaries and hospitals.[16] Poor Richard had been aware of what Pringle was preaching, and cited his thoughts on the need for fresh air before his printer, Franklin, had a chance to meet Pringle in person.[17]

While in Britain, Franklin chided some of his "backward" physician friends for only slowly recognizing the importance of removing foul air from hospital rooms. But Alexander Small, a Scottish surgeon, was not one of these men. Franklin had been discussing hospital ventilation with Small for some time, and from the outset the two men agreed on what had to be done. Small even composed a memorandum, probably early in 1777, largely reflecting Franklin's views on the subject.

The need for information, Small wrote, "has induced me to endeavor to recollect all I can of the many instructive conversations I have had upon these matters with that judicious and most accurate observer of Nature, Dr. Benjamin Franklin."[18] He continued: "Dr. Franklin justly concluded that, in crouded rooms . . . a current of air should be kept up in the lower part of the houses, to carry off what is thus affected."[19] He even included Franklin's instructions on how to make ventilators and flues more effective. And finally, to help allay fears, some examples of people who followed the guidelines were presented to show that even cold fresh air would not be detrimental to one's health. One reads: "Dr. Franklin mentioned an instance of a number of Germans, who, on their arrival in Pensilvania, were obliged to live in a large barn; there being at that time no place of residence, fit for them. Several small windows were made on both sides of the barn, under the eaves. These windows were kept constantly open, even during a severe frost in the winter; and this, without any detriment to the health of the Germans."[20]

The history of Small's memorandum is informative. He sent a copy to Sir John Pringle, whose enlightened outlook on hospitals was cited in his text.[21] Then, in 1788, with it still unpublished in English, Small showed his memorandum to members of the Royal Society of Edinburgh.[22] The Scots were no longer interested in publishing it in their society's *Transactions* because, as they told Small, his material was no longer new.[23] In retrospect, the Scottish reviewers were right. The ideas about fresh air that Franklin and Pringle had been promoting had spread all over Britain and throughout Europe by the 1780s.

Many physicians in the American War of Independence took the new, fresh air approach to hospital care seriously. Ebenezer Beardsley noted that troops quartered in warm crowded houses, garrets, and underground facilities were much more likely to get dysentery than soldiers exposed to circulating air. He subsequently made up his mind to remove the sick from their "putrid atmospheres" and expose them to more fresh air. Beardsley reported that this simple act markedly improved the chances the men had of recovering from the putrid fevers closely associated with hospital confinement.[24]

Not surprisingly, Benjamin Rush, who owed so much to Franklin, also promoted fresh air during the War of Independence. As a high-ranking medical officer, he visited military hospitals and was appalled by what he saw— and smelled. He attributed the unacceptably high death rate in these places for care and healing to overcrowding and one of its consequences, putrid air. Rush was particularly interested in curtailing typhus, which he thought was caused by human perspiration and respiration that permeated the air and made it unhealthy. Hence, he recommended treating the sick in private homes in rural areas, rather than in crowded hospitals, if at all possible.

Changes in thinking about hospital ventilation and fresh air were also taking place in France. Franklin helped by personally asking Jean-Baptiste Le Roy to help him translate Small's memorandum into French. Le Roy readily complied, having long maintained an interest in improving hospital conditions. Prior to this time, he had corresponded with Franklin on rebuilding the Hôtel Dieu, the old Paris hospital that had partially burned in December 1772. Le Roy hoped to give the building a new design, one that would be more beneficial to the patients.

In one of his letters, Franklin told Le Roy that "light covering and fresh Air continually changing" might help the sick. He further informed him: "Our Physicians have begun to discover that fresh Air is good for people in the Small Pox and other Fevers."[25]

As was the case in Britain, the reform movement to improve air quality in France concerned more than just hospitals. It involved all places of confinement from which tainted air could spread and poison the atmosphere. Historians Laurence Brockliss and Colin Jones put the fresh air movement in Paris in perspective. They wrote: "Attempts to ensure the better circulation of the air were focused in the city as a whole and in crowded and enclosed places (hospitals, prisons, meeting-halls, plus some private dwellings), and had important ramifications for town planning . . . and for domestic and public architecture. . . . The salubrious circulation of air, it was hoped, would relieve smells caused by social intercourse and human waste, and the public was assailed by a flood of writings and demonstrations of sundry experiments with bellows, vaults, fans, and the like."[26]

In summary, Franklin was not the only one bothered by sooty, smelly, and corrupted air. Nor was he the only one to recognize that fresh air could be healthy and invigorating. But what the most famous American of his day brought to the international medical community were some well thought out solutions. And, not to be overlooked, he had a large network of influential followers and dedicated admirers who looked upon him as a leader when it came to applying experimental natural philosophy to medicine—and these people understood the problem and how Franklin's suggestions might be put into action.

## NATURE'S SOLUTION

In his *History of Electricity*, which came out in 1767, Joseph Priestley described some observations and experiments from the previous year on how foul air was (or was not) affected by fire and other forms of "combustion."[27]

Franklin had encouraged Priestley to write this book, and prior to publication he carefully checked what the younger man had written.[28] The theory that stale or vitiated air could in some way be purified and restored intrigued both men, much as it did other natural philosophers at the time. As a minister, Priestley felt certain that God had provided a remedy for purifying noxious air so it could sustain life. And as an electrical scientist, Franklin hoped that Priestley would be able to cite experiments showing that electricity could refresh the air. But the data from numerous experiments suggested that this hypothesis, although intriguing, could not be supported.

During the fall of 1767, Priestley moved with his family from Warrington, where he was a tutor of languages at that city's academy, to Leeds, where he accepted a position as a minister. Being financially strapped, he lodged in a house adjoining "Jakes and Nell," a foul-smelling public brewery. The story often told is that Priestley was amazed to observe that the plants growing near the brewery were not thwarted or wilted. On the contrary, they seemed to thrive in the horrible air.

Hoping to learn more, in 1771 Priestley began to conduct some experiments on plants in different "atmospheres." He placed mint plants in bottles of choking "fixed air" (carbon dioxide) in a few of his studies. In others, they were placed in air that had been "injured" by a lighted candle, poisoned by leaving a mouse in a closed chamber until it died, or made unfit for respiration by exposing it to acid fumes. To his amazement, the plants exhibited an uncanny ability to return the ruined air to its original, breathable state. This was shown by the fact that healthy mice could live in the previously lethal atmospheres, provided plants had adequate time to cleanse them of their poisons.

That summer, Priestley sent a draft of his startling observations to Franklin, asking for his comments and additions. Franklin graciously complied, and other communications followed. To Priestley's delight, Franklin was so pleased with his research at Leeds that he made sure his findings were presented to the Royal Society in 1772 and published later that year in its *Philosophical Transactions.* Priestley's 117-page treatise bore the title "Observations on Different Kinds of Air," and it included some of Franklin's recommended changes, additions, and even wording.[29]

Between the first rough draft of this monumental paper and its printing, Franklin witnessed some of Priestley's experiments firsthand. On June 13, 1772, Priestley wrote to Franklin: "You make me happy by the near prospect of seeing you and Sir John Pringle at Leeds. I shall be intirely at liberty to receive you, and I hope you will contrive to stay as long as possible in the town and neighbourhood."[30] Priestley then told Franklin about some of the experiments that he was now conducting, whetting Franklin's appetite even more. During the third week of June 1772, Franklin and Pringle were in Leeds, where they saw some of Priestley's mint plants thriving in their poisoned atmospheres. They also witnessed some of his ingenious experiments with mice. When the amazed visitors said goodbye, they were convinced that plants could really purify the atmosphere. They congratulated Priestley and strongly encouraged him to continue his groundbreaking research.

Extracts of the Priestley-Franklin correspondence from this important time period illustrate how these two great figures of the Enlightenment grappled with new findings. They also show how they shared ideas for additional experiments that might shed even more light on God's remarkable remedy for spoiled air. Priestley penned some of his new findings to Franklin a week after Franklin and Pringle left Leeds. The letter was waiting for Franklin when he returned to Craven Street on July 14. "I have fully satisfied myself that air rendered in the highest degree noxious by breathing is restored by sprigs of mint growing in it," wrote Priestley.

You will probably remember the flourishing state in which you saw one of my plants. I put a mouse into the air in which it was growing on the Saturday after you went, which was seven days after it [the mint] was put in, and it continued in it five minutes without shewing any sign of uneasiness, and was taken out quite strong and vigorous, when a mouse died after being not two seconds in a part of the same original quantity of air, which had stood in the same exposure without a plant in it.

The same mouse that lived so well in the restored air was barely recoverable after being not more than one second in the other. I have also had another instance of a mouse living 14 minutes, without being at all hurt, in little more than two ounce measures of another quantity of noxious air in which a plant had grown. I have completely ascertained the restoration of air in which, tallow or wax candles, spirit of wine, or brimstone matches have burned out by the same means.[31]

In response to this letter, Franklin told Priestley that he hoped people would now do more to preserve trees. "I hope this will give some check to the rage of destroying tress that grow near houses, which has accompanied our late improvements in gardening, from an opinion of their being unwholesome. I am certain, from long observation, that there is nothing unhealthy in the air of the woods, for we Americans have every where our country habitations in the midst of woods, and no people on earth enjoy better heath, or are more prolific."[32]

Franklin was serious when he stated that most people believed that pockets of trees should be cut and woods avoided.[33] The notion was linked to the idea that trees impeded lower air movements and made the air moist, stagnant, and a haven for noxious effluvia and insects. The imperative, as most people saw it, was to clear the forests with their miasmas, stenches, and rot, and to cultivate or "civilize" the land.[34]

This view was clearly expressed by London physician John Woodward, who even pointed to the dangers faced by the early settlers in America: "The great Moisture in the Air was a mighty inconvenience and annoyance to those who first settled in *America:* which at that time was much overgrown with Woods and Groves. But as these were burnt and destroy'd, to make way for Habitation and Culture of the Earth, the Air mended and clear'd up apace."[35]

Franklin agreed with Woodward to a point. Cultivating the land occupied by marshes, insect-infected bogs, rotting trees, and green scummy swamps was a good idea. But he drew the line at felling all trees in and around cities and towns. He did not believe they caused or contributed to health problems and could find no reason to view them with a jaundiced eye. On the contrary, based on what Priestley was able to show experimentally, they appeared to cleanse, freshen, and purify the foul city air. Franklin went on to write: "I wish we had two Rows of them in every one of our Streets" to provide shelter, shade from the hot sun, and because they "improv'd [the] Health of the Inhabitants."[36] Unfortunately, his thoughts about trees fell largely on deaf ears, especially in America, where the burning and cutting continued with vigor as the population increased, the cities grew, and the farmers plowed ever greater tracts of land.

## UNDERSTANDING PHOTOSYNTHESIS

The note Franklin sent to Priestley, which included his thoughts on preserving trees, also contained a section that shows how laying out the facts derived from systematic experiments, when combined with good reasoning, could result in fundamental truths. "That the vegetable creation should restore the air which is spoiled by the animal part of it, looks like a rational system," Franklin wrote. "We knew before that putrid animal substances were converted into sweet vegetables when mixed with the earth, and applied as manure; and now, it seems, that the same putrid substances, mixed with the air, have a similar effect. The strong thriving state of your mint in the putrid air seems to shew that the air is mended by taking something from it and not by adding to it."[37]

In his 1772 article, Priestley concurred with Franklin's assessment that "the air is mended by taking something from it and not by adding to it." His exact words were: "Since the plants that I have made use of manifestly grow and thrive in putrid air; since putrid matter is well known to afford proper nourishment for the roots of plants; and since it is likewise certain that they receive nourishment by their leaves as well as by their roots, it seems to be exceedingly probable, that the putrid effluvium is in some measure extracted from the air, by means of the leaves of plants, and therefore that they render the remainder more fit for respiration."[38]

Franklin and Priestley were clearly on the right track. Leafy plants do take harmful carbon dioxide from the air, making it healthier for breathing. But this would prove to be only one part the story. They also return life-sustaining oxygen back into it. To his credit, Priestley would go on to describe the properties of oxygen in 1774, and he would isolate this gas two years later.[39] Nevertheless, Priestley never fully grasped the actions that were occurring at the chemical level.[40]

Two of Franklin's other friends, however, now stepped in to advance the work started by Priestley. One was Jan Ingenhousz[41] and the other was Antoine Laurent Lavoisier.[42] And like Priestley, both Ingenhousz and Lavoisier communicated with Franklin, telling him about their discoveries and insights.

While visiting London in 1779, the year in which he was elected to the Royal Society, the Dutch-born Ingenhousz became so intrigued with Priestley's discoveries that he moved to a quiet house in the countryside to conduct hundreds of experiments on plants and gasses. His major contribution was in fully recognizing the important role that sunlight played in the process.[43] He found that streams of "dephlogisticated air" (oxygen) bubbled from the green leaves when they were submerged in water and put into the light on a bright sunny day, but not when they were kept in the dark. When he burned a wax candle in the air released by the bubbles, he found that it burned with greater intensity than it did in ordinary air.

Ingenhousz published his *Experiments upon Vegetables* late in 1779, and dedicated the book to Franklin's and his mutual friend, John Pringle.[44] As soon as it came off the press, he sent a copy to Franklin, who was then in Passy, and later, when a French edition was published, he dedicated it to him.

Lavoisier first met Priestley in Paris in 1774. Priestley told him about the newly discovered gas that supported life and allowed a candle to burn even brighter. Lavoisier then replicated some of his experiments and conducted many new ones, some of which he showed to Franklin and discussed with him after he arrived in France. Lavoisier recognized that common air is a mixture, not an element, and that oxygen (his term) accounts for about one-fifth of the mixture.

When Lavoisier's improved *Traité Élémentaire de Chimie* (Elementary Treatise on Chemistry) was published in 1789, the scientist who considered himself a citizen of the republic of learning sent two copies to Franklin, who had now returned to Philadelphia. One was dedicated for the world's most distinguished public servant's personal library and the other for his American Philosophical Society, which had honored Lavoisier by electing him a foreign member.

Knowing that Franklin was close to dying when he received the book, Lavoisier wrote: "As you will see in the preface, I have tried to arrive at the truth by pursuing facts and by suppressing, in so far as possible, specula-tion, which often misleads and deceives us. We should follow the torch of observation and experience whenever possible. This approach, which has never been followed in chemistry, led me to organize my book in a way that is completely new, a way that makes chemistry appear quite like experi-mental physics. I sincerely hope you will have the time and strength needed to read the first few chapters, for I seek only your approbation and that of those learned men in Europe who are without prejudice in these matters."[45]


## PROPERTIES AND DANGERS OF MARSH GAS

Despite his lack of formal background in chemistry, Franklin conducted several of his own experiments on fresh and foul air in this era of great dis-coveries about airs and gases. Further, when Priestley called upon others to pursue his work on different kinds of air, and to come forth with new facts, Franklin responded. He told him about his own experiments on marsh gases, which were considered dangerous to one's health by both the laity and physicians.

Franklin had been fascinated by marsh gases for more than a decade when he penned: "When I passed through New Jersey in 1764, I heard it several times mentioned, that by applying a lighted candle near the surface of some of their rivers, a sudden flame would catch and spread upon the water, con-tinuing to burn for near half a minute." He explained that he "had no oppor-tunity of seeing the experiment," but that a friend told him that when the mud in some shallow water was stirred with a stick, bubbles would come forth, that would bust into a strong flame if put in contact with a candle. Franklin continued:

A Worthy gentleman who lives a few miles distance, informed me that in a certain small cove of a mill-pond, near his house, he was surprized to see the surface of the water blaze like inflamed spirits. I soon after went to the place, and made the experiment with the same success.

I have tried the experiment twice here in England, but without success. The first was in slow running water with a muddy bottom. The second in a stagnant water at the bottom of a deep ditch. Being some time employed in stirring this water, I ascribed an intermitting fever, which seized me a few days after, to my breathing too much of that foul air which I stirred up from the bottom, and which I could not avoid while I stooped in endeavouring to kindle it. The discoveries you have lately made . . . may throw light on this experiment, and explain its succeeding in some cases, and not in others.[46]

Priestley was engaged in a dispute with another physician when he received this note from Franklin in 1774. That physician, a Scot named Alexander, had just played down the dangers posed by marsh airs. Priestley, in contrast, had been finding that air rising from mud under stagnant, putrid water is typically "unfit for respiration." Priestley published his findings and thoughts about marsh airs in the *Philosophical Transactions* in 1774.[47]

The article following Priestley's paper was by Richard Price, who presented some powerful medical statistics from Switzerland. Price did not mince words: "The probabilities of life are highest in the most hilly parts of the province, and lowest in the marshy parish just mentioned. One half, of all born in the mountains, live to the age of 47. In the marshy parish, one half live only to the age of 25. In the hills one in 20 . . . live to 80. In the marshy parish, only one in 52 reaches this age."[48] Here was good statistical evidence that marsh air could be dangerous, even if Price did not delve into the issue of why. With data like these to ponder, choosing a healthy environment in which to live and work, and filling in or draining swampy areas with poor air quality, became even more meaningful to Franklin and those in his circle.

## THE CHAMPION OF FRESH AIR

Franklin used all of his talents when it came to improving the air and promoting the benefits of fresh air. His work involved building better stoves, fireplaces, and innovative ventilation systems to make homes and workplaces healthier. He also served as an advocate for improving air quality in crowded schools and hospitals. And he tried to show people through personal example that fresh air, even when cold or damp, can be stimulating to both mind and body, and therefore doubly beneficial.

Additionally, while in London Franklin involved himself in the discovery of what would later be called photosynthesis, by which plants purify the air. In doing so, he tried to show the importance of trees, which were being cut down in many areas as a health menace. Moreover, as an experimentalist, he even engaged in a few experiments on putrid marsh gases, the results of which he was happy to share with others, including the fact that he got sick while conducting his studies.

In a lighthearted moment, Franklin even wrote an essay on flatulence.[49] His logic was that since "a few stems of Asparagus" and some drugs "can alter the smell of the urine," and stale meat and onions can make human gas smell worse, it might be possible to "discover some Drug wholesome & not disagreeable, to be mix'd with our common Food, or Sauces, that shall render the natural Discharges of Wind from our Bodies, not only inoffensive, but agreeable as Perfumes." Might not the mineral lime in our food or a glass of water, he asked, help to make the smell less unpleasant?

Franklin drew on his great sense of humor while writing this piece, which he dedicated to Joseph Priestley. He even referred to it as no more than a "jocular Paper."[50] But he still managed to raise some interesting questions about ways to reduce the stenches that he viewed as embarrassing, offensive, bad for the environment, and unhealthy for others. Nobody of the time was more involved in promoting the benefits of fresh air and in thinking about ways to improve air quality than Benjamin Franklin.

# CHAPTER 11

# The Perils of Lead

I therefore sometimes heated my Case when the Types did not want drying. But an old Workman, observing it, advis'd me not to do so, telling me I might lose the Use of my hands by it, as two of our Companions had nearly done.

—Benjamin Franklin, recalling an event from 1724

During his stay in England, Franklin received a letter from Cadwalader Evans, the physician he had worked with in 1752 to treat C.B.'s hysteria with electricity (see Chapter 6). He had recently written to Evans to ask what books were now on the shelves of the library at Pennsylvania Hospital, in order to know what titles might still be needed. Along with his inquiry, which he had sent in 1767, Franklin had enclosed a treatise on lead poisoning as the cause of a serious epidemic in Devonshire, England, one associated with a painful colic.

The author of the treatise was Dr. George Baker, who had received his B.A., M.A., and M.D. degrees from Cambridge University in 1745, 1749, and 1756, respectively. Baker had started his career as a practitioner in Lincolnshire, but settled in London in 1761. By the time Franklin met him, he was a Fellow of the Royal Society, a member of the Royal Society Club, and a Fellow of the Royal College of Physicians. Franklin explained to Evans that he had just received the treatise "as a Present from the Author. It is not yet published to be sold, and will not be for some time, till the second Part is ready to accompany it."[1]

Franklin felt sure that Evans would be interested in Baker's new material, since Evans was knowledgeable about the "West India Dry Gripes," a New World colic that had also been associated with lead poisoning. Evans had previously observed the dry gripes while living in Haiti and Jamaica, had read Thomas Cadwalader's treatise on this colic, and was now treating patients in Pennsylvania Hospital for the intense stomach pains it caused.

For Baker, understanding the cause of the Devonshire colic also had personal significance. He had been born in this beautiful fruit-growing region of

# AN
# ESSAY,

Concerning the CAUSE of the

# ENDEMIAL · COLIC
OF
# DEVONSHIRE,

Which was read in the THEATRE of the
COLLEGE of PHYSICIANS, in LONDON,
on the Twenty-ninth Day of JUNE, 1767,

BY GEORGE BAKER,

Fellow of the COLLEGE of PHYSICIANS, and of the ROYAL
SOCIETY, and Physician to her MAJESTY's Houshold.

---

ἘΚ ΤΟΎΤΩΝ ΝΟΣΟΥΜΕΝ, ΟΙΣ ΚΑῚ ΖΩΜΕΝ.

PLUTARCH.

---

LONDON:
Printed by J. HUGHS, near LINCOLN's-INN-FIELDS.
M.DCC.LXVII.

*George Baker's (1772–1809) landmark* Essay on lead poisoning.

southern England in 1722. The area was renowned for its orchards, and apple cider had been a major product in its economy since at least the thirteenth century.[2] In the past, the colic, which tended to show up in the fall, had been attributed to many things, and a number of physicians pointed specifically to the cider. William Musgrave and John Huxham were two such physicians, and they suggested that unripe rough cider and overly sour and acetic pomace were the cause of the problem.[3]

Baker concurred that the cider was the likely culprit, but he was not sure why. Hence, with the mindset of an enlightened natural philosopher, he studied how the local cider was processed from start to finish, the records of patients admitted to the Royal Devon and Exeter Hospital between 1762 and 1767, and cider processing and hospital admissions in other areas. And he conducted a series of clever experiments to test his ideas. Baker's reasoned conclusion, backed by these experiments, was that the disorder that turned people into pallid ghosts with stomach pains and dangling hands stemmed from lead in the Devonshire cider.

Baker had discovered that the local cider makers had been using lead in just about every stage of their cider's production. Lead was present in the presses, the troughs, and the vats. His research showed that cider from the nearby counties of Hereford, Gloucester, and Worcester, which was manufactured without lead in the machinery, did not cause the colic. And, to make matters worse, he discovered that litharge (lead monoxide) was sometimes added to the Devonshire cider to reduce the drink's acidity and sweeten its taste.

Although Franklin could send only the first part of Baker's treatise on lead poisoning to Evans when he inquired about books contained in the Pennsylvania Hospital library, Baker soon completed his second tract. Both would be read before the London College of Physicians in 1767 and published in that society's *Medical Transactions.*[4] Over the next few years, Baker would present and publish several other scholarly papers on the Devonshire colic and lead poisoning in general.[5] And he would repeatedly write that he owed a great debt of gratitude to Benjamin Franklin for making him aware of crucial facts—facts that led him to a better understanding of the Devonshire colic and served as a reminder of the dangers of lead in general.

## THE EARLY HISTORY OF LEAD POISONING

Objects made with lead have been dated back to 6,000 B.C. in central Turkey, 3,800 B.C. in Egypt, and to 2,200 B.C. in Troy.[6] Mentioned repeatedly in the

Old Testament, the malleable metal was used in one form or another by biblical tribes for art, cosmetics, pipes, pots, utensils, currencies, paints, poisons, contraceptives, and even health-promoting medicines.

The rise of Athens was based in part on the wealth obtained from the nearby Laurion mines. Worked by a steady stream of slaves and convicts, who inevitably became too ill to function and required replacements, this mine produced large amounts of lead and small amounts of silver. The two metals were separated with a crushing, heating, and skimming technique called cupellation. To the Greeks of antiquity, the lead that rose up to the surface was the father of all metals. It was also associated with Cronus, the father of all gods, but the gloomiest of the deities as well.

Saturn was the Roman equivalent of Cronus, a fact that was not lost on Poor Richard, who wrote: "Saturn diseas'd with Age, and left for dead; Chang'd all his Gold to be involv'd in Lead."[7] The adjective "saturnine" has long been applied to individuals who become downcast, withdrawn, morose, and taciturn—all early symptoms of lead poisoning. But whereas Saturn was supposed to have devoured his sons—the analogy being to how molten lead can consume silver or gold—victims of lead poisoning tend to become impotent, producing few or no sons at all.

Some historians have argued that lead poisoning contributed to the decline of the Roman Empire.[8] They note that the late Roman emperors fathered few children and tended to be mentally unstable. Moreover, they point out that bone samples of well-to-do Romans have revealed unusually high levels of lead. Many affluent Romans did, in fact, cover their copper pans and storage vessels with pewter made from lead, drink water from lead pipes, and consume wine stored in lead-lined vessels and, in some cases, sweetened with lead additives.

The theory that lead played a role in the fall of Rome has its critics,[9] yet Pliny the Elder drew attention to the pale faces, shaking hands, sore eyes, and insomnia of the heavy wine drinkers in Rome. Two other acute observers, Galen and Vitruvius, also expressed serious concerns about the drinking water flowing into the city through leaded pipes.

Lead poisoning did not disappear with the downfall of the Roman Empire. Paul of Aegina, a Byzantine physician, described an epidemic of what appeared to be acute lead poisoning in seventh-century Italy. Further, Eberhard Gockel dealt with an outbreak of acute lead poisoning in the Duchy of Württemberg only a decade before Franklin was born.[10]

Gockel deduced that the local wines were the source of the epidemic in his region of Germany, and he decided to sample some of the suspicious wine himself. Within a short amount of time, he began to suffer what he called "atrocious colic pains." His continuing investigations of the wine revealed that the regional wine sellers were adding copious amounts of lead to their wines. They did this because the grape harvests had been bad, and trying to sell poor tasting wines would have hurt their reputations and been unprofitable. Concerned by Gockel's revelation and what further offenses could do to the regional economy, the lawmakers in Württemberg passed edicts to curtail further offenses, including threatening to put lawbreakers to death.

Gockel even suggested a chemical test for identifying lead in wines. If a wine had lead, he wrote, the addition of a few drops of sulfuric acid will cause a white precipitate (lead sulfate) to form at the surface.

## THE EFFECTS OF LEAD AND
## THE SCOPE OF THE PROBLEM

Lead poisoning can be associated with more than just the painful colic seen by Gockel. Another hallmark of the disorder is a graying of the complexion. It can also cause insomnia, fatigue, sensory, and intellectual changes. And it can result in tremors and palsies of the limbs. Franklin and his contemporaries referred to "the dangles" or "the drop," sometimes adding the adjective "wrist," "hand," "ankle," or "foot" before the noun. In advanced cases, hallucinations, delusions, and even convulsions may be seen.

Baker divided lead poisoning into acute and chronic types. Acute lead poisoning comes on rapidly, and the victim quickly knows that something is wrong and that help is needed. Generally, many people are affected at once, causing great concern among the laity, their physicians, and the civil authorities. Typically this form of the disorder has a suspicious source, such as the wine, even if the source might not be associated with lead at first.

In contrast, significant signs and symptoms of what Baker called his "chronic species" may take months or years to show themselves. "The first beginnings of it are slight," he wrote. "It steals on by slow progression. It is gradually, and in small quantities, accumulated in the constitution . . . and lays a foundation for irreparable mischief, before any alarm is taken."[11] Renal damage is one form of "irreparable mischief" that can take place very slowly from repeatedly ingesting low or moderate amounts of lead, and the unsuspecting victim may have no idea that what is happening to his or her kidneys could cause or contribute to gout, stones, and other problems.[12]

As a printer handling lead type every day, and because he had lead in his household, Franklin developed a personal interest in chronic lead poisoning. And as a respected physician, Baker was particularly interested in acute lead poisoning, since professional medical help was most likely to be sought by individuals and communities for this condition. Yet both Franklin and Baker were anxious to learn everything they could about both types of lead poisoning, because they were concerned and inquisitive individuals and also because they knew that lead was pervasive in eighteenth-century life.

During the 1760s, lead was a problem of enormous proportions, and one that was still not being adequately recognized by consumers, workers, governments, or physicians. Despite the best efforts of Gockel at the turn of the century, it continued to be added to inferior wines by unscrupulous dealers. After having drawn attention to lead in Devonshire cider, Baker would go on to gripe: "Notwithstanding the severe laws, which are still in force, both in France and in Germany, against the adulteration of wines, by the means of litharge, we still frequently find that the small French white wines, and the Rhenish and Moselle wines, bear marks of this most pernicious fraud."[13]

Baker would also damn the fortified wines that were being imported from southern Europe and that were very much in vogue at the time. The fortified wine group includes Ports, Madeiras, Málagas, and sherries. These sweet, syrupy, and more stable wines are made by adding thick grape spirits (brandy) to local wines. Here, he asked, "may not there be, either by means of fraud, or of accident in the wines, drunk at Madrid, a saturnine adulteration?"[14]

A modern chemical analysis of some late eighteenth-century fortified wines from Spain and Portugal that were shipped to England showed that Baker had every reason to be suspicious of the lead content of these more syrupy wines.[15] Their lead levels were found to be shocking high, most likely because of lead in their production (see Chapter 17).

Franklin, as noted by all of his biographers, was partial to these wines, suggesting he did not recognize that the danger they posed was considerably more extensive than a rare bad bottle here or there. Indeed, when describing his social life, historians write that he was particularly "fond of Madeira, and liked to gossip with his friend Strahan over the second bottle," and that, in France, "Old Madeira had a special place in his affections."[16] More precisely, we know that his wine cellar in France contained 216 bottles of Madeira but only 153 bottles of common table wine in 1782, which was well after Baker published his warning.[17] And by this time Franklin's body was already reeling from both gout and stones.

In addition to beverages being tainted deliberately or accidentally, some occupations, such as painting and plumbing, had considerable lead exposure. And lead or pewter (then containing about 25 percent lead and 75 percent tin) could be found in a myriad of household items for cooking or storing foods, including casserole pans and storage containers for milk. Lead was also present in glazes, crystal glass decanters, and even some candlewicks.

Even more troublesome, the saturnine element was being given to sick patients by their physicians. Practitioners were prescribing lead salts for hemorrhages, epilepsy, and diarrhea, and it was also utilized to produce abortions. Remarkably, swallowing lead "bullets" was sometimes recommended for cases of colic that might have been caused by lead. Because lead was eleven times the weight of water, one belief was that it could push blockages through the obstructed bowels. Cotton Mather mentioned the lead cure in *The Angel of Bethesda,* but then had the good sense to reject it as both silly and dangerous.[18]

Hence, while Franklin and Baker were sharing ideas in London, there was a great need to show people just how harmful the gloomy element of antiquity could be, and this meant not only the laity but also their learned physicians. But exactly how much did Franklin know about lead poisoning when he arrived in London in 1757, a decade before Baker discovered that lead was the cause of the Devonshire colic and became England's own expert on the subject?

## FRANKLIN'S KNOWLEDGE OF LEAD POISONING

Benjamin Franklin had learned about the dangers of lead while he was still a teenager. He would later recollect that there "was a general Discourse in Boston, when I was a Boy, of a Complaint from North Carolina against New England Rum, that it poison'd their People, giving them the Dry Bellyach, with a Loss of the Use of their Limbs." He explained, "The Distilleries being examin'd on the Occasion, it was found that several of them used leaden Still-heads and Worms, and the Physicians were of Opinion, that the Mischief was occasioned by that Use of Lead. The Legislature of Massachusetts thereupon pass'd an Act, prohibiting under severe Penalties the Use of such Still-heads and Worms thereafter."[19]

"An Act for Preventing Abuses in the Distilling of Rhum, and Other Strong Liquors with Leaden Heads or Pipes" was made into law in 1723. It was the first public health act in the colonies specifically designed to protect consumers.[20] And with stiff monetary penalties, it led to some reforms in the loosely controlled colonial rum industry, although there would still be abuses.

In 1745, Franklin printed physician Thomas Cadwalader's *Essay on the West-India Dry-Gripes* on his press in Philadelphia.[21] Although the work's title might suggest that Cadwalader was writing about a colic in the Caribbean, the disorder he was describing could occur anywhere people drank lead-tainted rum, such as the Carolina rum that had led to legislation in Massachusetts. The patients, Cadwalader began, "have a disease similar to the *Cholica Pictonum,* " referring to a disorder that had long plagued the residents in Poitou France. He added, "they are both attended with excessive griping Pains in the Pit of the Stomach and Bowels; violent and frequent Reaching to vomit; sometimes bringing up small Quantities of bilious Matter; at other times there is a Sensation, as if the Bowels were drawn together by Ropes. . . . This sore Malady usually degenerates into the Palsy, and a Deprivation of all Sort of Motion in the Hands and Feet."[22]

Cadwalader rightfully associated the colonial colic with its French counterpart, but he was vague about why the colonial rum had such pernicious effects, and he did not point specifically and unequivocally to the use of lead in virtually every stage of its production. Instead, when discussing causes, he told his readers to avoid strong, fresh rum punch, as well as highly seasoned meats, moist air, and excessive perspiration.[23]

Poor Richard included several entries on the "Dry-Bellyach" or dry-gripes in his *Almanack* before and after his aspiring printer published Cadwalader's essay. In 1734, he warned: "Drink Water, Put the Money in Your Pocket, and leave the *Dry-Bellyach* in the *Punchbowl.*"[24] In 1756, just before Franklin went to England, Poor Richard saw fit to include a medical prescription for sufferers of the dry-gripes: "Take sixty Drops of Tincture of Castor, thirty of liquid Laudanum, in an Ounce of Mint or other simple Water, sweetened to your Taste; take of this Mixture a Spoonful every Half Hour, till you find Relief," he suggested. Nevertheless, Poor Richard went on to tell his readers, "These remedies are said to be excellent in their Kind; but as a Case may be mistaken by the Unskilful, let me, tho' no Physician, prescribe something more, viz. Whenever you can have the Advice of a skilful Physician, Take that."[25]

In addition to gaining a deep respect for the potential dangers of rum made in stills containing lead parts, and paying attention to various treatments suggested for the dry-gripes, Franklin also developed a profound respect for manually handling lead before he set sail for England as a diplomat. The event that opened his eyes to the possibility of occupational lead poisoning occurred while he was still in his teens. It took place after he was stranded in

London, having never received the letters of credit promised by Governor Keith to purchase some printing equipment to start his own business.

In 1724, being in London, I went to work in the Printing-House of Mr. Palmer, Bartholomew Close, as a Compositor. I there found a Practice, I had never seen before, of drying a Case of Types (which are wet in Distribution) by placing it sloping before the Fire. I found this had the additional Advantage, when the Types were not only dry'd but heated, of being comfortable to the Hands working over them in cold weather. I therefore sometimes heated my Case when the Types did not want drying.

   But, an old Workman, observing it, advis'd me not to do so, telling me I might lose the Use of my Hands by it, as two of our Companions had nearly done, one of whom that us'd to earn his Guinea a Week, could not then make more than ten Shillings, and the other, who had the Dangles, but seven and sixpence. This, with a kind of obscure Pain, that I had sometimes felt, as it were in the Bones of my Hand when working over the Types made very hot, induced me to omit the Practice.

   At this juncture, Franklin still was not sure how the lead from the hot type was entering his body.

But talking afterwards with Mr. James, a Letter-founder in the same Close, and asking him if his People, who work'd over the little Furnaces of melted Metal, were not subject to that Disorder; he made light of any danger from the effluvia, but ascribed it to Particles of the Metal swallow'd with their Food by slovenly Workmen, who went to their Meals after handling the Metal, without well washing their Fingers, so that some of the metalline Particles were taken off by their Bread and eaten with it. This appeared to have some Reason in it. But the Pain I had experienc'd made me still afraid of those Effluvia.[26]

   Two decades later, when promoting his new Pennsylvania fireplaces, Franklin made sure he included the statement that "Iron does not, like Lead, . . . give out unwholesome Vapours." He supported his statement by describing the "general Health and Strength" of ironworkers and the results of experiments on birds forced to breathe fumes of iron (which did not hurt them) or fumes from lead alloys (which killed them). "When hot," stated Franklin unequivocally, lead "yields a very unwholesome Steam."[27]

   Hence, Franklin had a wealth of knowledge about lead poisoning before he sailed to England in 1757, where he met George Baker at the Royal Society and Royal Society Club. He knew about the dry-gripes, how lead could give printers like himself pain, tremors, and the dangles, and how lead fumes could kill birds. If we also consider additional information that Franklin might have picked up from various books, pamphlets, newspapers, and by word of mouth, he had to have been one of the most informed people anywhere when it came to appreciating and understanding the perils of lead.

## FRANKLIN AND BAKER JOIN FORCES

On July 13, 1767, Baker wrote that he had "waited on Dr. Franklyn to shew him the inclosed paper, which . . . is to be read this afternoon at the College of Physicians. If Dr. Franklyn has anything to object, or to add, Dr. B. will take it as a particular favour, if he will send his alterations to him in Jermyn-Street."[28]

Franklin might have been Baker's most important source about lead poisoning, and he would continue to help him put the colic in perspective in his series of papers. He originally pointed out to Baker that the signs and symptoms of the Devonshire colic were similar to those shown by painters and other workers susceptible to lead poisoning. Occupational lead poisoning was, without question, one of the important clues that Baker needed to understand what was happening in Devonshire. Franklin further assisted him by pointing out that the disorder he was investigating in England had its counterpart in the dry-gripes that made people double over and grip their stomachs in the North American colonies and West Indies.

Some of the ways in which Franklin helped Baker were revealed in a follow-up letter Franklin sent to Cadwalader Evans in 1768. After receiving Baker's first tract, Evans had written back to Franklin, thanking him for passing the piece on to him and noting that he was inclined to believe that Baker's Devonshire colic and the West India dry-gripes must be closely related.

The Symptoms in the dry bellyach of the West Indians, and North Americans, are nearly the same with those in the colic of Poictou and Devonshire, wherefore it may be worth enquiery, whether a similar cause has not some share in producing like effects.

The climate and general way of living, in the English and French Islands, are nearly the same, except that the latter use wine, or wine and water for common drink, and the former Rum punch. Among the French, I am informed, the Belly ach, is scarcely known; with us it is almost endemic—Now whether this difference is caused by any admixture of lead, in the composition of Still Worms [condensers] or to the well known propertys of inflameable spirits, to relax the tone of the alimentary canal, and subject it to spasms may be easily determined by Dr. Bakers experiment.[29]

On February 20, 1768, Franklin replied back to Evans that he had for a very long time believed that the various instances of the dry gripes or dry bellyache had but a single cause. Further, Franklin had informed Baker of what had happened when lead solders and pipes were used for distilling spirits in the New World:

In yours of Nov. 20, you mention the Lead on the Stills or worms of the Stills as a probable cause of the Dry bellyach among Punch Drinkers in our West India Islands. I had before acquainted Dr. Baker with a Fact of that kind, the general mischief done by the use of Leaden Worms, when Rum Distilling was first practiced in New England, which occasioned a severe Law there against them; and he has mentioned it in the second Part of his piece not yet published. I have long been of Opinion, that that Distemper proceeds always from a metallic Cause only, observing that it affects among Tradesmen those that use Lead, however different their Trades, as Glaziers, Type-Founders, Plumbers, Potters, White-Lead-makers and Painters.[30]

Baker was pleased to get Franklin's assistance, and he repeatedly referred to his help in his writings.

It seems not improbable that, if we had an opportunity of making an accurate inquiry, we might see reason to conclude, that the disease, called popularly the dry-belly-ach, which is common as well in the northern colonies of America, as in the islands of the West-Indies, ought to be referred wholly to lead, as its cause.

My suspicions, concerning this subject, have been greatly confirmed by the authority of Dr. Franklyn of Philadelphia. That gentleman informs me, that, at Boston, about forty years ago, leaden worms were used for the distillation of rum. In consequence thereof, such violent disorders were complained of by the drinkers of new rum, that the government found it expedient to enact a law, forbidding the use of any worms, except such only as were made of pure block-tin. This law having been enacted, the dry colic was much less frequently heard of than before.

But, the law was complied with only in part; for from that time to the present, instead of block-tin, they have used a pewter, containing a large portion of lead. Dr. Franklyn likewise informed me, that the colic of Poitou is not so frequent a disease in any of the colonies, as it was formerly; and that the reason, commonly assigned, is that the people now drink their punch very weak in comparison with that what they were formerly accustomed to, which used to be rum and water in equal quantities.[31]

Baker even included Franklin's eyewitness account of how printers suffered dangles and lost the use of their hands from heating and handling hot type. In this case, however, he did not mention Franklin by name. He merely spoke about "several cases, which have been related to me on good authority" and, in another place, coming from "an intelligent printer."[32]

Baker was especially excited to have the information about occupational lead poisoning that Franklin and two of Franklin's closest medical friends passed on to him. Franklin and John Pringle had gone to France in 1767, where Pringle had visited La Charité, the famous Paris hospital. Pringle obtained a list of all the patients who seemed to be hospitalized with signs and symptoms of lead poisoning. Franklin then went through the list, paying careful attention to the occupations of the men. It was discovered that the men hospitalized with the painful colic were employed in trades that exposed them to high levels of lead.

In addition, when Jan Ingenhousz visited Normandy, he found out that lead was not used in the machinery and vats for making cider there, and that there was no associated colic. But, he was informed, and Baker was able to add, "in the hospital at Rouen, there are generally many patients, under the colic of Poitou, such as potters, painters, and other workers of lead."[33]

Baker's treatise upset some cider makers and tradesmen in Devon, and it bothered some physicians with their own pet ideas about what caused the epidemic. But his scholarship and experiments were applauded by almost everyone else, much as Gockel's had been some seventy years earlier in Germany. Thus, with Franklin's help, Baker ushered in a fresh new appreciation of lead poisoning, telling people both how to try to prevent it and what should be done if the first signs and symptoms of it appear.

In terms of prevention, Baker wrote about household objects with lead and, for the first time, pointed to the unique dangers faced by children. He wrote that "a very common, but dangerous practice, ought not to have been passed over without notice: I mean that of painting toys made for the amusement of children. It is well known, that children are apt to put every thing, especially what gives them pleasure, into their mouths; and it therefore can hardly be doubted but that the disorders of the stomach and bowels, to which they are particularly subject, are multiplied by this practice."[34]

On the subject of treatment, Baker pointed to the importance of immediately preventing any more lead from entering the body. He noted that even people with occupational lead poisoning may overcome their problems with time and by avoiding further contact with the gloomy element. "Almost every day's experience," he wrote, "furnisheth physicians with examples of painters, and plumbers, and the other numerous artificers, employed either in manufacturing the several preparations of lead, or in applying them to their respective uses; who, after having suffered the most extreme torments from the colic of Poitou, are restored to health, and remain free from that disease, so long, at least, as they quit their usual business, or pursue it with greater caution."[35]

In part because of his greater understanding of lead poisoning, and because of his ability to communicate his findings so clearly and convincingly to other physicians and the public, Baker was appointed a physician-in-ordinary to the queen and then King George III himself. He was also made a baronet and was repeatedly elected president of the College of Physicians. His influential treatises are still regarded as classics in environmental science and medicine, although how Franklin helped him tends to be glossed over or not even mentioned.

## SEARCHING FOR SUBSTITUTES

Franklin continued to tell people about the dangers of lead after war broke out between England and the American colonies. Moreover, he engaged the expert opinions of chemists and other men of science to see if there might be safe substitutes for lead products, especially in everyday life.

In 1780, he obtained some advice from chemist Antoine-Laurent Lavoisier in France. Lavoisier had recently conducted some experiments on tin and lead, and he was describing the properties of these metals to his colleagues at the Académie Royale des Sciences when he was handed a piece of paper with a question on it. Franklin wanted to know if a safe way had been found to plate copper casserole dishes. Tinning them had long been in vogue, as tin took away the disagreeable copper taste and covered the repulsive blue-green verdigris on the surface, which was believed to be dangerous to one's health.

Nevertheless, Lavoisier explained to Franklin that most craftsmen used tin with a lot of lead in it, which he described as the equivalent of covering an existing poison with an almost equally dangerous different poison. What made more sense, he felt, was plating pans with pure tin or an extremely high-quality tin. Two problems, however, made this an uncommon practice, even in Paris. One was finding an honest, skilled craftsman to do high-quality work without a substitution, and the other was the cost. Lavoisier advised Franklin that, if he could find an honest worker, he should not haggle over the price.[36]

Franklin did not learn anything new from Lavoisier. George Baker had written almost the same thing more than a decade earlier in one of his tracts, in which he thanked Franklin for his help. He warned "that culinary vessels, lined with a mixture of tin and lead, may communicate pernicious qualities to acid foods," and he even stated that "Galen, in his first book *de antidotis*, complains of this as a dangerous mixture." Baker further realized "that it is much more difficult, as well as more expensive, to line vessels with pure tin only."[37]

## FURTHER SPREADING THE MESSAGE

A few years after supplying many pertinent pieces of information to Baker and sharing ideas with Evans, Franklin returned to lead poisoning in a letter to Joseph Galloway in Philadelphia. Galloway served as speaker of the Pennsylvania Assembly from 1766 to 1775, and he might have had a mild case of lead poisoning when Franklin sat down at his desk in London in 1772 to write back to him.

"The Dry Gripes are thought here to proceed always from Lead taken by some means or other into the Body," Franklin began. "You will consider whether this can have been your Case, and avoid the Occasion. Lead us'd about the Vessels or other Instruments us'd in making Cyder, has, they say, given the cruel Disease to many. Preparations of Lead us'd to sweaten prick'd [sour] Wine have done the same."[38]

Nevertheless, it was not Galloway but Benjamin Vaughan who was the recipient of the most informative of all Franklin's letters about lead poisoning. In 1785, Vaughan made his way to Southampton, where he met Franklin, then en route back to Philadelphia after a lengthy stay in France. The two men were delighted to see each other again, and they discussed many things, one of which was lead poisoning. A year later, Franklin completed a detailed letter on lead poisoning and sent it to Vaughan, at his request. It summarized a lot of what was known at the time, including his own contributions to that knowledge base.

"Dear Friend," he began, "I recollect, that, when I had the great Pleasure of seeing you at Southampton, now a 12 month since, we had some Conversation on the bad Effects of Lead taken inwardly; and that at your Request I promis'd to send you in writing a particular Account of several Facts I then mention'd to you, of which you thought some good use might be made. I now sit down to fulfil that Promise."

Franklin started by presenting the story of how North Carolina filed a complaint against New England rum, which resulted in legislation to outlaw lead in its production. "Inclos'd," he informed Vaughan, "I send you a Copy of the Acct, taken from my printed Law-Book." He next conveyed what he witnessed among the workers handling hot lead type, and how he developed pains in his own hands, while employed at Palmer's printing house. This was followed by some comments about the smelting operations he saw in Derbishire, and what this might be doing to the cattle that were feeding on the vegetation in the region.

Franklin went on: "In America I have often observ'd, that on the Roofs of our shingled Houses, where Moss is apt to grow in northern Exposures, if there be any thing on the Roof painted with white Lead, such as Balusters, or Frames of dormant Windows, &c., there is constantly a Streak on the Shingles from such Paint down to the Eaves, on which no Moss will grow, but the wood remains constantly clean and free from it. We seldom drink Rain-Water that falls on our Houses; and if we did, perhaps the small Quantity of Lead, descending from such Paint, might not be sufficient to produce any sensible ill Effect on our Bodies."

But, he told Vaughan, "I have been told of a Case in Europe, I forgot the Place, where a whole Family was afflicted with what we call the Dry Belly-ach, or *Colica Pictonum*, by drinking Rain-Water. It was at a Country-Seat, which, being situated too high to have the Advantage of a Well, was supply'd with Water from a Tank, which received the Water from the leaded Roofs. This had been drunk several Years without Mischief; but some young Trees planted near the House growing up above the Roof, and shedding their Leaves upon it; it was suppos'd that an Acid in those Leaves had corroded the Lead they cover'd, and furnish'd the Water of that Year with its baneful Particles and Qualities."

He also described what he had learned about patients in the French hospitals with lead poisoning. Most had been in trades with obvious lead exposure, yet he admitted that two well-represented groups had initially puzzled him, specifically the stonecutters and soldiers. "These I could not reconcile to my Notion, that Lead was the cause of that Disorder. But on my mentioning this Difficulty to a Physician of that Hospital, he inform'd me that the Stonecutters are continually using melted Lead to fix the Ends of Iron Balustrades in Stone; and that the Soldiers have been employ'd by Painters, as Labourers, in Grinding of Colours."

He concluded: "This, my dear Friend, is all I can at present recollect on the Subject. You will see by it, that the Opinion of this mischievous Effect from Lead is at least above Sixty Years old; and you will observe with Concern how long a useful Truth may be known and exist, before it is generally receiv'd and practis'd on."[39]

Franklin clearly had become even more knowledgeable about lead. Did it matter that he could not remember that the case of leaves affecting the drinking water collected from a roof actually took place in Amsterdam?

In retrospect, Franklin made several important contributions to the understanding of lead poisoning. He informed people that what had been considered a number of separate disorders often named after different places was really a single disorder with lead being the common cause. He was also a pioneer in understanding and warning people about occupational lead poisoning. And although he might not have fully appreciated just how much lead was in the fortified wines that were so popular in his day, he helped people see the dangers of lead in everyday life and how they could prevent lead poisoning by being wary and using good common sense.

Franklin did all of these things in his conversations with George Baker, who then wrote lengthy treatises on the subject, and in his letters, the most important of which went to Benjamin Vaughan, with the expectation that he would share it with the British medical elite. Working behind the scenes, what Franklin did was in accord with his personal goal to improve man's lot, and consistent with the methods, ideals, and optimistic outlook of the Enlightenment.

# PART III

# LE DOCTEUR
# IN FRANCE

# CHAPTER 12

# French Medicine and Health Imperatives

The rapid Progress *true* Science now makes occasions my Regretting sometimes that I was born so soon.
                    —Benjamin Franklin to Joseph Priestley, 1780

In 1780, while in France, Franklin received a letter from Dr. James Potter in New Fairfield, Connecticut. A year earlier, Potter had been elected president of "the first Medical Society in the thirteen United States of America Since their Independence." The American physician's main objective was to begin a "literary Correspondence" between his new society and the "Royal Medical Society in France, of which we have the pleasure to find that Doctr Franklin is a member."[1] Potter spelled out his aspiration to "His Excellency Benjamin Franklin . . . Plenipotentiary at the Court of France," and he politely asked him to translate his letter, if necessary, before presenting it to the French physicians. Whether Franklin translated the letter into French and what Potter heard back are uncertain. But what cannot be doubted is that Franklin served as an American link to the French medical community during his nine-year stay in France. Further, he readily disseminated important medical information from France to English-speaking physicians around the globe.

In this chapter we shall first look at the events that led Franklin to France in 1776, how the French received him, and how he settled in socially and politically. Then we shall turn to the societies and groups that he joined; organizations that allowed him to discuss advances in hygiene and medicine with some of the brightest French medical minds. Franklin, as will be shown, engaged himself in diverse problems with major social consequences, such as the spread of diseases from dead bodies, the causes of soaring child mortality, and malnutrition.

RELOCATING IN FRANCE

Franklin left England and returned to America during the spring of 1775. While sailing west, the first battles of what would become the American War for Independence were taking place at Lexington and Concord, not far from Boston. On his arrival in Philadelphia, he was informed of the deteriorating political situation and asked to represent Pennsylvania at the Second Continental Congress. He soon found himself on a committee headed by Thomas Jefferson to draft the Declaration of Independence.

Franklin pondered how the colonies might be represented in the new confederation. But his greatest concern was how to fight and pay for a war when there was little money and inadequate supplies. When the French signaled that they wanted to help in the fight, Congress asked Franklin, Silas Deane, and Thomas Jefferson to sail to France. After Jefferson requested to be replaced because of his wife's failing health, Arthur Lee, another Virginian, was sent as his replacement; John Adams, in turn, would replace Deane in 1778.

After a grueling trip to Quebec, a meeting with George Washington in Massachusetts, and a rejection of Howe's peace initiative on Staten Island, Franklin boarded his ship. He was seventy at the time and accompanied by two grandsons. One was Sarah's son Benny, aged seven, and the other was William's son Temple, aged seventeen, who would serve as his private secretary.

Franklin was not dressed like other diplomats when he arrived in Paris late in 1776. He wore a strange-looking marten fur cap from Canada, which permitted little of his thinning hair to show, and he donned dark clothes with no ornamentation, as if he were a Quaker. He also carried a walking stick rather than a ceremonial sword, and wore the spectacles of a philosopher. The French absolutely loved the image Franklin created. As described by Franklin biographer Carl Van Doren, "the French were looking for a hero who should combine the reason, wit, skepticism, and clarity of Voltaire with the primitive virtues celebrated by Rousseau, and they were sure they had found their hero in Franklin. . . . No one could have foreseen the outburst of enthusiasm. . . . Likenesses of him were so quickly and widely called for that before the middle of January it was fashionable for everybody to have an engraving of him over the mantelpiece."[2] In his assessment of Franklin's popularity in France, historian I. Bernard Cohen added: "But the chief foundation of this popularity was his enormous scientific fame. There is hardly a contemporaneous account of Franklin's renown in France that does not stress his having been a scientific celebrity."[3]

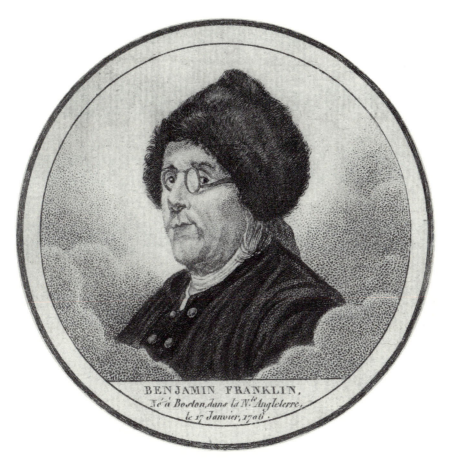

BENJAMIN FRANKLIN,
*Né à Boston, dans la N.<sup>le</sup> Angleterre,
le 17 Janvier, 1706.*

*Benjamin Franklin wearing his marten-fur cap and plain clothes. (Print courtesy of the American Philosophical Society.)*

Marie Antoinette, however, was not enthused by the cult that surrounded Franklin, who was, after all, a commoner. Her husband, Louis XVI, worried even more about Franklin being such a powerful symbol of democracy. The king, in fact, became so fed up with images and symbols of "Docteur Franklin" (never Monsieur) showing up everywhere he turned, that he even presented one Franklin worshipper with a Sèvres chamber pot. It had the famous American's face looking up from the inside.

After spending two months in Paris, Franklin moved to Passy, then a village surrounded by forests and vineyards just a half mile outside the city. He lodged in a wing of the Hôtel de Valentinois, a chateau that belonged to Donatien Leray de Chaumont, a shipping magnate and superintendent of the Hôtel Royale des Invalides, a Paris hospital. Franklin had ample room for his grandchildren, his guests, ministerial associates, and help. He even had basement space for a small printing press, from which he could print passports and other legal documents, as well as his philosophical writings. Monsieur Chaumont turned down his guest's offer to pay rent. He did, however, accept his American guest's willingness to fix the chimneys and install proper lightning rods on his magnificent estate.

## DIPLOMACY AND THE WAR

Franklin developed a good working relationship with the French prime minister, the Comte de Vergennes, who did not speak English, but understood European politics, the balance of power, French pride, and the fears of the monarchy.[4] He did his best to support the Americans with money and supplies, even when the war went badly. And things did go badly at first. Not only were the rebels poorly supplied and insufficiently trained, so many men were sick that the troops were often unable to fight effectively. In the first year of the war, ten times as many Americans died from typhus, typhoid fever, smallpox, malaria, dysentery, and respiratory infections than from bullets, shrapnel, or bayonets.[5]

Two factors made Franklin's mission even more difficult than it might have been, given how much the French hated the English and wanted to help ensure their defeat. One was Congress, which made impossible demands on the delegation and had little understanding of how business was conducted in France. And the other was the fact that the three American ministers often did not get along.

Franklin was particularly troubled by Arthur Lee, who had graduated from the Edinburgh medical school with honors and had built a successful medical practice in Virginia before joining him in France.[6] Lee had been elected into the Royal Society, had been considered for a medical school position by John Morgan, and was married to the sister of physician William Shippen, Jr. Yet Lee was so quarrelsome and at times paranoid that Franklin even questioned his sanity.

During the spring of 1778, a very angry Franklin picked up his pen to inform Lee that he had enough of his "Snubbing and Rebukes." He wrote that he had not expressed himself before out of "Pity for your Sick Mind, which is forever Tormenting itself, with its Jealousies, Suspicions and Fancies that others mean you ill." He added: "If you do not cure yourself of this Temper it will end in Insanity, of which it is the Symptomatick Forerunner, as I have seen in several instances."[7] After cooling off, however, he decided not to send this letter, although he later wrote of Lee: "That Genius must either find or make a Quarrel wherever he is. The only excuse for him that his Conduct will admit of, is his being at times out of his senses. . . . [I] am persuaded that if some of the many Enemies he provokes do not kill him sooner, he will die in a Madhouse."[8]

Following a very poor start to the war, the bickering ministers began to receive better news. Particularly significant was the victory at Saratoga, New York, in 1777. General Burgoyne's surrender effectively ended the threat from the north and isolated General William Howe's troops in Philadelphia. Now sensing that the Americans could defeat the British, the French agreed to recognize the new nation and to send their own troops and warships to help the rebellious colonists. They asked for some spoils of war, to be a part of any truce, and for a single minister plenipotentiary as befitting a recognized country. They let Congress know that Franklin was their choice, and he was given the position on September 14, 1778.

Three years later, Franklin was informed that General Cornwallis had surrendered at Yorktown, Virginia. The resignation of Lord North's conservative ministry followed, and with the change in government both sides began to talk peace. Franklin was asked to help draw up a peace accord, and he did so with John Adams and John Jay, who had also been in Europe serving the American cause. Thankful that the war was over, Franklin sent a letter to Joseph Banks, president of the Royal Society. "I join with you most cordially in rejoicing at the return of Peace," he began. "I hope it will be lasting, and that Mankind will at length . . . have Reason and Sense enough to settle their Differences without cutting Throats; for, in my opinion, there never was a good War, or a bad Peace."[9]

## THE ACADÉMIE ROYALE DES SCIENCES

Franklin's life in France was not just that of a diplomat, as was the case on his two earlier missions to England. When able, he took his carriage to Paris to attend meetings of the Académie Royale des Sciences. This elite society was formally established in 1666, shortly after the Royal Society, and its mission was likewise to promote useful knowledge, which included the application of new findings in science to the practice of medicine. Franklin became one of the organization's eight foreign associates in 1772, a high honor reflecting the esteem the French had for him, particularly as an electrical scientist.

Lavoisier was one of the leading figures in the Académie.[10] Like Franklin, he was involved in just about everything in the natural world, including mete-orology, electricity, gases, light, geology, and medicine. His brilliance had been recognized early, and he had been a member of the government-backed society since he was twenty-five. When Franklin arrived, Lavoisier was fol-lowing up on Priestley's work on plants and gasses, working on his new oxy-gen theory of combustion, and setting the groundwork for his new chemistry. He had also taken on the arduous project of improving the quality of French gunpowder, a matter of considerable interest to the Americans.[11]

Lavoisier had a well-equipped laboratory and his living quarters at the Arsenal, another structure Franklin helped make safe with lightning rods. Among the first demonstrations Franklin witnessed when he visited him there were some replications of Joseph Priestley's experiments on plants and gasses. Lavoisier's wife Marie Anne sometimes helped with the experi-ments—and her husband's English. Having studied painting with Jacques-Louis David, she even painted a portrait of Franklin to replace the painting taken by the British when they sacked his Philadelphia home.

The Arsenal was just one of several meeting places for the experimental natural philosophers associated with the Académie des Sciences. Another was La Muette, where Jean-Baptiste Le Roy operated the king's laboratory. Along with Jacques Barbeu-Dubourg, Le Roy was highly instrumental in translat-ing some of Franklin's communications on electricity into French. He now helped introduce Franklin to other men of science and medicine in Paris.

Jean-Paul Marat was one of the individuals that Franklin met through Le Roy.[12] Marat wanted to be a physician and he took some medical courses in Paris before moving to London in 1765, where he practiced for a decade. Marat received a degree from St. Andrews University in 1775, but unlike Franklin's 1759 honor, Marat's degree was in medicine and was purchased for ten guineas from the financially troubled university that he never visited. At this time, medical degrees could be obtained from Scottish universities in absentia, if one had letters of recommendation from two physicians, wrote a thesis, and paid a fee.[13]

Near the end of 1778, Marat contacted Franklin to ask if he would help him bring some new ideas about fire and light before the Académie Royale des Sciences. He then sent Franklin additional letters and invited him to see some of his experiments. Franklin walked away more impressed with Marat's instruments than he was with his questionable theory about a newly discovered fluid from hot objects that can be seen in the dark with special instruments.

A year later, Marat asked for Franklin's support again, this time because

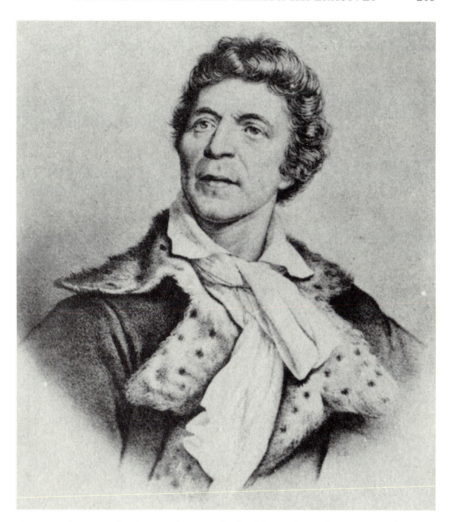

*Jean-Paul Marat (1743–1793), French physician, electrotherapist, and revolutionist.*

he felt sure that his latest experiments would overthrow Sir Isaac Newton's theories about the nature of color. Franklin used his painful gout, which was now flaring up more frequently, as an excuse not to get further involved with Marat, who hoped to become a member of the Académie. Rejected by the French scientific community and now politely rebuffed by Franklin, Marat began to spit venom at the government-backed societies and the scientific élite of the Ancien Régime. He even turned on Franklin, viewing him as a tool of the bankrupt French scientific establishment, although he still held him in high regard for his democratic ideals.

Not ready to give up his intellectual pursuits, Marat turned to medical electricity in the 1780s with a scientific approach that was refreshing, given the exaggerated claims that were being made at the time. He might have been the first Frenchman to conduct electrical experiments on animals to determine how electricity affected individual body parts. He then used his scientific findings to evaluate which human disorders might be treatable with electricity. In agreement with Franklin's position, Marat showed that electricity was by no means a panacea for everything. But breaking from Franklin, he thought that it could be quite helpful for the palsies. Marat's books on medical electricity were published in 1782 and 1784, and even included the idea of using electricity to stimulate growth in underdeveloped children.[14] To his delight, he won a prize from the Académie Royale de Rouen for his second treatise, on applied medicine.

Nevertheless, Jean-Paul Marat is best remembered today for his fanatical politics during the French Revolution that started in 1789. It was Marat as the zealous *Ami du Peuple* (Friend of the People), not Marat the medical scientist, who sent numerous "enemies of the state" to the guillotine during the Terror of 1793 and 1794. Among those beheaded was his enemy from the Académie and Franklin's close friend, Lavoisier. Marat's own life ended when Charlotte Corday, a member of a rival political party, stabbed him while he was taking a medicinal bath. Jacques-Louis David, the "Painter of the Revolution" who had earlier given art lessons to Madame Lavoisier, memorialized the event in one of his most famous paintings.

## SOCIÉTÉ ROYALE DE MÉDECINE AND PUBLIC HEALTH

In 1776, four years after joining the Académie Royale des Sciences, Franklin was invited to become a foreign associate of the Société de Médecine, which was then being organized. The two progressive French physicians who fought hardest for the new society were Joseph Lassone, its first president, and Félix Vicq d'Azyr, its Perpetual Secretary and a talented experimentalist after whom a structure in the brain would be named.

The new medical society made concerted efforts to increase practical knowledge, combat quackery, and utilize new findings to change public policy. The leadership stressed the scientific methods of the Enlightenment, including well-planned experiments, improved instruments, careful observations, and meticulous data collection. They also gave physicians very specific jobs. For example, Mauduyt de la Verenne was asked to evaluate medical electricity, which he did using Franklin's work as a starting point, while others were asked to analyze highly touted mineral waters or to record the weather and track diseases throughout the country.[15]

Lassone and Vicq d'Azyr strove to apply medical science to problems they felt had been neglected for too long. Among their concerns were hygiene, preventive medicine, mental illness, and the plight of children. They moved things along by holding public assemblies to discuss the more pressing issues, and by bringing key governmental officials into the organization. The Comte de Vergennes and Pierre Lenoir, the public-health-conscious *lieutenant-général de police*, were among the officials that became involved and worked with the Société de Médecine.

The members of the new society viewed a healthy population as France's greatest resource. With open eyes and noses, they knew that the time had come to deal with ugly city sites that had offensive stenches and seemed to be spreading sickness and death. In practice, this meant moving or "purifying" some of the old landmarks, draining marshes, and determining where new hospitals, cemeteries, and sewers should be located. For Vicq d'Azyr and his followers, such decisions had to be based on enlightened experimental science, not just on reason.

The matter became particularly pressing in 1780, when an epidemic broke out in Paris near the Cemetery of the Innocents. Under intense pressure, the government agreed to close the old city burial ground, and it ordered the decaying human remains and bones exhumed and moved out of the crowded city to a less densely populated location. It also ordered other cemeteries moved outside the city walls, as a part of a general effort to clean up the often-plagued city.[16]

Knowing the actions in Paris would be carefully watched throughout France, Vicq d'Azyr handed Franklin a copy of a manuscript that dealt with how long infection might remain in an exhumed dead body. What did Franklin think? Franklin responded on July 20, 1781, citing several examples to support the theory that people could catch infectious diseases from the dead, even after they had been buried for a very long time. "With respect to the length of time during which the Power of Infection may be continued in dead Bodies. . . . I would mention to you three Facts," Franklin penned in his letter back to Vicq d'Azyr.

While I resided in England, I read in a Newspaper, that . . . at a Funeral of a Woman whose Husband had died of the Small Pox 30 Years before, and whose Grave was dug so as to place her by his Side, the Neighbours attending the Funeral were offended with the Smell arising out of the Grave, occasioned by a Breach in her Husband's old Coffin, and 25 of them were in a few Days taken ill with that Distemper, which before was not in that Village or its Neighborhood, nor had been for the Number of years above-mentioned.

About the Years 1763 or 1764, several Physicians of London, who had been present from Curiosity at the Dissection of an Egyptian Mummy, were soon after taken ill of a malignant Fever, of which they died. Opinions were divided on this Occasion. It was thought by some that the Fever was caused by Infection from the Mummy, in which Case the Disease it died of must have been embalmed as well as the Body. Others . . . imagined the Illness of those Gentlemen might have had another Origin.

About the Year 1773, the captain of a Ship which had been at the Island of Tenerife, brought from thence the dried Body of one of the ancient Inhabitants of that Island, which must have been at least 300 Years old. . . . Two members of the Royal Society, one an eminent Physician, went to see that Body. They were half an hour in a small close[d] Room with it, examining it very particularly. The next Day they were both affected with a singularly violent Cold & attended with uncommon Circumstances and which continued a long time. On comparing together the Particulars of their Disorder, they agreed in suspecting that possibly some Effluvia from the Body, might have been the Occasion of that Disorder in them both.

Franklin's letter ended with a warning: "But as we do not yet know with Certainty how long the Power of Infection may in some Bodies be Retained, it seems well in such Cases to be cautious till farther Light shall be obtained."[17] In 1785, he would discuss the same fascinating topic with Jan Ingenhousz. He would tell his Dutch physician-friend, "Your Ideas of the long Conservation possible of the Infection of some Diseases, appear to me well-founded."[18]

## MASONIC CONNECTIONS

While in France, Franklin also joined a very different sort of society, the Loge des Neuf Soeurs (Lodge of the Nine Sisters), which also had medical connections. His induction into this Masonic group took place in 1778, sixty-one years after Freemasonry was founded in London to promote Enlightenment ideals.[19] Drawing heavily on the ancient rituals and symbols of the stone-cutting guilds, the Freemasons combined fellowship with civil service, while promoting religious and political tolerance. Franklin was more than familiar with Freemasonry; he had joined Philadelphia's Lodge of St. John in 1731 and he had become grand master of all Masonic lodges in Pennsylvania.

The Loge des Neuf Soeurs held closed meetings on an estate owned by Madame Helvétius, whose late husband was the *philosophe* Claude-Adrien Helvétius. Claude-Adrien wanted to build a lodge that would attract the greatest minds in philosophy, letters, and the arts, but he died before he was able to realize his dream. In 1771, however, his wife moved from Paris to Auteuil, where she established the lodge he dreamed of five years later. She named it after the nine muses of antiquity.

Franklin was the first American member of this elite lodge. Nevertheless, the Loge des Neuf Soeurs tended to be seen as a subversive organization by the church and the French monarchy, especially in its early years, because it worked in secrecy and seemed to be a haven for dangerous freethinkers. The philosopher and writer Voltaire, who returned to Paris in 1778 after almost thirty years in exile, was one such freethinker. Soon after Voltaire came back, Franklin went with the entire American delegation to visit him. Two months later, the returned exile was initiated into the Loge. Being eighty-four and frail, Voltaire entered the room holding onto Franklin's arm. Franklin was seventy-two at the time.

Franklin and Voltaire had great respect for each other. The French *philosophe* had erected a lightning rod on his house, and he had long been an ardent supporter of smallpox inoculations. In the 1720s, while in London, he even met Lady Mary Montagu and composed a philosophical letter "On the Insertion of Smallpox." Later on, he successfully convinced Catherine the Great and other notables in Russia to inoculate. And like Franklin, he had been dismayed by the slowness of the French to take action, at least until Louis XVI inoculated his children in 1774.[20]

Franklin and Voltaire, two of the truly great figures of the Enlightenment, met for the last time in 1778, at a public meeting of the Acádamie Royale des Sciences. They arrived at the same time and with strong urging from the crowd embraced and kissed each other on each cheek in the French style. "*Il faut s'embrasser à la française,*" wrote John Adams in his diary.[21] Voltaire died less than a month later.

The Loge des Neuf Soeurs mourned Voltaire's passing with tributes befitting the great philosopher. A year later, Franklin was appointed *Vénérable* or Grand Master of the Loge. His appointment and the reorganization of the Loge helped to placate the suspicious government, and the organization prospered under his direction.

Franklin's personal relationship with Madame Helvétius is of more than passing interest.[22] Although beautiful when young, Madame Helvétius was in her late fifties when Franklin arrived. Her backstabbing rivals compared her body to "the ruins of Palmyra," whereas Abigail Adams remarked that her outlandish behavior merely matched her frizzled, slovenly appearance. Franklin, nonetheless, found her attractive, in part because she could sing, paint, write poetry, and converse brilliantly. In addition, she attracted ingenious and interesting people to her estate, which he liked to refer to as "l'Académie d'Auteuil."

There, just five kilometers from Passy, Franklin was able to converse informally with Turgot, the Controller-General of Finances, whose interests went well beyond just financing the war. Turgot was also instrumental in the establishment of the Société Royale de Médecine as an instrument for fighting epidemics, and he was involved in chemistry and the "social sciences" (a term he coined). His Latin description of Franklin's greatness in two distinct areas would soon circulate throughout France and then around the world. Proclaimed Turgot, "Eripuit coelo fulmen, sceptrumque tyrannis" (He seized lightning from the sky, and the scepter from tyrants).

It was also at l'Académie d'Auteuil that Franklin met Denis Diderot and Jean Le Rond d'Alembert, the editors of the massive *Encyclopédie,* which was published between 1751 and 1772. This work covered all knowledge, and Voltaire, Rousseau, and Turgot were among its contributors. So many medical and hygienic topics required entries in this "central document of the Enlightenment" that they had to be covered by more than thirty physicians, surgeons, and apothecaries.[23]

The three most likely people to be present under Madame Helvétius's roof at any given time, however, were not Turgot, Diderot, or d'Alembert, but two liberal and highly stimulating abbés and an altruistic young medical student. The abbés whose company Franklin enjoyed were André Morellet, an economist and linguist, and Martin Lefebvre de la Roche, a librarian and classicist. The medical student was Pierre Jean Georges Cabanis, who was in his early twenties and undernourished when Madame Helvétius took him under her wing. Cabanis became almost like a son to Franklin and they spent considerable time discussing medical care. When Franklin wrote his famous bagatelle on the gout (see Chapter 17), Cabanis was there to look it over. And when Cabanis wanted to know about hospital care in America, Franklin was there to help.

In 1784, Cabanis completed his medical studies. He then set forth to reform French medicine, becoming the leader of a group called the "Idéologues." These men adopted an empirical approach to medicine, emphasizing what the physician could see and feel. They also were materialists—Cabanis even applied his materialistic philosophy to the production of mental acts.[24] As enlightened physicians, they also adopted utilitarian goals.

Perhaps spurred on by Franklin, Cabanis became particularly interested in hospital care and reform. His 1789 *Observations sur les Hôpitaux* led to his appointments as an administrator for Paris hospitals and as professor of hygiene at the Paris medical school. Prior to this time, Cabanis had introduced Philippe Pinel to Franklin and and others at Auteuil.[25] Although the story is complex, the conversations he had in Auteuil helped Pinel to realize just how badly the insane were being treated in the Paris hospitals. In 1793, after being placed in charge of the Bicêtre, the large Paris hospital for men, he removed the chains from some of the inmates who had been anchored to the walls for as long as three decades. In 1795, he did the same for the insane women at La Salpêtrière, the even larger hospital for women. Under Pinel's administrations, the emphasis changed from restraining mental patients to improving their hygiene, giving them exercise and, if possible, engaging them on projects.

Auteuil was a magnet for enlightened minds and a place where Franklin could enjoy himself and talk informally about what interested him, including medical treatments for the physically ill and the need to reform hospital care for the insane. The high death rate among children was also a major concern to French men of medicine at this time, and Franklin was appalled by what he heard and (upon entering Paris) could see with his own eyes.

## ON PEDIATRIC PRACTICES

Prior to the eighteenth century, child-rearing practices were left in the hands of parents. By mid-century, however, European physicians and reformers were calling for changes, and state officials were becoming more involved.[26] What occurred had a lot to do with the Enlightenment's emphasis on the welfare of every member of the family and the development of the middle class. But with an endless string of wars, it also reflected the needs of governments for more and stronger soldiers and better workers.

Books, pamphlets, and papers on parenting and child care were streaming off the presses when Franklin arrived in Paris in 1776.[27] The situation paralleled the "revolution" that was under way in England, where Steven Hales had first drawn attention to the plight of children by assailing the use of garments tight enough to affect a child's breathing and digestion.[28] In his treatise, which appeared in 1743, Hales also lashed out at ignorant nurses who tried to "close the Mold of the Head," oblivious to the fact that the cranium should not be fully fused in newborns.

Four years later, William Cadogan, who held a medical degree from Leyden, published his *Essay on Nursing*, which also questioned child-rearing methods.[29] Cadogan applauded the opening of the London Foundling Hospital in 1741, and he responded to the managers, who were then asking for instructions from the medical community on child care. Like Hales, he took aim at the swaddling clothes that restricted infants from moving, inadequate fresh air, low levels of cleanliness, poor nursing, and other practices that doomed children in the past. In 1754, Cadogan was appointed physician to the Foundling Hospital, where he and Franklin probably met on several occasions. We know that Franklin attended a benefit performance of *Messiah* at the Foundling Hospital in 1759. It was conducted by Georg Frideric Handel, its composer, shortly before he died.

Well aware of what was happening in England, French reformers were also beginning to call for changes. Lighter, looser fitting clothing was high on many lists. Jean-Jacques Rousseau was especially influential in promoting the idea that children should move about without restraints, while also advocating feeding babies mother's milk. To Rousseau, particularly in the introduction to his best-selling book *Émile*, which appeared in 1762, a return to more natural ways was long overdue.[30]

Having campaigned for fresh air so vigorously while he was in England, Franklin was pleased to see the changes in thinking about tight-fitting clothing that shielded the body from circulating air. He also favored having infants nursed by their own mothers, but here there was a major hurdle. Since ancient times, well-to-do mothers did not breastfeed their infants. And during the eighteenth century, the practice of giving newborns to wet nurses had become widely accepted in the great cities of Europe, even by middle-income families.[31]

The idea of using cow's or goat's milk as a substitute for mother's milk was not associated with appreciably better survival at this time. Animal milk could sour very quickly in the summer, and it was rarely fresh in the big cities. It also tended to be administered on dirty rags and sponges, virtually assuring the spread of disease.

Tragically, because many wet nurses were uneducated and unskilled and did not have good hygiene, a staggering percentage of the children entrusted to them died. William Cadogan, for one, was shocked to discover that, among children who were sent off for nursing, 75 percent died by age two, with mortality approaching 90 percent in some London parishes.[32] In France, Jean-

Charles Desessartz was equally appalled at how few Parisian infants made it past the toddler stage—if sent off for wet nursing.

Franklin had become aware of the statistics and the economic burdens that current child-rearing practices were placing on society. He discussed the need for new mothers to breastfeed and the frightening number of babies abandoned by poor and unmarried women with both French physicians and governmental officials.

He also wrote to George Whatley in London, fostering an international exchange of information. Whatley was responsible for running London Foundling Hospital. Hence, he was very interested in what foreign organizations and governments were doing to help deal with the soaring number of dying and abandoned children. In fact, he was under considerable pressure at the time to reduce the explosive inflow of admissions to his own institution. There were more children than the hospital could handle.

In 1784, Franklin informed Whatley: "A Subscription is lately set on foot here to encourage and assist Mothers in Nursing their Infants themselves at home; the Practice of sending them to the *Enfants trouvés* [foundling hospitals] having risen here to a monstrous Excess, as, by the annual Bill, it appears they amount to near one Third of the Children born in Paris. The Subscription is likely to succeed, and may do a great deal of good, tho' it cannot answer all of the purposes of a Foundling Hospital."[33]

A year later, he sent Whatley more statistics on how many children were being abandoned in Paris. The number "thrown on the Public," he pointed out, had grown from 10 percent at the beginning of the century to about 50 percent at the present time. Lamented Franklin,

Is it right to encourage this monstrous Deficiency of natural Affection?

A Surgeon I met with here excused the Women of Paris, by saying, seriously that they could not give suck. . . . He assured me it was a Fact, and bade me look at them, and observe how flat they were on the Breast; "they have nothing more there," said he, "than I have on the back of my hand." I have since thought that there might be some Truth in his Observation, and that, possibly Nature, finding they made no use of Bubbies, has left giving them any. Yet, since Rousseau, with admirable Eloquence, pleaded for the Rights of Children to their Mother's Milk, the Mode has changed a little; and some Ladies of Quality now suckle their Infants and find Milk enough.

May the Mode descend to the lower Ranks, till it becomes no longer the Custom to pack their Infants away, as soon as born, to the *Enfans Trouvés,* with the careless Observation that the King is better able to maintain them. I am credibly inform'd that nine-tenths of them die there pretty soon, which is said to be a great Relief to the Institution, whose Funds would not otherwise be sufficient to bring up the Remainder.[34]

Franklin went on to tell Whatley about new actions being taken by the French government, including passing a law that called for examining and licensing nurses involved with child care. He concluded his letter by stating: "I wish Success to the new Project of assisting the Poor to keep their children at home, because I think there is no Nurse like a Mother (or not many), and that, if Parents did not immediately send their Infants out of their Sight, they would in a few days begin to love them, and thence be spurr'd to greater Industry for their Maintenance."[35]

The idea that breastfeeding would enhance the bonding between the mother and her child was just beginning to be discussed seriously when Franklin sent this letter. The older ideas behind breastfeeding were quite different, usually stressing the benefits to the mother. One held that breastfeeding gave the mother immunity against cancer. A different notion, which at least placed the emphasis on the child, was that the baby would acquire the personality and physical characteristics of the person who did the nursing, a chilling thought, especially to some socially prominent families.

Although pediatrics would not become a specialized branch of medicine until the mid-nineteenth century, the child was beginning to be "discovered" in the great cities of Europe during the late eighteenth century. Franklin had strong opinions on the subject of child care, but his real contribution to the movement was that he helped stimulate open discussion on the subject by disseminating important information. Through his efforts, concerned physicians and administrators in different countries gained perspective and acquired a better idea about the scope of the problem, and about actions that were being taken elsewhere to do something about it.

## PREVENTING MALNUTRITION

During the 1770s Antoine Augustine Parmentier, who had lived on potatoes while being held by the Prussians as a prisoner of war, and Antoine-Alexis Cadet de Vaux, another French pharmacist and his disciple, began to apply enlightened science and reasoning to bread making. France had recently experienced a devastating wheat crop failure, and prizes were being offered for the best ways to ward off malnutrition in children and adults in the future.

Individually and in various combinations, the two men tried oats, buckwheat, corn, and potato flour in the breads they made. During the fall of 1778, Cadet de Vaux sent Franklin some inexpensive potato bread to try. He hoped that the highly visible American visitor would approve of his *pain de pommes de terre* and set a shining example for others to try it. Franklin must have been impressed, because Lavoisier and he subsequently attended a special feast at the Boulangerie de l'Hôtel Royal des Invalides, where the new potato bread made its official debut. Every course was made of potatoes for the gala occasion.

This was an important event because French had long looked askance at the potato, since it was a member of the nightshade family and therefore potentially poisonous. Some French peasants even believed it caused leprosy. Thus, even though potatoes had been cultivated by the Incas and then transported to Europe by the Spanish conquistadors, there were still places in the western world where people were not about to grow them, much less eat them.

Franklin, in contrast, had no fears about potatoes, having eaten them in America where they were not stigmatized like they were in France. Potatoes were so inexpensive and easily obtained in the colonies that Poor Richard even recommended using them for treating burns: "Beat or scrape Irish Potatoes to a soft pulpy Mass; mix some common Salt finely powder'd; and apply it cool to the Part. When it grows warm or dry apply a fresh Quantity."[36]

Franklin not only thoroughly enjoyed his meal made entirely of potatoes, he showed no signs of food poisoning or leprosy afterward. Moreover, as hoped for by Parmentier and Cadet de Vaux, he now began to tout the health attributes of the potato, in addition to its good taste and economics. In part because Franklin was involved, the French began to treat the potato with considerably more dignity. Administrators started serving the inexpensive but nutritious food in hospitals, charity houses, and prisons, and it began to grace more plates. In other countries, people soon took notice.

By setting a real-life example, endorsing the potato, and informing people about the acceptance of the potato in America, Franklin helped prevent further outbreaks of malnutrition. He also helped to bring to tables around the world an easily grown health food, one that we now know contains many essential vitamins and minerals. His actions in this domain further illustrate the breadth of his medical activities while in France. In fact, to Franklin's fertile mind, even hot-air ballooning had medical ramifications.

## BALLOONING AND ITS MEDICAL POTENTIAL

Despite the ongoing fighting and the bitterness that followed the American War for Independence, Franklin still managed to communicate with members of the Royal Society in London. John Pringle had headed this body until 1778, when George III forced him out by for favoring Franklin's pointed lightning rods over blunt ones, a dispute that prompted the remark that while a king might change the law of the land, he could not change a law of nature. Joseph Banks replaced Pringle, and although he was more in tune with the king and his advisors, he was just as determined to keep the lines of communication open.[37] In 1782, a year before the Treaty of Paris was signed, Franklin penned Banks, "Be assured, that I long earnestly for a Return of those peaceful Times, when I could sit down in sweet Society with my English philosophic Friends, communicating to each other new Discoveries, and proposing Improvements of old ones."[38]

Through Banks, Franklin kept the Royal Society informed about hot air ballooning, the craze that began in France in 1782 when the Montgolfier brothers showed that a bag filled with heated air could rise high above the ground. Franklin was not present for this historic event in the south of France, but he did attend the memorable launch of César Charles' silk balloon filled with "inflammable gas" (hydrogen) in Paris in August 1783. Franklin informed Banks: "A little Rain had wet it, so that it shone, and made an agreeable Appearance. It diminish'd in Apparent Magnitude as it rose . . . and soon after became invisible, the Clouds concealing it. The Multitude separated, all well satisfied & much delighted with the Success of the Experiment, and amusing one another with Discourses of the various Uses it may possibly be apply'd to, among which many were very extravagant. But possibly it may pave the Way to some Discoveries in Natural Philosophy of which at present we have no Conception."[39]

Franklin also gave Banks some details of the upcoming flight at Versailles.[40] It would involve a Montgolfier balloon thirty-eight feet in diameter "at the Expense of the Academy." He informed him that Monsieur Pilâtre de Rozier asked the Académie's permission to go up with the balloon, but was discouraged from doing so. After the flight, he told Banks that "The Basket contain'd a Sheep, a Duck, & a Cock," but no human passengers.[41]

The first manned balloon was launched in Passy on November 20, 1783. A day later, Franklin wrote to Banks, "When it went over our Heads, we could see the Fire which was very considerable. . . . They say they had a charming View of Paris & its Environs, the Course of the River, &c. One of these courageous Philosophers, the Marquis d' Arlandes, did me the Honour to call upon me in the Evening after the Experiment with Mr. Montgolfier the very ingenious Inventor. I was happy to see him safe."[42]

Franklin kept his thoughts about the utility of ballooning largely to himself, but only at first. "When we have learnt to manage it," he told Banks, "we may hope . . . to find use for it, as men of science have done for magnetism and electricity, for which the first experiments were matters of amusement."[43] And when asked what good could possibly come from ballooning, he initially responded: "Eh, à quoi bon l'enfant qui vient de naître?" meaning "What good is a newborn baby?"

Still, Franklin was thinking hard about practical uses for the balloon right from the start. He thought they might provide a means of reconnaissance and they might speed the mails, the latter thought stemming from his years as a colonial postmaster.[44] Given his concern for healthy foods, he also postulated that they might be used to prevent spoilage. A tethered balloon could be sent into colder air to preserve foods, such as meats, that might spoil at ground level. Alternatively, people could send up water and bring down ice for preserving meats and other foods, thereby also lowering the risk of dangerous food poisoning.[45]

A second idea with ties to medicine stemmed from the poor condition of his own body. Like others at the time, he thought that balloons might be used for travel. But what he further saw was a way to move disabled people from one place to another. A person like himself, who might no longer be able to walk between towns or endure the bouncing of a horse-drawn carriage because of painful gout or stones, or a wounded person, might now be transported smoothly and comfortably.

In 1780, two years before the balloon craze had even been launched, Franklin had written to Joseph Priestley to tell him about a premonition. "The rapid Progress *true* Science now makes," he wrote, "occasions my Regretting sometimes that I was born so soon. It is impossible to imagine the Height to which may be carried in 1000 years the Power of Man over Matter. We may perhaps learn to deprive large Masses of their Gravity & give them absolute Levity, for the sake of easy transport."[46]

Franklin now contemplated attaching the balloon to a man or a horse on the ground; the thought being that, with a fair breeze, they would be able to "run in a straight line across Countries as fast as that Wind, and over Hedges, Ditches, & even Waters."[47] And he also thought that it would be just a matter of time before people would invent "some light handy Instruments to give and direct motion," so there might not even be a need for the balloon to be tethered.[48]

Following his return to America in 1785, Franklin received word from Le Roy that his wife and several other ladies had traveled safely across the French countryside at a height of almost four hundred feet in a nontethered balloon.[49] Two years later he confided in Le Roy: "I sometimes wished I had brought a balloon from France, a balloon sufficiently large to raise me from the ground. In my malady it would have been the most easy carriage for me."[50]

Franklin was not exaggerating. His bladder stone made traveling terribly difficult for him, even before he left France for America. This was clearly the case in 1784, when he was called upon by the French government to investigate Franz Anton Mesmer's claims about animal magnetism, the subject of the next chapter.

CHAPTER 13

# The Folly of Mesmerism

Questo è quel pezzo
Di calamita,
Pietra mesmerica
Ch'ebbe l'origine
Nell' Alemagna
Che poi si celebre
Là in Francia su.

(This is that piece
Of magnet,
That stone of Mesmer
Who originated
In Germany
And then became so famous
In France.)

> —*Cosi fan Tutti*, 1790, opera by Wolfgang Amadeus Mozart,
> libretto by Lorenzo da Ponte

$T$he major episode of medical significance during Franklin's tenure in France, and indeed one of the most important in terms of psychology, psychiatry, and medicine, involved mesmerism, the best remembered healing fad of the century. The movement's leader, the flamboyant Franz Anton Mesmer, claimed he was endowed with special powers that could make sick people better. But many natural philosophers, including Franklin, doubted his ability to manipulate invisible cosmic forces.

## MESMER AND HIS THEORY

Franz Anton Mesmer was born in 1734 in Iznang, a town in the south of Germany near Lake Constance.[1] He first studied theology and philosophy at the Jesuit University of Dillingen in Bavaria, where he also became interested in mathematics and physics. He then transferred to the University of

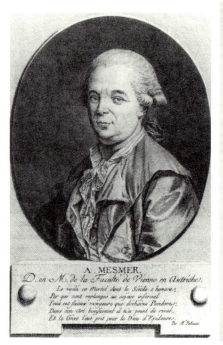
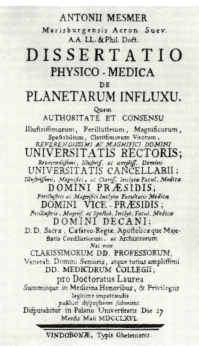

*Franz Anton Mesmer (1734–1815) and the cover of his medical dissertation.*
*(From Frank A. Pattie,* Mesmer and Animal Magnetism *[Hamilton:*
*Edmonston, 1994]; permission courtesy of Edmonston Publishing.)*

Ingolstadt, later to become the University of Munich, and afterward to the
University of Vienna. After studying law, he went into medicine.

The controversy surrounding Mesmer began with his 1766 medical dissertation, *De Planetarum Influxu* (On the Influence of the Planets) (see Figure 35, right). Not only was its subject matter archaic and mystical, but he
stole some of his basic ideas from earlier writers without giving them credit.[2]
One of his sources was Paracelsus, the father of iatrochemistry, who had
written about planetary influences on the body early in the sixteenth century.

Another of Mesmer's sources was Richard Mead, personal physician of
Sir Isaac Newton and Queen Anne, and later vice-president of the Royal
Society. Mead had pondered how the sun and the moon might affect the
body and cause poor health in *A Treatise Concerning the Influence of the Sun
and Moon Upon Human Bodies, and the Diseases Thereby Produced*, which
was published in Latin in 1704.[3] He informed his readers that the sun and
moon can affect the atmospheric pressure, and that this in turn can influence

the amount of nervous fluid in the body. "This powerful action of the moon is observed not only by philosophers and natural historians, but even by the common people . . . [and] that births and deaths chiefly happen about the new and full-moon, is an axiom even among women," wrote Mead.[4]

The same basic idea can be found in the writings of Nicholas Culpeper, a mid-seventeenth-century physician who reasoned: "If you do but consider the whole universe as one united body, it will seem strange to none but madmen and fools that the stars should have influence on the body of man. . . . Every inferior world is governed by its superior, and receives influence from it."[5] Jan Baptista Van Helmont, another respected physician from the seventeenth century, also hypothesized that cosmic forces could influence the physiology of the body.

Mesmer used the term "animal gravity" for the cosmic force in his earlier writings, but changed his term to "animal magnetism" in 1775. His two basic contentions were that there is an imperceptible fluid that can be found throughout the cosmos, and that every object can influence every other object because of it. The sun can affect the planets, the planets can influence each other, and the moon can change the earth's tides via this force. The human body is no exception; the moon and the other heavenly bodies can also affect it.

Up to this point, Mesmer drew heavily on the writings of Mead, Culpeper, and other physicians, as well as on Newton's concept of a gravitational force. Invisible forces and fluids had, in fact, become something of an obsession in the eighteenth century. In the words of historian Robert Darnton, "Mesmer's contemporaries . . . were surrounded by wonderful, invisible forces: Newton's gravity, made intelligible by Voltaire; Franklin's electricity, popularized by a fad for lightning rods and by demonstrations in the fashionable lyceums and museums of Paris; the miraculous gases of the Charlières and Montgolfières that astonished Europe by lifting man into the air for the first time in 1783. . . . In fact, there were enough fluids, sponsored by enough philosophers, to make an eighteenth-century reader's head swim."[6]

Mesmer tried to relate his invisible force to some of these other forces. He explained that his subtle but powerful force had, under different circumstances, been associated or equated with gravity, fire, light, and magnetism. And of particular interest to Franklin, he also thought that electricity might be no more than some sort of a subspecies of animal magnetism.[7]

Mesmer further hypothesized that physical problems, ranging from a stomach pain to a sudden loss of speech, might be caused by overly viscous fluids and blockages, which was again nothing new. But he deviated from his iatromechanical predecessors when he stated that a gifted physician could control the invisible force to overcome these bodily abnormalities and restore the internal harmony.

Singling out specific types of illnesses was not necessary according to Mesmer's new way of thinking. There was, he believed, only one disease, and it had to do with obstructions and internal imbalances. The physician needed just a single remedy, one that would open the channels for a proper redistribution of the fluids. By skillfully manipulating his newly discovered yet invisible force, a qualified therapist could treat colic, hemiplegia, convulsions, tremors, headaches, and other problems.

In 1774, Mesmer turned to iron magnets for controlling the subtle force. The first patient he treated in this manner was Franziska (Franzl) Oesterlin, who suffered from convulsions with toothaches, earaches, vomiting, and fainting. Reduced to "skin and bones," the twenty-nine-year-old woman with hysteria remained under his care for more than two years. Mesmer recalled: "It was on July 28, 1774, that my patient having suffered another of her attacks, I placed three magnets on her, one on the stomach and one on each leg. Almost immediately she began to show severe symptoms. She felt painful volatile currents moving within her body. After a confused effort to find a direction, they flowed downward to her extremities. Alleviation followed and lasted for six hours. A repetition of the attack on the following day caused me to repeat the experiment, with the same success."[8]

Soon after helping Franzl Oesterlin with his magnets, Mesmer began to believe that the powerful cure really resided in his great ability to control the magnetic force. Stroking a patient and even moving his hands without touching that person could work just as effectively as physical contact with an iron magnet. Moreover, he could communicate the magnetic effluvia to a rod, water, food, glass, and even someone's pet—and these objects would now have the same effect on the patient as a real magnet, which he became convinced was merely a conductor of animal magnetism.

## MESMER IN PARIS

Father Hell, the distinguished Austrian astronomer who had introduced Mesmer to magnets, had difficulty with Mesmer's revelation. He was convinced that Mesmer's new cure was not based on a special gift but on the patient's imagination.[9] Mesmer scoffed at the notion, arguing that his ability to treat infants and even comatose patients proved that mental factors like suggestion and imagination could not account for his new cure.

Anxious to demonstrate his special powers to the establishment, Mesmer contacted Franklin's friend Jan Ingenhousz, who was then serving Maria Theresa and the royal family in Vienna. Ingenhousz was not in the least impressed with Mesmer's demonstrations or with his talk about some people being particularly magnetic. He had discovered that Franzl Osterlin did not respond to hidden magnets, but only to people or objects she believed had been magnetized. Ingenhousz subsequently became one of the harshest critics of Mesmer and his theory.

Ingenhousz's influence at the Austrian court helped push Mesmer out of Vienna. The precipitating event was a well-publicized but failed attempt by Mesmer to cure Maria Theresa Paradis, who had been "totally blind" since she was three. Various doctors had tried to cure her with leeches, purgatives, and even electric shocks to her eyes. But she was unresponsive and became even more depressed, occasionally having bouts of delirium. Taking pity on the young girl, Empress Maria Theresa provided funds for her to have music lessons, which allowed her to become a popular clavichord player, organist, and singer. At a later date, Wolfgang Mozart would compose his Concerto in B-flat specifically for her.[10]

Mesmer took on the case, and in 1777 the teenaged girl regained her sight. But the seemingly hysterical Fraulein was less than ecstatic. Restored vision made her life very confusing and much too complicated to handle. Consequently, she began to suffer more fainting spells, convulsions, and crying episodes. When her musical career plummeted, putting her royal pension in jeopardy, her parents whisked her away from Mesmer—and she quickly relapsed back into the world of the blind.

Believing that Mesmer had single-handedly ruined both her goddaughter's nerves and technique, Empress Maria Theresa demanded an end to "all this nonsense" later in 1777. Denounced by the imperial family, under fire from Ingenhousz and the physicians of the establishment, accused of fraud, and castigated by the conservative church, Mesmer abandoned Vienna for Paris.

Ingenhousz sent a note to Franklin in 1778, the year Mesmer arrived and settled in the fashionable Place Vendôme. He warned Franklin: "I hear . . . the Vienna conjuror Dr. Mesmer is at Paris, that he has been presented to the Royal academy, that he still pretends a magnetical effluvium streams from his finger and enters the body of any person without being obstructed by walls or any other obstacles, and that such stuff, too insipid for to get belief by any old woman, is believed by your friend Mr. Le Roy."[11]

Mesmer asked Charles-Nicolas Deslon to help him with his practice.

Deslon was *docteur régent* of the Faculté de Médecine and *premier médecin* of the Comte d'Artois, one of the two brothers of King Louis XVI. Having Deslon at his side increased his visibility and brought him into contact with the aristocracy. It also allowed patients to be treated in his clinic, since foreign physicians could practice only with governmental approval. Mesmer had been denied official authorization but Deslon, being French, did not need it.

Mesmer moved his fashionable and highly successful practice to Créteil, six miles away from the city, after it became clear that he needed more space to treat patients, and that most members of the Parisian academies wanted nothing to do with him or his theories. His new facilities were made to order.

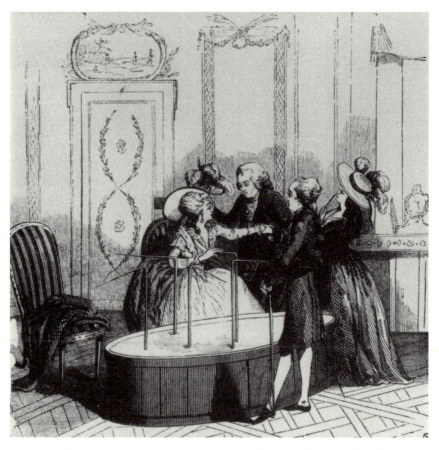

*A mesmerist treating a woman at a* baquet *with iron rods projecting from the tub. (From Frank A. Pattie,* Mesmer and Animal Magnetism *[Hamilton: Edmonston, 1994]; permission courtesy of Edmonston Publishing.)*

His large séance room accommodated four oak tubs, or *baquets,* each more than four feet in diameter and about a foot high. They contained bottles of personally magnetized water, surrounded by wet sand and bits of iron filings or glass powders. Jointed iron bars jutted out through holes in the lids of the tubs. He also had smaller rooms for dealing with patients individually, and facilities to help some treated patients recover.

Tall, imposing, and charismatic, Mesmer recognized that his own appearance and demeanor could enhance the effects of his treatments. He wore a flowing lilac taffeta robe with fine lace trim. He also set the tone with various rituals and testimonials, subtle lighting, astrological symbols, and mirrors that he believed would intensify the magnetic interactions. His final touch was some music from a piano, or even better, the eerie sounds of a glass armonica, a then-popular musical instrument invented by Franklin (see Chapter 14). Nothing was overlooked; everything was carefully monitored for effect.

The patients that went to Mesmer's clinic were instructed to touch the bars extending from the baquet to the afflicted parts of their bodies. The therapist would also touch, stroke, or point to those body parts with his hand or an iron wand. With groups of twenty and thirty patients, a rope was looped around those people next to the *baquet* and extended to others behind them. Mesmer also had patients hold a neighbor's thumb and touch a neighbor's knees as additional ways of transmitting the invisible fluid across clients.

Consistent with medical thinking at the time, Mesmer strove to achieve a "crisis" in his patients. This dramatic turning point sometimes manifested itself with convulsions or fainting. The crisis could be so overpowering that some patients would have to be taken to a special padded room. When groups were involved, a cascade reaction might be seen, with one patient going into crisis, then followed by others around him or her in fairly rapid succession.

Less often recognized is that Mesmer often supplemented his magnetism with more conventional medicines. He bled some patients, prescribed emetics, told them to take warm or cold baths, and altered their diets. He claimed, however, that these traditional treatments were prescribed because they affected the conduction of animal electricity. In this way, conventional medicines were integrated into his highly theoretical framework.

All told, Mesmer's clinic treated more than one hundred paying patients a day at the height of his popularity. There were men and women, children and adults, soldiers and financiers, and patients from every level of society.

Some had hysteria and obvious mental problems; many suffered from strokes, gout, and other physical disorders. Yet Mesmer, who had become extremely wealthy, was never really satisfied. More than anything else, he still wanted official recognition for his discovery.

## FRANKLIN AND MESMER

It is easy to understand why Mesmer would have wanted to befriend Franklin while both men resided in France. In his eyes, Franklin was a person of great intellect and a scientist the recalcitrant establishment would listen to and respect. Thomas Jefferson, Franklin's successor, would write that there was "more respect and veneration attached to the character of Dr. Franklin in France than to that of any other person, foreign or native."[12] Franklin's support for his theories, Mesmer knew, would boost his standing among the medical elite. But in addition, Mesmer believed that Franklin and he had more ideas in common than the most famous American in Europe was then realizing.

Anxious to discuss his theory with Franklin, and hoping to secure his backing, Mesmer invited him to his residence in 1779. A note from Mesmer reads (in translation): "It is with great eagerness that I would be honored to see you as well as Madame Brillon on the day that you indicated. . . . I would be flattered if I could put you in a position to acknowledge the reality and the usefulness of my discovery and demonstrate to you my deep respect."[13]

The details of what transpired in 1779 are fuzzy. But when Madame Brillon later described her conception of heaven to her neighbor Franklin, she specifically excluded Mesmer. "In paradise we shall be reunited," she wrote, "never to leave each other again! We shall live on roasted apples only; the music will be composed on Scotch airs; all parties will be given over to chess; . . . Mr. Mesmer will content himself with playing on the harmonica, without bothering us about electrical fluids; ambition, envy, pretensions, jealousy, prejudices, all these will vanish at the sound of the trumpet."[14]

Mesmer might have brought up his belief that his animal magnetism and Franklin's electricity share certain features—perhaps that they are different products of a single force permeating the universe. He might also have suggested that both Franklin and he had discovered fundamental truths that could benefit the sick, that they were both great saviors of mankind. But Mesmer clearly underestimated Franklin's skepticism. Franklin had taken Ingenhousz's earlier warning seriously, and he left Mesmer convinced that his magnetic theory was fanciful and not rooted in solid scientific evidence.

A month later, Mesmer invited Franklin to meet and dine with him again. He now wanted Franklin to witness some cures, possibly for the second time. "The desire that you have shown to learn about the advantages that one can derive from the discovery of animal magnetism," Mesmer wrote, "makes me hope that you will have the kindness to assure yourself of the reality of the cures that I have made. Besides the illnesses that you have seen, I have several others that have conditions that will amaze you; I shall have the honor of presenting them to you next Friday the 3rd of this month at noon."[15] Just what Franklin actually witnessed on his first visit is not clear, and whether the two men met again is also uncertain.

Franklin's doubts about Mesmer and his theory continued to grow after Mesmer sent him his *Précis Historique* in 1781. His continuing skepticism can be appreciated from a letter written in March 1784 to La Sablière de la Condamine. "As to the Animal Magnetism, so much talk'd of," began Franklin, "I am totally unacquainted with it, and must doubt its Existence till I can see or feel some Effect of it. None of the Cures said to be perform'd by it have fallen under my Observation; and there being so many Disorders which cure themselves and such a Disposition in Mankind to deceive themselves and one another on these Occasions . . . I cannot but fear that the Expectation of great Advantage from this new Method of treating disease will prove a delusion."

He continued: "That Delusion may however and in some cases be of use while it lasts. There are in every great rich City a Number of Persons who are never in health, because they are fond of Medicines and always taking them, whereby they derange the natural Functions, and hurt their Constitutions. If these People can be persuaded to forbear their Drugs in Expectation of being cured by only the Physician's finger or an Iron Rod pointing at them, they may possibly find good Effects tho' they mistake the cause."[16]

Mesmer's troubles had intensified by the time Franklin sent this letter. In fact, he had moved to the Belgian resort of Spa in 1782 rather than endure further humiliation in France. The Académie de Médecine had rejected his theory of animal magnetism, and he had been unable to secure the blessings of the Faculté de Médecine, which oversaw medical education. Nor could the new Société Royale de Médecine be swayed from its negative assessment, and its secretary, Vicq d'Azyr, acting as a medical policeman, had done everything in his power to drive Mesmer out of the country as a fraud. Adding to his woes, Deslon had broken away from him and had opened his own clinic.

Nonetheless, Mesmer did have some supporters. One was fellow Austrian Marie Antoinette, who offered him a large stipend to stay in Paris. In addition to the queen, he also had the backing of the Loge de l'Harmonie, which became the Société de l'Harmonie Universelle and spawned many affiliates.[17] Organized by Nicholas Bergasse and Guillaume Kornmann in 1782, this organization was a stock company with more than four hundred paying members in Paris alone. To Franklin's surprise, his grandson Temple joined this organization, although he would later tell his famous grandfather, that he had little faith in magnetism.

In America, the Marquis de Lafayette was the best-known member of this society, and Mesmer personally asked him to introduce animal magnetism into North America. Lafayette complied and wrote about it to George Washington on May 14, 1784, informing the war hero and future first President, "A German doctor named Mesmer, having made the greatest discovery about animal magnetism, has trained some pupils, among whom your humble servant is considered the most enthusiastic. . . . Before leaving I will obtain permission to let you into Mesmer's secret, which, you can count on it, is a great philosophical discovery."[18]

Lafayette did not have the blessing of Marie Antoinette's husband, Louis XVI, who asked him, "What will Washington think when he learns that you have become Mesmer's chief journeyman apothecary?"[19] And Washington adroitly chose not to get involved. Washington's mind was not changed when Lafayette personally handed him a letter from Mesmer on November 25, 1784. Instead, the American leader was more responsive to Franklin, who could not have been more opposed to such quackery, and to Jefferson, who was in full agreement with his countryman Franklin.

## "FRANKLIN'S" COMMISSION

For Franklin, everything that had to be said about Mesmerism had just appeared in a published report that stands as a landmark in medicine and psychology. On March 12, 1784, the king had called for a formal commission to investigate Mesmer's controversial theory and cure. Baron de Breteuil, a minister whose responsibilities included keeping public order in Paris, had just explained the need for a proper assessment of animal magnetism to the monarch.[20] Louis XVI consented for several reasons. One was that he learned that Mesmer was planning to set up an academy and a hospital with public money. But more important, the monarch was concerned about the associated secret societies. Some of the ringleaders of the cult, he was told, seemed intent on weakening governmental control over French science and medicine, and word was spreading that they were promoting even more subversive ideas.[21]

Four prominent physicians from the Faculté de Médecine were appointed to the official commission: Jean-François Borie, Charles-Louis Sallin, Jean d'Arcet, and Joseph-Ignace Guillotin. To them, the status of traditional medicine was at stake. Five learned men, four of whom had worked on electricity, were then added from the Académie des Sciences: Benjamin Franklin, Jean-Baptiste Le Roy, Jean-Sylvain Bailly, Gabriel de Bory (who died and was replaced by Michel-Joseph Majault), and Antoine-Laurent Lavoisier. These men were guided by facts born of experimentation, and they understood how Mesmerism was a challenge to the laws of nature that they worshipped.

Franklin, the only foreign member of the commission, was chosen because of his integrity, experimental acumen, perspective, and exceptional reasoning ability. He also carried international credentials. In addition to being a member of important élite organizations in France, he was a member of learned societies in London, Philadelphia, Edinburgh, Padua, Turin, Rotterdam, Göttingen, and elsewhere. Reflecting on the composition of this committee, the late Stephen Jay Gould of Harvard University once wrote: "Never in history has such an extraordinary and luminous group been gathered together in the service of rational inquiry by the methods of experimental science. For this reason alone, the *Rapport* . . . is a key document in the history of human reason."[22]

The king, however, was not finished. Three weeks later he approved a second committee, to be made up of five members of Vicq d'Azyr's Société Royale de Médecine, which also wanted a say in the matter. Compelled to leave no stone unturned, the king also sanctioned a "secret" inquiry to determine whether the Mesmerists were taking advantage of women. The French monarch had been informed that the majority of patients were women, and it was widely believed that women have more sensitive nerves than men do, as well as "more lively and more easily excited" imaginations. Even more disconcerting, the practitioner was said to gaze at times at the woman's face and enclose her knees within his own, and at times he might even touch erotic parts of the sensitive female body, producing *titillations délicieuses*.

The public *Rapport des Commissaires*, the most important of the three documents, was completed in August 1784.[23] Franklin, having served as the president of this commission, signed his name above the others. Consequently, this report is often referred to as the Franklin Commission Report. But some scholars believe that his friend Lavoisier may have played an even larger role in determining the path the commission followed and in writing the document.

Estimates are that 20,000 copies of the Franklin Commission Report were sold soon after it was issued. Summaries of the report quickly appeared in *Gentleman's Magazine* and the *London Medical Journal*. The demand for the document was so great in the English-speaking countries that Benjamin Vaughan, Franklin's old friend in London, printed an English edition in 1785.[24] Temple, who was bilingual and had been a member of the Loge d'Harmonie, helped him.

In the introduction to the English translation, we read: "M. Mesmer refused to have any communication with these gentlemen; but M. Deslon, the most considerable of his pupils, consented to disclose to them his principles, and assist them in their enquiries."[25] After presenting this pertinent bit of information, the commissioners summarized the principles of animal magnetism and described how they used instruments to test the physical part of Mesmer's theory. Specifically, the investigators used an electrometer to try to detect his magnetic force. But the needle did not budge. This finding did not support Mesmer's theory, but since the instrument might not have had the sensitivity to pick up Mesmer's subtle force, it did not disprove it, either.

Nevertheless, the commissioners recognized that a number of patients showed what appeared to be crises during the séances. "Some of them are calm, tranquil, and unconscious to any sensation; others cough, spit, are affected with a slight degree of pain, a partial or an universal burning, and perspirations; a third class are agitated and tormented with convulsions. The convulsions are rendered extraordinary by their frequency, their violence, and their duration. As soon as one person is convulsed, others presently are attacked by that symptom. The commissioners saw examples of this kind, which lasted upward of three hours. . . . Nothing can be more astonishing than the sight of these convulsions."[26]

Curing a patient, however, did not prove that animal magnetism existed. Expectations, suggestion, and time could play roles, as Franklin had long emphasized. What followed on the pages of the report can rightfully be thought of as the first systematic use of the methods that would later be adopted by psychologists to investigate how the human mind can be manipulated and even tricked. Even by today's standards, the deceptions and logic employed by Franklin, Lavoisier, and the other commissioners are exemplary.

The commissioners started by going to Deslon's clinic once a week for more than three months to be magnetized. One at a time, they sat around the *baquet* and held an iron rod while Deslon or one of his associates tried to magnetize them. But nothing much happened. "Not one of the commissioners felt any sensation, or at least none which ought to be ascribed to the action of the magnetism."[27] The number of treatments changed from once a week to three days in succession, "but their insensibility was the same, and the magnetism appeared to be perfectly impotent."[28]

Partly because the highly regarded president of the commission was suffering from gout and a painful bladder stone that made traveling for him difficult, Deslon agreed to conduct some additional experiments at Franklin's residence in Passy. Franklin took full advantage of the opportunity. It is believed that he designed and oversaw some of the critical experiments that took place there, and he served as a subject in a few of them.

One set of experiments involved seven lower-class sick people chosen by Deslon. The widow Saint-Amand was asthmatic, dame Anseaume had a swelled lump on her thigh, François Grenet had a tumor in one eye, dame Charpentier had a ruptured abdomen, and the like. Interestingly, there were also two children: six-year-old Claude Renard, who was consumptive (tubercular), and nine-year-old Geneviève Leroux, who had a convulsive movement disorder "resembling that which is called St. Vitus's dance."

Anseaume, Saint-Amand, Leroux, and Renard felt nothing as Deslon carefully applied animal magnetism to their ailing bodies. In contrast, Grenet, who was blind in one eye, felt some pain, but it was in his healthy eye. Because dame Charpentier experienced pain and faintness and Joseph Ennuyé felt some weak sensations, the results provided a very confusing and contradictory picture. Four people were unaffected, one (Grenet) was questionable, and two might have been affected as expected by Deslon.

The commissioners decided to learn more by turning to more affluent people—individuals that also had more education and were more worldly. Madame de Bory and Monsieur Romagni were unaffected. The same was true for Franklin, his grandsons, a member of his staff, and a visiting American military officer. "The commissioners, even those who have had their nerves most irritable, . . . have felt none of those sensations, which were experienced by the three patients of the lower class."[29]

The evidence continued to suggest that those people who felt the effects of the treatment had high expectations and vivid imaginations. "It was necessary to destroy or confirm the suspicion they had formed and to determine to what degree the power of the imagination can influence our sensations," wrote the commissioners. "It must be demonstrated whether it can be the cause, in whole or in part, of the effects attributed to the magnetism."[30]

One of the experiments Franklin now oversaw was described in the Introduction. It involved a twelve-year-old boy hand-chosen by Deslon, because he was so susceptible to animal magnetism. As noted, he was instructed to embrace several trees, in order to see if the tree secretly magnetized by

Deslon would have any unusual effects on his body. The boy began by per-spiring and coughing at the first tree, and complained of a headache at the second. His head pains intensified at the third tree. And at the fourth, he went into a crisis and passed out. This tree, however, was twenty-four feet away from Deslon's magnetized tree. "The result of this experiment is entirely contradictory to the theory of animal magnetism," wrote the commission-ers. "The crisis was the effect of no physical or exterior cause, but is to be attributed solely to the influence of the imagination."[31]

Other experiments, including some at the Arsenal, where Lavoisier lived and worked, produced comparable results. One involved a susceptible woman, who had been blindfolded and was led to believe that Deslon was in the room magnetizing her, when he was not. She shuddered and felt pain within three minutes and went into a crisis shortly thereafter. The mirror image of this experiment had Deslon supposedly magnetizing a susceptible patient from behind a door. Even when he was not present, the patient showed visible changes. When the reverse experiment was conducted on the same woman, one in which Deslon tried to magnetize her without her knowing it, nothing happened.

The inescapable conclusion was that suggestion and imagination could account for every effect that Mesmer, Deslon, and their loyal followers had been attributing to animal magnetism. When a patient's imagination was not in play, there were no effects, and when the imagination was unleashed, there were cures and wonders to behold. The instructions, dress, rituals, mirrors, music, design of the *baquet,* and the esteem the patients had for the therapist all contributed to what happened—but only for those patients who believed in the practitioner and the miraculous new cure.

Franklin and his cohorts concluded: "The experiments which we reported, are uniform in their nature, and contribute alike to the same deci-sion. They authorize us to conclude that the imagination is the true cause of the effects attributed to the magnetism. . . . If the symptoms are more con-siderable and the crisis more violent at the public exhibition, it is because var-ious causes are combined with the imagination, to operate, to multiply and to enlarge its effects. . . . This agent, this fluid has no existence. . . . The mag-netism is no more than an old falsehood."[32]

## AFTERMATH

The unanimous opinion expressed in the Franklin Commission Report drew different reactions from the two leading proponents of animal magnetism.

At the end of the report we read: "M. Deslon is not much adverse to the admission of these principles. He declared in our session held at the house of Dr. Franklin the 19th of June, that he thought he might lay it down as a fact that the imagination had the greatest share in the effects of the animal magnetism. . . . He remarked to the commissioners that the imagination thus directed to the relief of suffering humanity, would be a most valuable means in the hands of the medical profession. Persuaded of the reality of the power of the imagination, he invited the commissioners to embrace the opportunity which his practice afforded to study its procedure and its effects."[33]

Deslon was, however, inwardly disappointed. He believed that lengthier treatments were needed for some of the patients to be cured, and he had hoped that the commissioners would have concentrated more on the cures than on the physics of the theory. In fact, although he recognized and even praised the importance of suggestion, he remained unconvinced that the commission had really disproved the existence of animal magnetism.[34] Unfortunately, he did not have the opportunity to try to cure sick souls with his new understanding of suggestion. He was expelled from the Faculté de Médecine right after the report came out, and he died soon afterward.

Mesmer, in contrast, did not accept the report, period. He viewed the document as inherently biased and politically motivated, and vigorously contended that it was not a good test of his theory. As he saw it, the men that controlled the leading scientific and medical institutions under the watchful eyes of the king and his ministers were biased against him, since they had the most to lose. Moreover, he was infuriated by the fact that the commissioners had based their conclusions on treatments performed by his traitorous, incompetent former assistant. In his frenzy, Mesmer made a number of offers and appeals. One was to magnetize a horse, which he felt would prove convincingly that animal magnetism does in fact exist. His critics ignored the horse offer. They also brushed off his sudden willingness to have his practices examined by yet another commission, albeit under a different set of rules.

Not about to give up, Mesmer tried to revitalize animal magnetism, a move that led to more charges and a flurry of pamphlets from both sides. But he was up against very formidable opponents in France, where the government now orchestrated a public opinion campaign against him. Not helping matters was a popular new play called *Les Docteurs Modernes,* which poked unrelenting fun at him, his followers, and his movement.

Mesmer spent his later years visiting England, Italy, Austria, Switzerland, and Germany, with only brief visits back to France. He died peacefully in

1815 in Meersburg, Germany. The terms "magnetic personality" and "mes-merized," which are so much a part of today's vocabulary, still remind us how influential he had been in his day.

As for Franklin, even while working on reports discrediting Mesmer, he knew that no person or commission could put an end to medical quackery. He expressed this thought in letters to two individuals who had known mes-merism first hand. One was his grandson Temple and the other was Jan Ingenhousz.

The letter to Temple was composed right after the commission had fin-ished its work. Here Franklin wrote: "The Report is publish'd and makes a great deal of talk. Everybody agrees that it is well written; but many wonder at the Force of the Imagination describ'd in it, as occasioning Convulsions &c. and some fear that Consequences may be drawn from it by Infidels to weaken our Faith in some of the Miracles of the New Testament. . . . Some will think it will put an End to Mesmerism. But there is a great deal of Credulity in the World, and Deceptions as absurd, have supported them-selves for Ages."[35]

The Ingenhousz letter followed a year later, in 1785. In it Franklin grieved: "Mesmer continues here and has still some Adherents and some Practice. It is surprising how much Credulity still subsists in the World. . . . And we have now a fresh folly."[36] A well-meaning Mesmer disciple, the Marquis de Puységur, was now promoting magnetic sleep (somnambulism), another medical fad that had Franklin scratching his head, but one that would also lead to hypnotism as a useful tool in medicine.

Poor Richard, had he still been writing almanacs, would have agreed with Franklin's words about medical foolishness, quack remedies, and mistaken causes. In 1732, two years before Mesmer was even born, he had written: "He's the best physician that knows the worthlessness of the most medi-cines."[37] Wit, humor, and crystal ball aside, Franklin's alter ego knew exactly what he was talking about in the very first edition of his *Almanack*—and his words remain pertinent today.

CHAPTER 14

# From Music Therapy to the Music of Madness

There may be various reasons for the scarcity of armonica players, principally the almost universally shared opinion that playing it is damaging to the health, that it excessively stimulates the nerves, plunges the player into a nagging depression, and hence into a dark and melancholy mood.

—Friedrich Rochlitz, 1798

On July 13, 1762, just prior to departing England, Franklin penned a letter to Father Giambatista Beccaria, a professor of natural philosophy and the most ardent supporter of his electrical science in Italy.[1] Beccaria had sent a new treatise on electricity to Franklin, and Franklin used the occasion to tell him about his latest invention, the glass armonica. It was his gift to people who loved music, and he expected it to revolutionize the playing of musical glasses.

What neither man knew at the time was that Franklin's glass instrument would be associated with medicine in two very different ways. For some, its strange music would be looked upon as a way to lift one's spirits, to soothe the angry, and to heal the sick. But for others, it would be closely tied to frayed nerves and even insanity. The unusual charms of armonica music and even its use in music therapy became apparent to Franklin soon after he invented the glass instrument in England. The association with madness would take on a life of its own while he was in France, and it would have a lot to do with Mesmer.[2]

## MUSICAL GLASSES

The Greeks recognized that tapping cups and jars of various sizes with their fingers, sticks, or even pebbles could produce distinct musical sounds.[3] The ancients also realized that filling matched containers with different amounts of liquid could produce different notes.

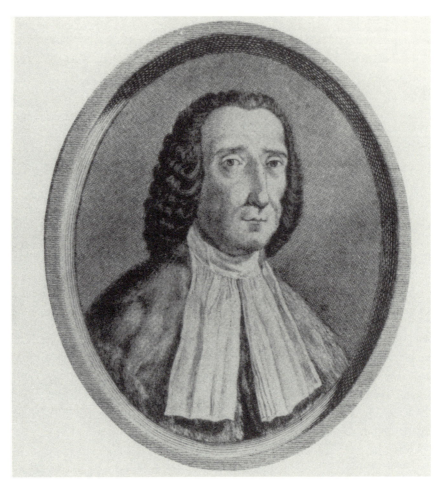

*Giambatista Beccaria (1716–1781), who Franklin wrote to about his glass armonica in 1761.*

During the thirteenth century, when Westerners began to explore the world, they found that musicians in the Middle and Far East played glass bowls. It was not until well into the fifteenth century, however, that the first references to musical glasses appeared in Western books on music. In Franchino Gafori's *Theoria musicae*, which was published in 1492, there is even an illustration of a person tapping glasses filled with different amounts of liquid.[4]

Galileo wrote about an alternative way of making sounds with glass in 1638. In his *Two New Sciences*, he discussed how rubbing moist fingertips on the rims of water glasses could produce different tones.[5] Toward the end of the century, wine glasses were being played with some frequency at small social gatherings, where music lovers were charmed by the sounds.

During Franklin's own century, musical glasses and their players achieved much higher status. In the hands of Christian Gottfried Helmond and others, they began to be used as concert instruments. The eighteenth-century literature abounds with references to the "verrillon," which could be accompanied by violins, basses, and other concert instruments. The verrillon (from the French *verre*, meaning glass) was a table on which a set of glasses filled with precise amounts of liquid could be set. The musician's job was to strike the glasses with a long stick to elicit desired notes.

Early in the 1740s, Richard Pockrich learned to play the verrillon. This free-spirited Irishman first tapped his glasses and then learned to rub their rims with his moistened fingers to produce more drawn out, celestial sounds. In 1746, Christoph Willibald Gluck played a concerto at the new Haymarket Theatre in London that utilized a *Glasspiel* made of twenty-six glasses "tuned with spring water."[6]

In 1761, Miss Ann Ford, a popular performer on the musical glasses, published a pamphlet on how to play wineglasses "in a few days, if not a few hours."[7] Five years later, and perhaps even more telling of how popular music glasses had become, Oliver Goldsmith referred to them in his best-selling novel *The Vicar of Wakefield* with these words: "The two ladies threw my girls quite into the shade, for they would talk of nothing but high life, and high-lived company; with other fashionable topics, such as pictures,

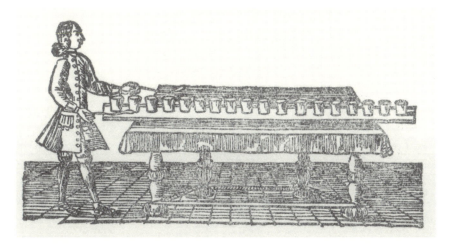

*The verrillon, a musical instrument that used a set of glasses filled with different amounts of liquid.*

taste, Shakespeare, and the musical glasses."[8] Franklin's own glass instrument already had a large following when Goldsmith, who had trained in medicine at Edinburgh, published these telling lines in 1771.

## FRANKLIN'S ARMONICA

Josiah Franklin played the violin and had a good singing voice. Following in his father's musical footsteps, Benjamin learned to play a number of instruments, including the viola da gamba, the harp, the Welsh harp, the bell harp, the harpsichord, the spinet, the Chinese gong, and a type of xylophone.[9] He might also have played the violin and the guitar, and he definitely enjoyed singing. But it was his interest in electricity that led him to glass music.

In 1758, Franklin made a trip from London to Cambridge to see Edmund Delaval, a talented electrical scientist and the first of his nominees for membership in the Royal Society.[10] There he discovered that Delaval owned a set of musical glasses that he played masterfully. Thomas Gray, who heard Delaval play in 1760, wrote: "We heard Delaval the other night play upon the water glasses, & I was astonish'd. No instrument that I know has so celestial a tone. I thought it was a Cherubim in a box."[11]

In the letter describing his new instrument to Father Beccaria, Franklin mentioned both Pockrich and Delaval. He explained: "Mr. Puckeridge, a gentleman from Ireland, was the first who thought about playing tunes, formed from these tones. He collected a number of glasses of different sizes, fixed them near each other on a table, and tuned them by putting into them water, more or less, as each note required. The tones were brought out by passing his fingers round their brims." But, he continued, "Mr. E. Delaval, a most ingenious member of our Royal Society, made one in imitation of it, with a better choice and form of glasses, which was the first I saw or heard. Being charmed with the sweetness of its tones, and the music he produced from it, I wished only to see the glasses disposed in a more convenient form."[12]

Franklin's armonica utilized twenty-three soda-lime "hemispheres" of different diameters, each with a hole in the base. The bowls were assembled on an iron spindle from largest to smallest, with a small piece of cork between each one. The spindle was then placed horizontally in a tapered wooden case. A flywheel attached to a foot treadle allowed the player to rotate the bowls while touching them with fingers on one or both hands. Franklin explained to Beccaria that the "instrument is played upon by sitting before the middle of the set of glasses . . . turning them with the foot, and wetting them now and then with a spunge and clean water." He then added: "The advantages of

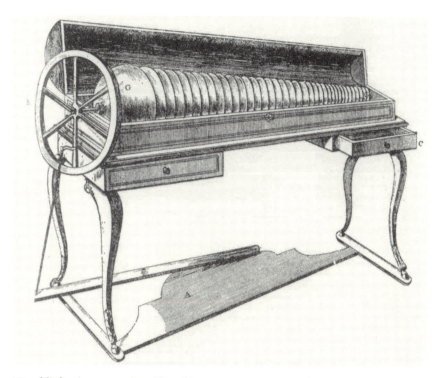

*Franklin's glass armonica (from his* Papers *10: 126–130).*

this instrument are, that its tones are incomparably sweet beyond those of any other; that they may be swelled and softened at pleasure by stronger or weaker pressures of the finger, and continued to any length; and that the instrument, being once well tuned, never again wants tuning. In honour of your musical language, I have borrowed from it the name of this instrument, calling it the Armonica."[13]

Franklin probably began working on his armonica right after seeing Delaval. In a letter dated April 1761, Thomas Penn informed James Hamilton, the new governor of Pennsylvania, that Franklin was wasting time "in philosophical, and especially in electrical matters, and musical performances on glasses."[14] At a later date, Franklin defended his behavior to Cadwallader Colden, writing: "While in England, *after my chief Business was over,* I amus'd myself, with contriving and bringing to a considerable Degree of Perfection, a new musical instrument, which has afforded me and my Friends a good deal of Pleasure."[15]

By the end of 1762, the armonica was already being built commercially in London. Franklin was so pleased with his latest invention that he even took one with him to America later that year. In the *Autobiography of Leigh Hunt* we read: "I have heard Dr. Franklin invented the Harmonica, he concealed it from his wife till the instrument was fit to play; and then woke her with it one night, when she took it to be the music of angels."[16]

Franklin's daughter Sally, who was trained on the harpsichord, soon began to play it. During the winter of 1763, she received some Scottish songs from Janet Dick, the fourteen-year-old daughter of Sir Alexander Dick, the eminent physician who housed and entertained Franklin in Edinburgh in 1759. Later that year, Franklin informed Sir Alexander: "I play some of the softest Tunes on my Armonica, with which Entertainment our People here are quite charmed, and conceive Scottish Tunes to be the finest in the World."[17]

On December 27, 1764, the *Pennsylvania Gazette* announced a concert at the Assembly Room in Lodge Alley. The venue was to be "a Variety of the most celebrated Pieces now in Taste, in which also will be introduced the famous Armonica, or Musical Glasses, so much admired for the great Sweetness and Delicacy of its Tones." A few months after the Philadelphia event, there was an armonica concert at Raleigh's Tavern in Williamsburg, Virginia. George Washington paid 3 shillings 9 pence to hear it.

The Europeans were even more fascinated by Franklin's armonica. In Britain, Miss Marianne Davies emerged as the first lady of the new instrument. She filled concert halls in England, sometimes with her sister Cecilia singing to the music, and she referred to Franklin as her benefactor. Davies then began a concert tour of Europe. She was applauded in Ireland, Italy, France, and Germany, where Franklin had become "as famous among German musicians for his harmonica as among German electricians for his lightning rod."[18]

By the mid-1760s, Davies was in music-hungry Vienna, where Gluck, one of the most ardent promoters of glass music, was the chapel-master. Empress Maria Theresa and the royal family fell in love with the new music and with Davies' artistry. Maria Theresa's fifteenth child and youngest daughter, Marie Antoinette, even took lessons on the armonica from Marianne Davies, having no idea that its inventor would later appear in her royal court as an American ambassador to France.

The Mozarts were in and out of Vienna at this time, and it was here that they first heard the glass armonica. The same can be said for Franz Anton Mesmer, who lived in Vienna and was entranced by the unusual instrument. Mesmer loved music and he had already mastered the violin, cello, and clavichord. After meeting the Mozarts, Mesmer commissioned Wolfgang to write

*Bastien und Bastienne,* an opera that was first performed during the fall of 1768.[19] Thereafter, the Mozarts remained in contact with Mesmer.

In 1773, Leopold Mozart sent a letter to his wife, telling her "The Mesmers are all well and in good form as usual. Herr von Mesmer, at whose house we lunched on Monday, played to us on Miss Davies's Harmonica or glass instrument and played very well. It cost him about 50 ducats and is very beautifully made."[20]

Three weeks later, Leopold informed her: "Do you know that Herr von Mesmer plays Miss Davies's harmonica unusually well? He is the only person in Vienna who has learnt it and he possesses a much finer instrument than Miss Davies does. Wolfgang too has played upon it."[21]

But although Mozart enjoyed playing Mesmer's armonica as a teenager, he did not compose for it until 1791, a year after Franklin had died. The event that stimulated him to pick up his pen was an armonica concert given in Vienna by Marianne Kirchgässner, who had been blind since age four. He was so inspired by her performance that he composed his Adagio and Rondo for Glass Harmonica, Flute, Oboe, Viola and Cello (K. 617) and Adagio Solo for the Glass Harmonica (K. 356) specifically for her.[22]

The attraction that the armonica had for Mesmer and the Mozarts reflected its broad appeal. It has been estimated that several hundred compositions were written with a part for Franklin's armonica by the end of the century. More followed early in the nineteenth century. Ludwig van Beethoven, for example, would write an armonica piece for *Leonora Prohaska,* a tragic play by Friedrich Dunker, in 1815.

## MUSIC THERAPY

Glass music, perhaps more than any other kind, was already associated with an uncanny ability to affect people when Franklin came forth with his armonica. One of the tales known to Franklin involved Richard Pockrich.

Mr. Pockrich, in his brewery near Island-bridge, happening one day to be seized by bailiffs, thus addressed them: "Gentleman, I am your prisoner, but before I do myself the honour to attend you, give me leave as an humble performer of musick, to entertain you with a tune." . . . In the meantime, he flourishes a prelude on the glasses, and afterwards displays his skill thro' all the pleasing turns and variations of the Black Joke. The monsters, charm'd with the magic of his sounds, for some time stand at gaze. At length, recovering their trance, thus accost the Captain: "Sir, upon your parole of honour to keep the secret, we give you your liberty. 'Tis well, playing upon the glasses is not more common: if it were, I believe our trade would find little employment."[23]

Franklin never denied that music, and especially glass music, could have powerful effects on people's emotions and health. He might even have read Richard Browne's *Medicina Musica, or, A Mechanical Essay on the Effects of Singing, Musick, and Dancing, on Human Bodies*, which was published in 1727.[24] But even more likely to have caught his eye was Richard Brocklesby's *Reflections on Ancient and Modern Music, with the Application to the Cure of Diseases*, a treatise dated 1749.[25] Brocklesby was an influential London physician whose clientele, like that of Franklin's close friend John Fothergill, included the rich and the famous.

Franklin also learned how glass music could affect people from personal experience. Soon after arriving home in 1762, he used his armonica to great advantage to ease the strain of a potentially heated meeting with Ann Graeme, the wife of Thomas Graeme, a fashionable Philadelphia physician, who had worked with Franklin on several projects. Franklin's son William had proposed marriage to the Graemes' daughter Elizabeth in 1756, before he went with his father to England. "Betsy" had accepted his proposal, with the provision that he would not engage in factional politics. But while abroad, "Billy" lost interest in her. Prior to coming back to America, he married Elizabeth Downes, whose father owned a sugar plantation in Barbados.

The inevitable meeting with Betsy's mother that Benjamin Franklin had been dreading took place in his Philadelphia home. Hoping to soothe Mrs. Graeme and to keep things under control, he first entertained her with some light tunes on his armonica. The strategy of relaxing her with armonica music before turning to discuss what Billy did to her daughter was successful. Tempers did not flare and Ann Graeme left the Franklin residence with a calm demeanor.

Realizing that Shakespeare was right when he wrote, "music oft hath such a charm to make bad good" (from *Measure for Measure*), Franklin also recommended listening to armonica music to Debby. His wife was justifiably dejected when he was whisked back to London on his second diplomatic mission so soon after having returned home. Hoping to lift her spirits, he told the woman who had earlier thought she had heard "the music of angels," "Let Sally divert you with her Music. Put her on Practicing on the Armonica."[26]

Franklin took music therapy to a higher level in 1772. His patient was Princess Izabella Fleming Czartoryska, who was prone to depression and hysteria. The princess was the openly unfaithful wife of Adam Kazimierz

Czartoryski, a wealthy Polish nobleman, the foreign affairs minister under Czar Alexander I, and a patriot.[27] The prince is still remembered as one of the men who brought the Enlightenment to Poland, and even before he joined the Loge des Neuf Soeurs, he had become a devoted follower of Franklin and his ideas.[28]

Franklin first met the prince and his twenty-six-year-old wife in London.[29] "I was ill, in a state of melancholia, and writing my testament and farewell letters," the princess recalled. "Wishing to distract me, my husband explained to me who Franklin was and to what he owed his fame. . . . Franklin had a noble face with an expression of engaging kindness. Surprised by my immobility, he took my hands and gazed at me saying: *pauvre jeune femme* [poor young woman]. He then opened a harmonium, sat down and played long. The music made a strong impression on me and tears began flowing from my eyes. Then Franklin sat by my side and looking with compassion said, 'Madam, you are cured.' Indeed that moment was a reaction to my melancholia. Franklin offered to teach me how to play the harmonium—I accepted without hesitation, hence he gave me twelve lessons."[30]

The reference to the "harmonium" in this translated passage of how the Polish princess was treated by Franklin can be questioned. The harmonium is a small, manually pumped reed organ with a keyboard that did not make its debut in Europe until 1842. More likely, Franklin lifted this melancholic woman's sprits with his armonica (also incorrectly referred to as his "harmonica" in many books and letters), the musical instrument that he adored and most loved to demonstrate at this time.

Unfortunately, the effects of Franklin's music therapy were short-lived. Within a year, the Polish princess went from being happy and entertaining a lover again to being stricken with "attacks of nerves" and fainting spells. Izabella Czartoryska even attempted suicide. After more failed love affairs, the birth of an illegitimate son, and the deaths of two of her children, she developed hysterical palsy. This time she was treated with therapeutic electricity, which appeared to have more lasting effects.

Whether Franklin recommended the electrical treatment based on his colonial experience with hysterical case C.B. (see Chapter 6) is not clear. Interestingly, no mention is made of the princess in any of his known letters. Franklin does not even tell us why he thought music might have been helpful in her case. But, as with medical electricity for hysterics, two basic possibilities have to be considered, one physical and the other mental.

In the physical realm, many eighteenth-century physicians believed that musical vibrations and exercises could stimulate the nerves and increase the circulation, both of which might produce a better frame of mind. Thomas Cadwalader expressed the idea that music could act as a stimulant in his *Essay on the Dry-Gripes,* which Franklin published in 1745, writing "every Stroke of a musical Instrument causes an Undulation of the Air, which giving some Degree of Concussion to the Fibres of the Body, without overstraining them, produces a brisker Circulation of the Blood; and consequently invigorates the Nerves, and lessens the Viscidity of the Fluids. . . . It might perhaps be applied to very noble Purposes . . . it may, by acting on the Solids, be the means of regulating our Passions."[31]

The second possibility is that Franklin used his armonica to effect a cure based on nothing more than suggestion. He might have thought that it would first soothe or charm the princess, taking her mind off what was disturbing her, much as it did for Ann Graeme. Once relaxed, if not intoxicated by his glass music, he could complete his masterful deception, telling the princess in just so many words that she had been cured.

In his commentary on this case, Z. J. Lipowski (who also translated the Polish) wrote: "It may seem exaggerated to regard Franklin as a precursor of modern brief psychotherapy on the basis of one sketchy anecdote. Yet one cannot fail to be impressed by his remarkable display of the very elements of such therapy which are essential to its success. Empathy and warmth, sensitivity and genuine interest, a confident attitude and a touch of suggestion ("Madame, you are cured"), and reinforcement (twelve sessions or "Lessons"), are all key ingredients. In addition, Franklin was a famous older man and seemed to have an air of self-confident yet kind authority about him. None of these characteristics was likely to be lost on the perceptive younger woman."[32]

## MADNESS AND THE ARMONICA

Elkanah Watson, a young American entrepreneur who visited Franklin in France during 1781, provides us with an engaging vignette of a relaxed Franklin with his armonica.

I dined and spent the evening with Franklin, at Passy. He asked me if I knew he was a musician, and then conducted me across the room to an instrument of his own invention, fixed as a harpsichord. On my intimating a wish to see him perform, he immediately placed himself before it with his habitual condescension, touching the ends of his fingers on a moistened piece of sponge, and commenced playing with his right foot, bearing upon a treadel fixed in the manner of a spinning wheel, which turned a set of musical glasses . . . so as to produce all of the requisite tones. He touched the edges with the ends of his fingers, playing a Scottish pastoral tune, in sweet delicate melody, which thrilled me to my very soul."[33]

We also have some wonderful images from Franklin about how much he enjoyed playing the armonica for his coquettish neighbor in Passy, Madame Brillon, who was accomplished on the harpsichord and pianoforte (Boccherini dedicated six sonatas to her). In one of his letters, Franklin wrote: "In forty years, I shall have time to practice on the armonica, and perhaps I shall play well enough to accompany you on your pianoforte. From time to time we shall have little concerts . . . And we shall pity those who are not dead."[35]

From these communications it might seem hard to believe that others were beginning to have very different emotions about Franklin's armonica. But at the same time, some performers, town officials, and laymen were beginning to look upon it and its music with suspicion, fright, and outright terror. A few of these individuals probably knew Shakespeare's famous words about music having charm. A smaller number would have known that the Bard then went on to warn that music can also "provoke to harm."

Some of the early critics of the armonica were bothered by its strange, high-pitched, otherworldly sounds. "Its social effects were such as no other instrument whatever has produced. Its tones could . . . make women faint; send a dog into convulsions; make a sleeping girl wake screaming through a chord of the diminished seventh, and even cause the death of one very young," wrote Karl Leopold Röllig of Hamburg in 1787.[35]

To some of Röllig's contemporaries, what had happened to several musicians who played the instrument day after day was even more disconcerting. Marianne Kirchgässner, the blind musician whose armonica performances inspired Mozart to write for the instrument, died a horrible death that "was attributed to deterioration of her nerves caused by the unusually piercing vibrations of the instrument."[36]

The talented Marianne Davies, who had been the toast of Europe, also fell ill. In January 1778, she was taken to Paris "on account of health" by her mother and sister.[37] Cecilia sent a gracious note to Franklin notifying him of the situation, and Franklin politely invited the entourage to join him for dinner. Nevertheless, his invitation to join him at Passy was declined. Marianne Davies told others that Franklin's armonica was the cause of her health problems.

Mozart's death at thirty-five only added to the negative perception. The composer seemed to come down with a strange illness within a few months of starting to compose for the armonica. Was this just another coincidence? Was the armonica in some way the cause?

Three years before Mozart died, Johann Christian Müller had even issued a stern warning to readers of his new instructional manual for the armonica. He advised: "If you have been upset by harmful novels, false friends, or perhaps a deceiving girl then abstain from playing the armonica—it will only upset you even more. There are people of this kind—of both sexes—who must be advised not to study the instrument, in order that their state of mind should not be aggravated."[38]

Friedrich Rochlitz, writing for *Allgemeine Musikalische Zeitung*, was even more poignant a few years later. He contended that there "may be various reasons for the scarcity of armonica players, principally the almost universally shared opinion that playing it is damaging to the health, that it excessively stimulates the nerves, plunges the player into a nagging depression, and hence into a dark and melancholy mood, that it is an apt method for slow self-annihilation. . . . Many (physicians with whom I have discussed this matter) say the sharp penetrating tone runs like a spark though the entire nervous system, forcibly shaking it up and causing nervous disorders."[39]

In response to fears that the vibrations from physical contact with the glasses could be damaging to one's nerves, a few inventors tried to modify the instrument or how it might be played. One such person was the critic Röllig. He worked on constructing a keyboard for the armonica. Others also tried this innovation, which made the armonica a bit like a harpsichord, but this "improvement" repeatedly failed.

This fact was not lost on Franklin, who mentioned it in a letter to the Comte de Salmes in 1785.

"I received the Letter . . . respecting the Application of Keys to the Harmonica as contriv'd by Abbé Perno; and requesting to know if any thing of the kind had been done in Paris, London or elsewhere. When I was in London, about 12 years since, Mr. Steele an ingenious Musician there, made an Attempt of that sort; but the Tones were with Difficulty produc'd by the Touch from the Keys, and the Machinery in Playing made so much Noise and Rattle, as to diminish greatly the Pleasure given by the Sound of the Glasses; so that I think the Instrument was never completed. The Duchess of [unclear word] at Paris about the same time endeavor'd to obtain the same End, and has not yet laid aside the Project, tho' it has not hitherto perfectly succeeded. Baron Feriet of Versailles, began to work on the same Idea about the Time I receiv'd your Letter. . . . I hoped soon to have given you an Account of his Success; but I begin to doubt it.[40]

A keyboard was not the only idea that was bandied about. Another way of distancing the player from the vibrating bowls was with a violin-like bow.[41] Here too, despite the best efforts of a number of inventors and others, the innovation failed.

## THE MESMER EFFECT

The contention that armonica music could fray nerves and leave people in a state of permanent insanity was enhanced by Mesmer's association with the glass instrument. Mesmer, after all, often played it at his séances. The way that it affected his clients, and the fact that some of his patients seemed to be mentally unstable, made outsiders more than a little uncomfortable. In addition, Mesmer played the instrument for his own enjoyment, and to many people he appeared even more deranged or mad than some of his patients seemed to be.

Mesmer actually played his armonica in his therapy sessions for two reasons that he related to his new theory of medicine. First, he felt that it created the special ambience he wanted his patients to experience in his clinic, just as did his robe, the lighting, and the manner in which he decorated his baquet rooms. As put by music historian A. Hyatt King, "there seems little doubt that Mesmer used his mastery of the highly emotional tones of the harmonica to induce a receptive state in his patients."[42]

Even more important, he believed that music, particularly armonica music, could enhance the flow of his invisible magnetic force into and throughout the body. From this second perspective, it contributed directly to the removal of blockages and was an integral part of the cure. When writing about his theory and its application, Mesmer listed a number of "Propositions." That animal magnetism "is communicated, propagated, and intensified by sound" is stated under Proposition 16 in his 1779 *Mémoire*.[43]

There are many detailed descriptions of how people were affected by Mesmer's armonica music. "Mr. Mesmer's house is like a divine temple," wrote Jean-Jacques Paulet in his *Mesmer Justifié* in 1784. "There are magnetized bars, closed tubs, wands, ropes, magnetized flowering shrubs, and musical instruments including the harmonica, whose piping stirs one guest, causes slight rambling in another, laughter and tears in others."[44] Another report dealt with a client who, like Franklin, suffered from gout. Mesmer began by pressing his finger against the part of the patient's body that hurt, producing a tingling that followed his finger as he moved it over the skin. "Mr. Mesmer then seated him near the harmonica; he had hardly begun to play when my friend was affected emotionally, trembled, lost his breath, changed color, and felt pulled toward the floor."[45]

Mesmer's armonica music even affected Deslon, who had long suffered stomach pains and was thought to have an *embarras* (obstruction) in his head. One biographer of Mesmer tells us: "Mesmer experimented on him—apparently not very seriously—by playing on the glass harmonica or the piano and conveying animal magnetism to him. Deslon was obliged to beg for mercy about the music, presumably because of the discomfort caused by the charge of animal magnetism which it carried."[46]

Music historian King contends that it was none other than "Mesmer, who next to Marianne Davies, probably did more than anyone else to spread its [the armonica's] fame."[47] King probably should have added "and infamy," given how people were beginning to feel about Franklin's instrument during the 1780s. And popular perceptions were not about to improve.

## THE PHANTASMAGORIA

To some entrepreneurs, and even to some famous composers, the armonica had become the perfect instrument to frighten people. Could there be a better instrument for conveying images of madness? And what sounds could be better for conjuring up mind-deranging images of the supernatural or of death itself?

The master of optics and illusions at the end of the eighteenth century was Étienne-Gaspard Robertson, a smart, creative, and a shrewd businessman who knew how to promote his artistry.[48] He specialized in chilling horror shows for adults, using magic lantern slides and other devices. Robertson's crowning achievement was the *fantasmagorie* (phantasmagoria in English). Its name derived from the Greek *phantasma,* meaning phantom, and *ago-ereuein,* meaning to speak in public.

Robertson's first full-scale production took place in Paris a few years before the eighteenth century ended. By skillfully projecting his slides on invisible screens, walls, or even smoke, and by doubling them up and changing them at opportune times, he terrified people. He had ghosts, frightful witches, and other horrible figures increase and decrease in size, move forward and backward, and then vanish into the ground after having slowly arisen from their eerie tombs.

Robertson knew how to enhance the effects he wanted. He did things like locking his paying audience in a dark room and giving nightly shows in the crypt of an abandoned Capuchin convent. He also provided terrifying opening words and tales about death, ghosts, and the supernatural. And, with the lights blown out and the audience perhaps watching a heart-stopping witches' Sabbath, he added just the right music. Hidden from sight, his armonica player completed the effect, causing some women to faint right in their seats.

Robertson's shows were so good that he soon had competitors. One was Paul de Philipstal, whose shows in London's Lyceum Theatre also dazzled audiences. Given the outcome of the American War of Independence, and how many conservative Londoners felt about Franklin, the magic lantern illusion that his audiences seemed to enjoy most was "the head of Dr. Franklin being converted into a skull."[49]

In the context of what people were now thinking, it is easy to understand why Domenico Donizetti chose to include a part for the glass armonica in his immensely popular opera, *Lucia di Lammermoor.* Donizetti wanted to use the glass instrument in the crowning highlight of his masterpiece, the mad scene. But in part because the instrument now had such a frightening reputation, Donizetti was unable to find a good armonica player when his opera was scheduled to make its debut in the 1830s, and he had to rewrite the part for several flutes.

## LINGERING QUESTIONS

There are many reasons for the demise and almost complete disappearance of Franklin's armonica from the stage by Donizetti's time.[50] One was the irrational fears stemming from writers claiming that its sounds could wake the dead, destroy the nerves of both players and listeners, cause premature births, and even trigger convulsions.

Another was the belief that people could use the instrument to exploit unsuspecting citizens. Mesmer's use of the armonica at his séances showed how it allowed him to control other people. In this regard, when Franklin agreed to serve on the commission that discredited mesmerism in 1784, he might have helped to kill his own progeny. If the association had not been made earlier, people now learned how the armonica had been used by one of the best known symbols of madness as the curtain began to come down on the Enlightenment.

The high costs of buying and maintaining an armonica did not help. Nor did changing tastes, as Classicism gave way to Romanticism. Franklin's glass armonica, with its soft ethereal notes, found itself on the wrong side of the curve as the demand for more powerful orchestral pieces continued to increase. But whereas such factors have to be considered in any history of the armonica, two medical questions remain. Could the health problems of Marianne Davies and the other armonica players have resulted from lead poisoning due to the type of glass used? And did Franklin really believe that the vibrations from his glass instrument could cause nerve damage?

Although some people have raised the possibility that the glass used in the instrument had a high lead content, and therefore might have contributed to the nervous problems that some armonica performers suffered late in their careers, the evidence for this is scanty at best. The armonica players were not involved in the manufacturing or grinding of leaded glass, which could have posed a real danger, and the glasses used might not even have been leaded. Franklin, for example, used soda-lime glasses in his original instruments.

Even more important, the glasses were empty. They were not filled with an acid that might have leached some lead into the solution and onto the fingers of the performer. Thus, even if some of the early players developed chronic lead poisoning—and this is speculative at best—it is much more likely that they derived it from the tainted wines they were drinking, or perhaps from other sources, and not from the spinning glasses they were touching.

As for how Franklin reacted to the fears that began to be associated with his musical instrument in the 1780s, all available evidence would suggest that that he did not take the mass hysteria seriously. He continued to play his own armonica into his twilight years, showing absolutely no signs of shattered nerves or mental instability resulting from the vibrations. Had he entertained even the slightest doubt about the health risks of his armonica, he would have stopped its production and warned people. But Franklin did not do either of these things. Instead he encouraged his daughter, his friends, and the children of those he loved dearly to enjoy his creation. Even in his final years, while others were assailing his armonica, he never looked back on his instrument with any regret.

To Franklin, the myths that sprung up about his armonica were just another example of the gullibility of the human species. As far as he was concerned the issue was not worth a pamphlet or even a letter to set the matter straight. He had far more important things to do in his remaining years than to enter the bizarre concert hall of the absurd, including attending to his own health problems.

# PART IV
# OLD AGE, ILLNESSES, AND THE DOCTOR'S DEATH

CHAPTER 15

# Bifocals and the Aging Inventor

I am happy in the invention of Double Spectacles, which, serving
for distant objects as well as near ones, make my Eyes as useful to me
as ever they were.

—Benjamin Franklin, 1784

The previous set of chapters on Franklin's medical forays in France made brief mention of two of his health problems. One was his painful gout, which was flaring up with increased frequency and intensity. When it attacked, it was difficult for him to walk or stand for extended periods of time. He even turned to his gout as an excuse to avoid having to meet any more with Jean-Paul Marat. The other problem was his bladder stone, which was growing enormous by the time he was asked to evaluate Mesmer's claims. His stone was even more of an impediment than his gout, because it steadily grew larger and made riding in even a horse-drawn carriage painful. It was primarily for this reason that a number of tests of Mesmer's theories took place in Passy, where he was residing, rather than in Paris, where the royal academies of science and medicine were located.

These were not the only health problems that Franklin faced in France, although they were the two most debilitating. He also had a nasty itchy, flaky skin condition that he called the "Scurf." His skin problem was by no means life threatening, but it annoyed, embarrassed, and distracted him. In addition to these three disorders, Franklin's body was showing some of the usual changes that would be expected for a man in his seventies. In this domain, Franklin's eyes were no longer those of a young man. He needed glasses and, judging from his letters, increasingly stronger reading lenses. He had also become quite unsteady on his feet.

Given his chronic illnesses and increasing physical problems, it is easy to understand why Franklin asked Congress on several occasions for permission to retire from public office and head home. Considering the needs of government, in addition to whether he would even be able to endure a trip across the Atlantic, it is also easy to understand why he was not optimistic about ever seeing Philadelphia again. Franklin's letters show just how low his expectations of setting foot in his homeland were during the 1780s. For instance, he sent a note to George Washington in 1780 in which he wrote, "I must soon quit the Scene, but you may live to see our Country flourish, as it will amazingly and rapidly after the war is over."[1] Four years later, he confided to Samuel Mather: "I long much to see my native place, and to lay my bones there. . . . And now I fear I shall never have that happiness."[2] Even after he finally received Congressional permission to return home in the summer of 1785, he questioned whether he had the health and stamina to endure the trip.

In the five chapters comprising this section of the book, we shall look in more detail at Franklin's medical problems. Examining what he knew and did about his own disorders is informative in multiple ways. First, it allows us to get a better feel for clinical medicine late in the eighteenth century. Second, it shows us how Franklin, as a patient, worked hand-in-hand with his physicians to understand and treat his infirmities. Third, it reveals how he experimented with his own body and then shared what he was able to discover with others. Fourth, it provides us with a better understanding of the philosopher's personal thoughts about popular medicines, restoring health, and coping with the ravages of time. And fifth, not to be overlooked, it shows us just how sharp Franklin's mind was in his senior years, even when his body was giving way.

Plato had philosophized that a need or a problem encourages creative efforts to meet the need or solve the problem. People today are inclined to say that necessity is the mother of invention. Poor Richard somehow missed the opportunity to print this catchy aphorism in his *Almanack*. But his talented creator would have been in full agreement, especially in his senior years when he needed creative solutions to engage more easily in some of his most important daily activities.

This chapter deals largely with Franklin's eyes: his understanding of how vision can decline with age, his need for corrective lenses, and his invention of bifocals. His bifocals did not improve his vision any more than did his previous glasses, but not having to change glasses every time he looked up from his reading material to gaze at something further away made it easier for him to function. From this larger perspective, bifocals were just one of his inventions for dealing with the challenges of aging. Another, as we shall see later in this chapter, was his "Long Arm" for reaching objects high on shelves. Notably, both inventions stemmed from personal needs. But other people would adopt them and marvel at their everyday utility, in addition to praising the creative mind that gave birth to them.

## GLASSES BEFORE FRANKLIN

There were eyeglasses well before the eighteenth century, but who invented them is a mystery complicated by false leads, myths, fictitious characters, regional motives, and nationalism.[3] What we do know is that glass itself is at least 4,500 years old. It began with the Phoenicians, after which it spread throughout the Middle East.

In 1847, Sir Austen Layard discovered a polished, rock crystal lens while excavating an archaeological site in Nineveh, Iraq.[4] But this lens, which is thought to be from 650 B.C., did not have the right focal length to be held in front of an eye to enhance vision, nor the clarity to be put on top of written material to magnify it clearly. More likely, Layard discovered a decorative item or perhaps an early burning glass, a lens used to start fires, melt writing on wax tablets, and cauterize wounds.[5]

There is also little to suggest that the Greeks and Romans, who definitely made burning glasses, manufactured special lenses for reading. Cicero, who lived during the first century B.C., wrote to his friend Atticus that, in his advanced age, he was no longer able to read. His solution was to hire scholars or to use educated slaves to read to him. His contemporary, Seneca the Younger, used mirrors and a globe filled with water to magnify writing that had become too small for him to read.

Large reading spheres, specifically lenses put directly above written material to make letters appear larger, began to appear in the thirteenth century. They were probably the first real visual aids and were initially ground from beryl (beryllium), a semiprecious green stone, and from sections of quartz called "pebble." The problem with them, however, was that they were heavy and bulky. The demand for more practical devices led someone to attach a smaller lens to a handle, so it could be held in front of an eye. A matched pair of magnifying lenses with two handles riveted together followed this notable advance. The earliest paired lenses still used minerals, and some were framed with brass or iron.

Carlo Roberto Dati, a scholar who lived in Florence in the seventeenth century, wrote a *Veglia* or essay that can be translated as *The Invention of Eyeglasses, Is it Ancient or Not; and When, Where and by Whom Were they Invented?* He pointed out that Fra Giordano di Rivalto had presented a sermon in February 1306, in which he stated: "It has been less than 20 years since the art of making spectacles was discovered." Fra Giordano added that he had met the inventor, but he did not divulging his name. Consistent with this dating is a note from Sandro di Pozo written in 1289. "I am so debilitated by age that without the glasses known as spectacles, I would no longer be able to read or write," he wrote. "These have recently been invented for the benefit of poor old people whose sight has become weak."[6] Scholars agree that eyeglasses made their debut late in the thirteenth century.

Although the first eyeglasses might have come from Pisa, Venice emerged as the capital for the young industry. During the fourteenth century, edicts from the high court of Venice specified that only good crystalline glass could to be used; ordinary white glass was no longer good enough for Venetian lenses. When Nicolas of Cusa published his book on corrective lenses in 1541, Florence had become another major manufacturing site for glasses, and there were concave corrective lenses as well as convex ones on the market.[7]

By this time there was a rapidly growing demand for eyeglasses, thanks to the development in the printing industry. The landmark event occurred in 1440, when Johannes Gutenberg of Mainz began printing Bibles on his transformed winepress. In less than a century, there were at least 1,000 printers in more than two hundred locations throughout Europe. People now had access to more affordable Bibles and, in the spirit of the Renaissance, a desire to learn to read secular material as well. For individuals with less than perfect vision, most notably the older segment of the population, mass-produced, inexpensive lenses, or higher quality eyeglasses, seemed like a godsend. The market for the printed word and the market for spectacles would now grow together.

## FRANKLIN ON VISUAL AIDS

Franklin once philosophized: "Almost all Parts of our Bodies require some Expence. The Feet demand Shoes; the Legs, Stockings; the rest of the Body, Clothing; and the Belly a good deal of Victuals. Our Eyes, tho' exceedingly useful, ask, when reasonable, only the cheap Assistance of Spectacles."[8] Franklin wrote these lines late in life, but he had known for a long time that vision tends to deteriorate as people age. He also knew that the change typically is more severe for reading and examining objects close by than for seeing things at a distance. Although presbyopia, or an age-related loss of vision for material positioned close to the eyes, might not be a disaster for a farmer, a salesman, or a sailor, it could be one for a printer, a writer, or a civil servant expected to read documents. Franklin was, of course, all of the above.

Painted portraits and verbal descriptions reveal that Franklin had worn spectacles for reading and writing since he was in his thirties. But whereas eyeglasses had long been the mark of a learned man, many people in the

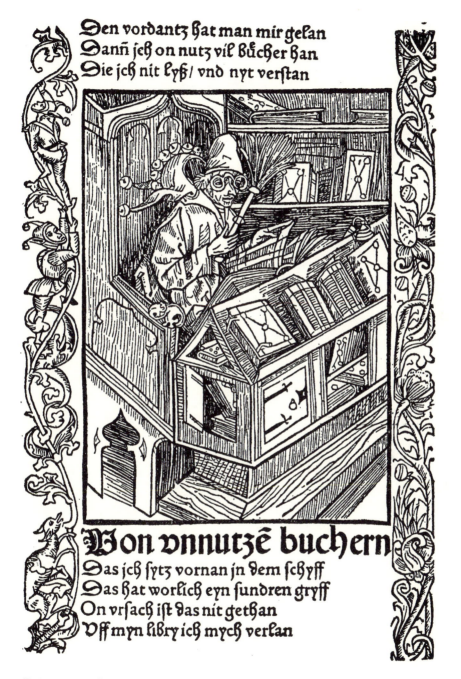

Den vordantz hat man mir gelan
Dann ich on nutz vil bücher han
Die ich nit lyß/ vnd nyt verstan

## Von vnnutzē buchern

Das ich sytz vornan jn dem schyff
Das hat worlich eyn sundren gryff
On vrsach ist das nit gethan
Vff myn libry ich mych verlan

*"The Scholar," a woodcut by Sebastian Brandt from 1494.*

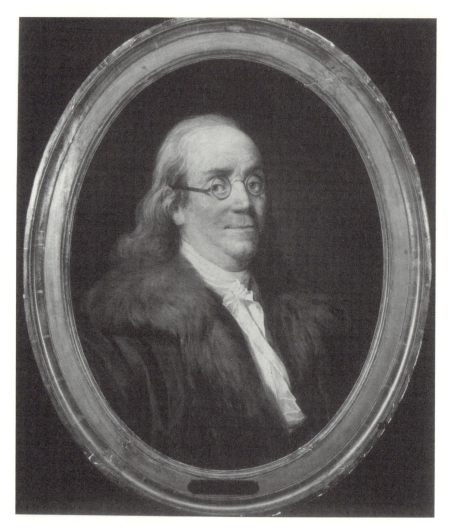

*Franklin wearing ordinary glasses. Portrait by Van Loo. (Courtesy of the American Philosophical Society.)*

eighteenth century shied away from them for personal and other reasons. The fact that Franklin wore eyeglasses and had them on when he entered Paris set an example for others to follow and helped increase their popularity. But there were notable exceptions, including Louis XVI, whose distance vision was so poor that he often had to rely on voices to identify the people in his court. Perhaps because Franklin, a foreign commoner with a disturbing cult following, made it a habit to show off his glasses, he was adamant about not gracing his own royal nose with a similar ornament.

Ordering glasses was fairly easy by this time, even for ordinary citizens. Eye charts were available, and oculists and peddlers set up some basic guidelines to fit buyers who could not be present to try out the glasses. The critical factor in such cases was the age of the client. One set of rules called for a convex glass of 2.0 degrees for a person between thirty and forty years of age; 2.5 degrees, if between forty and fifty; and on up to more than 5.0 degrees for an individual over eighty.[9] Of course, if the buyer were present, simple trial and error would be used for fine-tuning the selection of the lenses and for choosing from among several possible frames.

A person of means had still another option. By purchasing an entire set of lenses, he or she could increase the strength of the lenses as needed, while journeying into old age. Franklin was financially well off when he served his country in England and France, and he liked to chose his own reading glasses rather than simply following an age-related prescription. Hence, he would have been the kind of buyer who would have considered purchasing full sets of lenses. In fact, he bought several complete sets of lenses for a few other people. In 1771, he sent his favorite sister, Jane Mecom, "a Pair of every Size of Glasses from 1 to 13" from England. He instructed her to "take out a Pair at a time, and hold one of the Glasses first against one Eye, and then against the other, looking on some small Print. By trying and comparing at your Leisure, you may find those that are best for you, which you cannot do well in a Shop, where for want of Time and Care, People often take such as strain their Eyes and hurt them."[10]

Later in the same letter, Franklin revealed that he was fully aware of the possibility that the two eyes may not have identical needs, which would have been another reason not to buy glasses solely on the basis of age. "I advise your trying each of your Eyes separately," he told his sister, "because few Peoples Eyes are Fellows, and almost everybody in reading or working uses one Eye principally, the other being dimmer or perhaps fitter for distant Objects."[11] He also warned Jane, almost assuredly from personal experience, that she should be prepared to encounter more changes in her vision as she continued to grow older. "When you have suited yourself, keep the higher numbers for future Use as your Eyes may grow older," were his words.[12] He then advised her to give the weaker lenses that she would no longer need to a younger friend, rather than sending them back to him.

Franklin wrote a second letter on the same day to "my good and dear old Friend" John Bartram, the botanist who first envisioned an American Philosophical Society. At the time, Bartram was lamenting that "I cant know my own children [at] 3 foot distance & I write with trouble & must hold my face within 2 or 3 inches of the paper."[13] "Perhaps you have not Spectacles that suit you," Franklin wrote back.[14] And to help out, he also sent Bartram a complete set of thirteen pairs of lenses with instructions similar to those given to his sister.

Six months after sending Jane Mecom and Bartram their spectacles, Franklin composed a follow-up letter to his sister. He wanted to make sure that she tried to restore her vision only to where it had been. He warned her that people who try to do too much with corrective glasses will "hasten the time when still older Glasses will become necessary."[15]

## BIFOCALS

Franklin's fame in the field of optics never rested on how he selected glasses for himself or others in need, his knowledge about difference between the eyes or how vision might change with age, or the fact that he helped popularize spectacles in France and elsewhere. Rather, his lasting fame rests on his solution to a problem that was annoying to a person, namely himself, who was already committed to corrective lenses. Simply put, he did not like taking his glasses off every time he had to look up at a person who had come into the room while he was reading. Even worse, he found it bothersome to have to carry two sets of glasses, and then to have to keep switching between them, as he shifted his gaze from written material to something happening farther away.

One solution to the on-off problem came during the sixteenth century when opticians began to replace large, round reading lenses with smaller lenses that were oval in shape. With a set of smaller lenses, a farsighted person could simply look over the top rim of the glasses to see distant people, trees, or mountains with greater clarity. Nevertheless, this seemingly simple solution was far from perfect. First, low objects at a distance required tilting the head pretty far down, which could be socially awkward and even uncomfortable. And second, some people who needed corrective lenses for reading also had poor distance perception. Franklin was one such person, which is why he could not just look over the top of his reading lenses to see distant objects clearly. Instead, he had to keep switching between two sets of glasses, a cumbersome and at times inconvenient thing to do.

Wanting to simplify things, Franklin asked a skilled oculist to construct a set of spectacles with horizontally split lenses. At the time, the idea of combining lenses of different powers in a single frame had some history. But the divided lenses described by instrument makers Johann Zahn in 1683 and

Christian Gottlieb Hertel in 1716 were not intended to be everyday spectacles.[16] They were either trial lenses or just composite drawings showing two different lenses in a single illustration for convenience.[17] There is nothing to suggest that Franklin knew about these drawings when he came forth with his compound lenses for daily use. Rather, his idea of combining lenses to correct two visual defects at once seemed to originate with him.

The bottom half of each of Franklin's eyepieces might have been made by cutting one of his convex reading lenses in half. But given his statement that "few Peoples Eyes are Fellows," it is more likely that he instructed his chosen oculist to cut each of the two convex lenses from his reading glasses in half. As for the top half of the split lenses, since he complained about being farsighted, they also had to be made from convex lenses, but these lenses, cut from his distance spectacles, had to be of lesser strength.[18]

Exactly when Franklin had the idea for bifocals is not known, but they first appeared on his nose while he was in France struggling to read lips while also attending to his food or the written word. The first indication that we have to suggest that he was having bifocals made comes from a note dated 1779.[19] It was sent to Franklin in Passy by H. Sykes, who made glasses in Paris from 1776 to 1785. Sykes described himself as "Optician: Privilégié du Roi," and wrote that he "cut" a second pair of spectacles for Franklin—an unusual term to use if he were simply grinding lenses. He further informed Franklin that he had "been Unfortunate, for I have broke and Spoilt three Glasses." These additional words, along with his high price of eighteen francs for a set of glasses, are believed to suggest an order for bifocals. But whether a usable pair of bifocals resulted in 1779, or even a year later, is uncertain.

In 1784, however, Franklin mentioned wearing his useful "double Spectacles" to George Whatley, the philanthropist who served as treasurer of the London Foundling Hospital. He told Whatley that "Your Eyes must continue very good, since you can write so small a Hand without Spectacles. I cannot distinguish a Letter even of Large Print; but am happy in the invention of Double Spectacles, which, serving for distant objects as well as near ones, make my Eyes as useful to me as ever they were."[20]

Franklin provided Whatley with a full description of his bifocals and the logic behind their construction a year later. He explained: "I imagine it will be found pretty generally true, that the same Convexity of Glass, through which a Man sees clearest and best at the Distance proper for Reading, is not the best for greater Distances. I therefore had formerly two Pair of Spectacles, which I shifted occasionally, as in travelling I sometimes read, and often wanted to regard the Prospects. Finding this Change troublesome, and not always

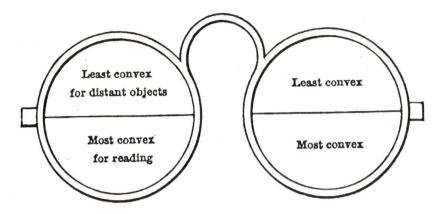

*Franklin's 1785 drawing of his "double spectacles" or bifocals with his handwriting replaced by type. (Courtesy of the Library of Congress.)*

sufficiently ready, I had the Glasses cut, and half of each kind associated in the same Circle, thus." Here Franklin included a drawing of his bifocals.

He went on: "By this means, as I wear my Spectacles constantly, I have only to move my Eyes up or down, as I want to see distinctly far or near, the proper Glasses being always ready. This I find more particularly convenient since my being in France, the Glasses that serve me best at Table to see what I eat, not being the best to see the Faces of those on the other Side of the Table who speak to me; and when one's Ears are not well accustomed to the Sounds of a Language, a Sight of the Movements in the Features of him that speaks helps to explain; so that I understand French better by the help of my Spectacles."[21]

The earliest known portrait of Franklin wearing his bifocals dates from the same year as the detailed letter to Whatley. Maryland-born portrait artist Charles Willson Peale, sometimes called the "Artist of the Revolution," painted and signed his name to this masterful work of art in 1785. As a portrait painter, Peale was personally enthused by Franklin's new glasses. Their construction allowed him to look at a person posing for a portrait some distance away and then immediately attend to a small detail on the canvas just in front of him. Bifocals, Peale concluded, were a far better idea than fusing or hinging one set of small glasses above the other, which was what some Londoners were now beginning to try, perhaps because of negative feelings about Franklin stemming from the American War of Independence.

About three years after painting Franklin's portrait, Peale wrote in his diary that he liked Franklin's glasses so much that he even made his own bifocals.

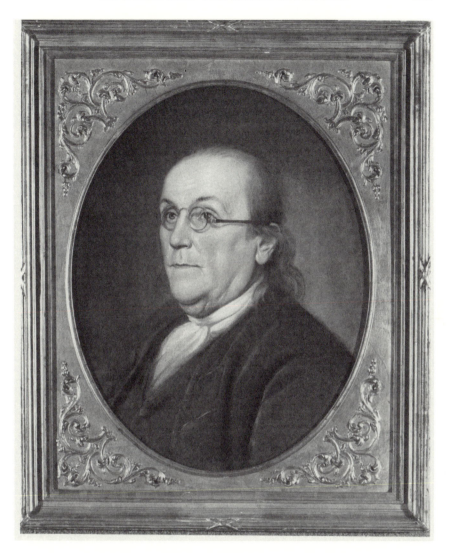

*Franklin wearing bifocals. Painted in 1785 by Charles Willson Peale.*
*(With permission of The Pennsylvania Academy of Fine Arts.)*

"Bought 2 pr. Spectacles one of 9 Inch focus & the other of 18, I cut the Glasses of both pr. And put the longest focus above and the shorter below in each frame, so that I have 2 pr. Of Spectacles which will serve for near or greater distance."[22]

Peale was not the only artist of the post–Revolutionary War era to adopt Franklin's split lenses. Sir Joshua Reynolds in England, and Benjamin West, who had moved from Philadelphia to England to become the favorite painter of George III, were two other artists that began to wear them.[23]

Thomas Jefferson, who went to France in 1784 and served as Franklin's replacement, was among the diplomats and scholars that began to order bifocals. He wrote to Peale: "I have adopted Dr. Franklin's plan of half-glasses of different focal distances, with great advantage."[24] Jefferson actually wrote several letters praising Franklin's bifocals, and this one was dated March 1807. The records show that Jefferson had previously written a note to John McAllister, Senior, the most respected optician in Philadelphia. "You have heretofore furnished me with spectacles, so reduced in size as to give facility to looking over their top without moving them," Jefferson began. "This is a great convenience, but the reduction has not been sufficient to do it compleatly. . . . Those who are obliged to use spectacles know what a convenience it would be to have different magnifiers in the same frame. Dr. Franklin tried this by semicircular glasses joined horizontally, the upper and lower semicircles of different powers, which he told me answered perfectly. I wish to try it, and therefore send you a drawing."[25]

Jefferson was the third President of the United States when he first put on his bifocals, and he was the first head of state to wear them. When asked about his new glasses, he always gave Franklin full credit for the practical invention that was now making his and other active lives so much easier.

## THE LONG ARM

As previously noted, another physical problem that Franklin faced as he entered his eighth decade of life was that he had become increasingly unsteady on his feet. As a result, he no longer wanted to risk climbing ordinary ladders to reach books and objects out of his reach. His desire to reach objects on the shelves in his personal library led him to invent a chair with arms that could be converted into a more secure sort of step ladder. But the chair-ladder posed two problems. One was that it still involved some climbing, and the other was that it did not allow the user to reach objects fairly high up.

Franklin's second solution to the reaching problem was his "Long Arm."[26] The "arm" was basically a lengthy stick with opposing end pieces. He called them the "Thumb" and the "Finger," consistent with the idea that his invention worked like a very long arm with a functional hand at the end. All he had to do was pull the "Sinew"—which was no more than a cord—and the hand piece opened and closed.

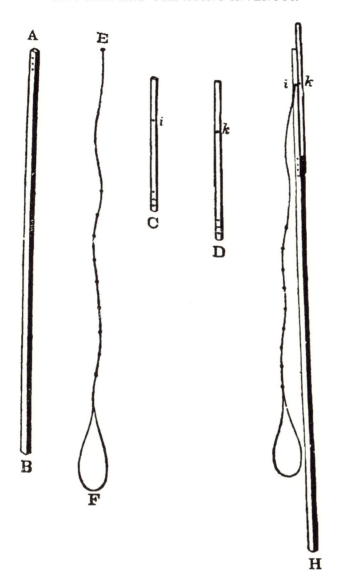

*The long arm Franklin invented for reaching books and other objects on high shelves.*

This simple and inexpensive device allowed Franklin to grasp books and other objects well out of his reach without worrying about slipping or falling several feet to the ground. Nevertheless, Franklin did not publish his description of the long arm in his lifetime; he stated that he was not even sure it was worthy of presentation at the American Philosophical Society. But he did send a description of his new prosthetic device to a few select friends. In his letters he attested to its "practical Utility" and how it could serve a handicapped person.

Today, devices based on Franklin's original design are widely used in libraries, stores, places of business, and homes—whenever people want to get small items that are out of reach. For the most part, even individuals who have no difficulty climbing ladders are using them, because they are so convenient. But they are also serving the sick and elderly, much as they served Franklin in the final years of his life.

Franklin invented or modified other household objects to make his life easier after he returned to America with his various disabilities. Like his bifocals, chair-ladder, and long arm, some also had a lot to do with his love of books and the printed word.

One was a shoe-shaped copper tub that was fitted with a special device to hold reading material safely above the water. At the time of this invention, he was being advised to take long medicinal baths. But rather than just passing his time in a tub, he viewed his baths as perfect opportunities to catch up on some reading—provided he could keep his books, pamphlets, and papers dry and positioned in front of his eyes. He also invented a chair with a large, foot-controlled fan attached to it. It allowed him to read more comfortably on blistering summer days in Philadelphia.

All of these inventions reveal just how well Franklin's intellect and creativity held up while he was in his late seventies and early eighties. He effectively employed his inventive genius to deal with the twin demons of aging and chronic illnesses that were now conspiring against him. But although Franklin's inventions made him more comfortable and allowed him to function better, they were not cures. In the next chapter, we shall see how closely Franklin worked with several of his learned physician friends to try to cure one of his chronic diseases, his persistent and annoying skin rash.

CHAPTER 16

# Skin and "Scurf"

> When you are sick, what you like best is to be chosen for a Medicine
> in the first Place; what Experience tells you is best, is to be chosen in
> the second Place; what Reason (i.e. Theory) says is best, is to be
> chosen in the last Place. But if you can get Dr. Inclination, Dr.
> Experience and Dr. Reason to hold a Consultation together, they
> will give you the best Advice that can be given.
>
> —*Poor Richard's Almanack*, 1736

On January 29, 1777, Jan Ingenhousz wrote a letter from his desk in Vienna to Franklin in Passy. "My journey to Ratisborn is fixed upon the 10 or 12 of April, if nothing hinders me, where I will inoculate the two sons of the Reigning Prince of Tour [Thurn] and Taxis, after which I should be very glad to take a trip to Paris and to have the great satisfaction of seeing you," he told his old friend.[1] Paris was not the final destination for the Austrian royal physician; it was a stop en route to London. Ingenhousz had been invited to address the Royal Society. In addition, he wanted to spend time with John Pringle, the English physician who had done so much to help him launch his highly successful medical career.

As it turned out, Ingenhousz did not perform the smallpox inoculations when he thought he would or even where they had first been planned. The inoculations took place a few months later in Trossingen, a town in the Swabian Alps. Consequently, he did not arrive in Passy until October 1777. Still, Franklin could not have been happier to see him.

The discussions between the two men inevitably turned to the overworked American minister's health problems. At the time, the expectation was that sick patients of means and sound mind would talk with their physicians, describing their aches and pains in reasonable detail. The patient's own information was considered more important than the physician's examination, which was usually perfunctory and restricted to gross signs that could be seen with the naked eye. Few physicians systematically touched and probed, and the key tools of the trade, such as the stethoscope and ophthalmoscope, were later developments. Hence, the ideal patient was one who could provide some oral history about a problem and then discuss how changes in his or her daily regimen might have exacerbated it or, even better, produced some improvements.

What Franklin did that set him apart from most patients was to provide Ingenhousz with as detailed a description of the state of his body as he possibly could—and not just in their conversations. He also handed him a collection of notes written as if he, Franklin, were a trained practitioner objectively examining another person, not his own body.[2] The material far exceeded what any eighteenth-century physician would have expected.

## FRANKLIN'S NOTES

Franklin wrote that "the patient" was first bothered with his annoying skin condition in 1774, while he was still in England.

He found a small Spot on his Head cover'd with a dry Scurff, which when rubb'd off from time to time, left always a Moisture on the Part that form'd another Scurf. This continuing some Months, and seeming to extend itself, alarm'd him, and he consulted Sir J.P. [John Pringle] who prescrib'd a Water to wet the Part and some Pills, which Prescription was follow'd, and the Disorder by slow Degrees quitted that Spot, but after some time shows itself in other Parts of the Head.[3]

The greater part of the Year 1775 he was almost every day 10 to 12 Hours of the Day employ'd in Business of Consultation with many other persons *sitting* in a closed room, and had no Leisure for Exercise. During this time the Disorder spread, and affected his Head in a Number of small Spots under the Hair, the Scurf tho' taken off from time to time by the Comb, returning continually.

Toward the End of Winter of 1776, he set out on a Journey of 500 Miles [to Quebec], of which the greater Part was perfom'd in a small open Boat, where he was kept sitting without Exercise for many Days. During this Journey which continu'd from the Middle of March to the Beginning of June, he was afflicted with a Succession of Boils, sometimes two or three together, each when heal'd leaving round about it Spots of the same Scurff, which obstinately continu'd, being renew'd after every Removal. At this time his Leg's swell'd in the Small, and Impressions made by the Finger would continue long. This Swelling went away on his Return home, but the Boils continu'd to harass him.

In November 1776 he made a long Sea Voyage [to France], in which the Disorder sensibly increas'd, and the Boils became more frequent. Part of each Arm, and of each side, the Small of his Back, and Parts of his Thighs and Legs, became cover'd with the Scurff, which became very troublesome, itching sometimes extreamly, and when rubb'd or scratch'd off, would spot his Linen with Blood.[4]

Franklin further described how he sought professional help in France for his itchy rash, scaling, and occasional boils.

He consulted a Physician, who prescribed Belloste's Pills, and an Infusion of a Root called *Patience*, or the Rhubard of the Parisians. This Prescription was followed some time, till the Mouth began to have an unusual Quantity of Water in it, and the Teeth to be a little loosened. The Disorder was not diminished, but appeared not to increase.

He has for some time omitted taking those Pills, but uses the warm Bath twice a Week, staying in the Water each time near two Hours, which are employ'd in rubbing off the Scurff when softened by the Water, and so clearing the Skin. The Disorder has now visibly diminish'd; for in many Places after the Scurff has been thus repeatedly rubb'd off, it does not return in such Substance, and at length ceases to return, leaving the Skin soft and natural. But the Amendment is slow; and it is apprehended, that on a Discontinuance of the Bathing, it may return and increase as before.[5]

Belloste's pills, which Franklin had taken for a while, were introduced by Augustin Belloste, who was well known in medical circles at the start of the century. He served as physician to the Duchess of Savoy and was the author of *Le Chirurgien de l'Hôpital*, which appeared in 1695. The main ingredient in his pills was mercury, an agent known to have severe side effects. Franklin was smart enough to stop taking the pills as soon as he began to experience problems with his teeth. Had he continued to ingest more mercury, he would have endangered himself and might not have lived to receive Ingenhousz.

As for his second medicine, rhubarb, it had long been used as a laxative. For the humoral theorists, it had been a means of evacuating excessive humors; for iatrochemists, it had been a way to drive toxins from the body; and for the new mechanically oriented physicians, it provided a gentle way to remove intestinal blockages, real or imagined. Rhubarb tended to be recommended for more than just clearing the bowels during the eighteenth century. Notably, it was also being employed for difficult skin conditions.

Having provided Ingenhousz with the history of his "Scurf" (or "Scurff") and how he had been treating it, Franklin now presented his visitor with even more written observations about the flaking on his skin.

The Scurf appears to be compos'd of extremely thin Scales one upon another, which are white, and when rubb'd off dry, are light as Bran. When the Skin is clear'd in the Bath, it looks red, and seems a little elevated above the sound Skin that is around the Place, but it is not sore: And in a few Hours after, it becomes dry, and feels stiffened as if it were with the first thin Coat of the new Scurff.

The Substance of this Scurff when dry is close and strong. The fine Lamina seem to be formed one under another, and not to make an united thick Substance by adhering together. In rubbing them off they separate, like Talc, each having a Polish that shines.[6]

After presenting this report, Franklin noted that "the patient's" skin condition finally appeared to be improving.

His Head is now almost clear of the Disorder, as are also his Legs and Thighs, and it seems diminish'd on his Arms. But it holds its ground on the Small of his Back and his Side. There were in the Heighth of it some small Spots on his Hands and face, but they have quite disappear'd.

His health is otherwise good. He feels on Comparison no Diminution of his Strength, but is capable of bearing Labour as he was at 50. His Legs particularly seem stronger since the Swelling [presumably gout] left them, and he can walk without much Weariness. His Digestion is good.[7]

Finally, "the patient" wrote out some questions. One reads: "He wishes to be inform'd whether this troublesome Disorder may not be of Service to him in other Respects?"[8] The belief at the time, which will be examined in more detail in the next chapter, was that some disorders might actually be beneficial, because they could protect the patient from considerably more debilitating or life-threatening diseases. That was why Franklin first asked this question and only afterward asked three follow-up questions: "Whether it be safe to cure it? If so, what are the Medicines to be used? And what ought to be his regimen?"[9]

Franklin handed Ingenhousz his written notes, hoping to get some immediate suggestions. He also asked Ingenhousz if he would be kind enough to show his material to John Pringle when he went to London, since Pringle was a close and knowledgeable friend, and had treated Franklin earlier. With both Ingenhousz and Pringle on the case, he felt sure he would get the best professional advice available.

## FOOD, EXERCISE, AND THE RASH

Franklin also kept a personal journal of his health that provides more information about the history of his stubborn skin condition—particularly how it seemed to be affected by diet and exercise.[10] In his conversations, Franklin would have provided Ingenhousz with many of these details, perhaps with his visitor taking notes. One journal entry informs us that his rash first came to his notice in 1773, right after he had made a month-long trip to Ireland.

On my Return I first observ'd a kind of Scab or Scurff on my Head, about the Bigness of a Shilling. Finding it did not heal, but rather increas'd, I mentioned it to my Friend, Sir J.P. who advis'd a mercurial Water to wash it, and some physic. It slowly left that Place but appear'd in other Parts of my Head. He also advis'd my abstaining from salted Meats and Cheese, which Advice I did not much follow, often forgetting it.

In 1775 I went to America. On the Passage I necessarily eat more Salt Meat than usual with me at London. . . . I went to Canada. On the Passage I suffer'd much from a number of large Boiles.

In my Passage to France Nov. 1776 I lived chiefly on Salt Beef, the Fowls being too hard for my Teeth. But being poorly nourish'd, I was very weak on my Arrival; Boils continu'd to vex me, and the Scurff extending over all the small of my Back, on my Sides, my Legs, and my Arms, besides what continued under my Hair, I apply'd to a Physician.[11]

It was this unnamed physician who now recommended Belloste's pills and the rhubarb infusion. After Franklin abandoned both recommendations, he tried a hot bath twice a week, two hours at a time, which provided some relief.

## NEW RECOMMENDATIONS FROM LONDON

We do not know what Ingenhousz prescribed for Franklin. But we do know that he took Franklin's handwritten notes to London to solicit John Pringle's valued opinion. On March 6, 1778, Ingenhousz wrote back to Franklin to inform him that their mutual friend had slipped and suffered a head injury that would postpone a discussion about his case by several weeks. Following Pringle's recovery, Ingenhousz met with him at least three times to discuss Franklin's skin condition.

Ingenhousz, who was fluent in several tongues, but not a good speller of English, explained to Franklin that Pringle felt that "the disordre of the skin seems to be reather a benefit and a critical discharge of some sharpness in the blood. . . . Therefore he thinks that the best Advice is to Continue beathing in warm water, and, for to keep up boddily strength and to prevent being relaxed by it, to take every day one dragm of the bark two hours before dinner or at bed time. If the Stomach should not bear it, it would be prudent to begin by half a dragm. As to the diet, he thinks that it will be good to abstain from smoaked and salted meat and fish, and from some food known to affect the skin, when diseased, as porck, eal, leavers [livers] of fishes &c."[12]

Ingenhousz's letter continued with the suggestion that Franklin might want to try a mineral water cure. "He thinks with me that bathing in sulphureous waters . . . would kleen the skin of those eruptions still better than common water. But those springs do not exist everywhere. Our friend thinks, that *Dr. Charles Le Roy*, who has written upon artificial baths, would be the best man to consult in case of necessity, for it is possible, and even easy to imitate Sulphureous waters with *hepar sulphuris* added to it."[13]

Dr. Charles Le Roy was the younger brother of Jean-Baptiste Le Roy, the skilled experimental natural philosopher who Franklin spent considerable time with in France. Charles had just returned to Paris from Montpellier, the southern French city renowned for its medical school. He was well published and had distinguished himself as a chemist, a physician, and a professor of medicine before heading north to Paris.

In addition to these recommendations, Pringle and Ingenhousz sent Franklin a few medicines from London. But Franklin might not have taken them. He remained shy about new concoctions and felt that the affair was "not pressing," especially since he was seeing further signs of improvement.

To Franklin's relief, his skin condition resolved by the summer of 1778. Franklin was not sure why it disappeared, writing: "I observ'd that there was no Redness under the Scurff, if I took it once off it did not return. I had hardly bath'd in those 3 Months, I took no Remedy whatever and I know not what to ascribe the Change to, unless it was the Heat of the Summer, which sometimes made me sweat, particularly when I exercis'd."[14]

Unfortunately, his happiness was short lived. During October, the affliction started to come back. Despondent, and postulating that the changing weather might be playing a causal role, he could do little more than "wish the Cool Weather may not bring on a return of the Disorder."[15]

Some brief entries in Franklin's diary from 1778, 1779, and early 1780 provide us with updates about his frustrating skin condition:

Oct. 4. The Itching continues, but somewhat abated.

Oct. 12. The Itching has not return'd; the Scurff continues to diminish.

Jan. 14, 1779. At length the Itching return'd, and a new Set of Eruptions of scurfy Spots appear'd in many Parts of my Body. My Back had never been entirely clear'd and the Scurf began to increase there and extend itself. But it is not yet so bad as it had been, and it seems to spare the Parts that were before affected, except in my Back.

Feb. 28, 79. The Disorder on my Skin has continu'd augmenting.[16]

The next entry, for Jan 16, 1780, is the most informative of all. It reads: "I have enjoy'd good Health ever since the last Date. Towards the End of the Summer most of the Disorder in my Skin disappeared, a little only remaining on my left Arm, a little under each Breast, and some on the small of the Back. I had taken at different times a good deal of Dr. Pringle's Prescription; but whether that occasion'd the Amendment, or whether it was the Heat of the Summer as I suppos'd in October 1778, I am uncertain. The disorder seems to be now increasing again, and appears upon my hands. I am otherwise well; my Legs sound; To-morrow I enter my 75th Year."[17]

## SO WHAT DID FRANKLIN HAVE?

Physicians today can only wish that their patients would be as informative as Franklin, who knew how to write an excellent case history with detailed descriptions, and who even tracked how his diet and changes in the weather may have affected his condition. Moreover, he kept his learned physicians apprised of changes in his condition. In 1788, six years after Pringle died, he even penned a note from his home in Philadelphia to Jan Ingenhousz on the recurrence of his "Scurf" and how it remitted when his gout came on.

"You may remember the cutaneous malady, I formerly complained of, and for which you and Dr. Pringle favoured me with prescriptions and advice," Franklin began. "It vexed me near fourteen years, and was, the beginning of this year, as bad as ever, covering almost my whole body, except my face and hands; when a fit of the gout came on, without very much pain, but a swelling in both feet, which at last appeared also in both knees, and then in my hands. As these swellings increased and extended, the other malady diminished, and at length disappeared entirely."[18]

But what exactly was the skin condition that Franklin was describing in this letter and in previous notes and letters; the occasionally itchy rash that he referred to as the "Scurf" or "Scurff"? The Oxford English Dictionary provides a clue. The first entry under "Scurf" informs us that this term appeared in print about a thousand years ago. It referred to "a morbid condition of the skin, esp. of the head, characterized by the separation of branny scales, without inflammation." The term was originally used for a skin condition of humans and animals.

Two of the most commonly consulted medical dictionaries from Franklin's time, James' and Motherby's, do not list "Scurf";[19] nevertheless, the slightly later *Hooper's Medical Dictionary* does include an entry, which reads: "Scurf. Furfura. Small exfoliations of the cuticle, which take place after some eruptions on the skin, a new cuticle being formed underneath during the exfoliation."[20] Returning to Motherby's medical dictionary, a reasonably good description of what Franklin seemed to have can be found appear under "Furfurosi." The entry reads: "Those patients are so called who are affected with a sort of scurf or scaliness on the head, which upon combing discharge a scaly substance like bran, whence the disease is called furfures, an furfuratio; though some call it porrigo and afrrea nubes."[21]

Surprisingly, other than the occasional comment that Franklin had a skin condition or a cutaneous infection, almost nothing has been written about his "Scurf" or "Furfurosi." William Willcox and his associates who edited Franklin's writings, however, did try to probe deeper, consulting Dr. Marguerite Lerner, a professor of dermatology at Yale University Medical School.[22] Lerner's conclusion was that Franklin probably had some type of psoriasis, a common skin condition characterized by red patches and dry, silvery scales, often on the scalp, face, elbows, knees, palms, and soles. Psoriasis is associated with skin cells reproducing faster than normal and accumulating on the surface, where they flake off as other take their place.

Following up on what Willcox did, the author showed several dermatologists associated with major university medical centers Franklin's letters, journal entries, and diary statements. The consensus was that psoriasis is a very reasonable candidate, and probably the most likely candidate, for Franklin's unsightly, flaky skin.

The cause of psoriasis is still not fully understood. Recent research suggests that the disorder involves the T cells, which are a part of the immune system. It has been shown that abnormal T cell activity can trigger inflammations and cause excessive skin cell reproduction. In about one-third of the cases, the problem seems to be inherited, but in the remainder other factors appear to be involved.

Hence, Franklin's "Scurf" could have been no more than a stubborn case of psoriasis. This disorder can be affected by the climate in some sufferers, consistent with what he discovered about his condition. Also noteworthy is the fact that some people with psoriasis report that certain foods may worsen their scaling and flaking, although not all people have the same food triggers. Franklin tracked how his diet might have affected his scaling, and he and his physicians believed that salty meats and alcohol might have made it worse.

Food and drink have been much more firmly tied to the two more serious disorders that Franklin had in his senior years, and which were very common in the eighteenth century: gout and stones. In the next chapter, we shall see that Franklin was very knowledgeable about how gout could be affected by meat and wine, and that he made dietary modifications when his gout flared up. But even more interestingly, we shall discover that he was not as determined to cure his painful gout as he was to get rid of his annoying, flaky skin condition, which unbeknownst to him, may have made his gout worse.

# CHAPTER 17

# The Gout as Your Friend?

I continue well, except for a little Gout, which is perhaps not more a Disease than a Remedy.
                                                        —Benjamin Franklin, 1783

Gout is a metabolic disorder characterized by sodium urate deposits in the joints. Typically, the joints of the extremities are most affected, and the great toe is usually the worst off of all. The result is a succession of localized pains with swelling and redness, which can make walking difficult and, in severe cases, almost impossible. Benjamin Franklin, like so many people in the eighteenth century, knew the clinical manifestations of gout firsthand.

## AN ANCIENT DISORDER

Gout received considerable attention in classical antiquity.[1] The Hippocratic physicians believed that it resulted from a humoral condition, usually too much bile or an overabundance of thickened phlegm. They had different names for gouty accumulations in different parts of the body. When the disorder involved the foot, as it often did, it was called *podagra*, a term meaning "foot-grabber."

Celsus, Arataeus, and Galen were among the numerous authors to write about gout in the Roman period. Celsus pointed out that many Roman emperors, with their rich diets and propensity for excessive drinking, suffered from gout. Arataeus suggested that the condition might be inherited, and added that a gout sufferer could still win an Olympic race, but only during a period of remission. Galen contended that venery, in addition to overeating and overdrinking, might cause it. Thus, in ancient times we have the idea that gout may result from rich foods, too much love, and excessive wine drinking. The Greeks imagined Aphrodite being seduced by Dionysis, whereas the Romans changed the names of gout's parents to Venus and Bacchus. Notably, both agreed that the joint swelling and pain could be kept at bay by limited wine intake, less love, and bland diets.[2]

Colchicum was one of the many herbals used to treat gout in antiquity. It gets its name from Colchis, a temperate region on the Black Sea where *Colchicum autumnale* (meadow saffron) was harvested.[3] But neither the Greeks nor the Romans suspected that this plant had specific anti-gout properties. To the ancients, colchicum was just another purgative for ridding the body of harmful matter. The subsequent idea that colchicum might have specific properties for fighting gout and other arthritic diseases seems to have emerged with Alexander of Tralles, a physician from the mid-sixth century. He recommended it to gout sufferers along with less wine and fewer "dainty dishes." Its popularity, however, decreased over the ensuing centuries, in part because it could upset the stomach and even prove fatal. When it was "rediscovered" in the sixteenth century, gout sufferers with the means to buy colchicum, strangely enough, preferred to wear it around their necks.

The word "gout" was first used in its modern sense by Randolfus of Bocking, a Dominican monk of the thirteenth century who suffered from *gutta quam podagram vel artetican vocant* ("gout which is called podagram or arthritis").[4] Because Randolfus seemed to be helped when he wore the boots of a bishop, he recommended bishop's boots as his treatment of choice. A related cure from this period of deep religious convictions was a pilgrimage to a church or a shrine, such as the tomb of Thomas à Becket, the destination of the pilgrims in Chaucer's *Canterbury Tales*.

Gout was thought to affect men more than women, adults more than the young, and the rich more than the poor well before and through the Renaissance. The tale of the spider and Mr. Gout, an early personification of the disorder, has been told from the ninth century on. Adopted by Petrarch in 1338 and by Jean de la Fontaine in 1668, it deals with gout's predilection for the rich.[5]

Richard Hawes, a Cambridge graduate and "useful preacher," included one version of the story in *The Poore-Mans Plaster-Box*, his popular medical handbook from 1634.[6] It begins with Mr. Gout meeting a spider. With night falling, they

came to a poore man's house, which the Gout took up for his lodging, for he being always a lazy companion, would not go further; but the spider being more nimble, went to a rich man's house, and there took up his lodging for the night. The next day they met again and discussed how the night went. "Mine," said the gout, "was the worst as ever I had, for I had no sooner touched the poor man's legs, thinking there to take my rest, but up he gets, and to thrashing he goes, so that I had no rest the whole night." "And I," said the spider, "had no sooner begun to build my house

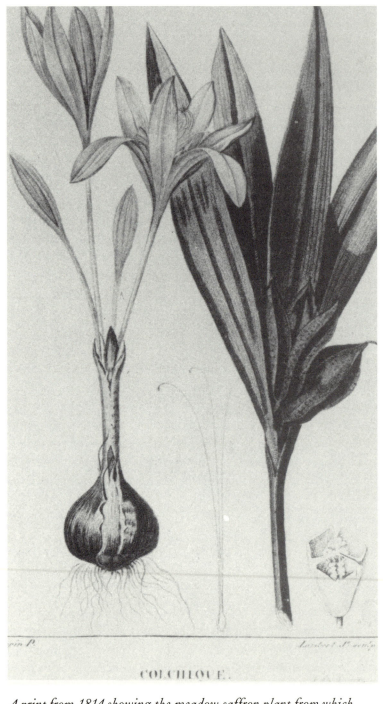

COLCHIQUE.

*A print from 1814 showing the meadow saffron plant from which colchicum is derived.*

in the rich man's chamber, but the maid came with a broom, and tore down all my work, and so fiercely did pursue me, that I had so much ado to save my life, as ever I had."

"Seeing it is so, then," said the Gout, "we will change lodging, I will go to the rich man's house, and thou shalt go to the poor man's." They both were well content, and did so, and found such ease and rest in their lodging, that they resolved never to remove, for the spider built and was not troubled, the Gout he was entertained with a soft cushion, with down pillows, with dainty candles, and delicate broths. In brief, he did like it so well, that ever since he takes up his lodging with rich men.[7]

At the time of Hawes's book, numerous rich men were known to be gout sufferers.[8] In Florence, Cosimo de' Medici, Piero il Gottose (Peter the Goutty), and Lorenzo the Magnificent had gout. In the sixteenth century, Holy Roman Emperor Charles V had it, as did his son Phillip II of Spain. Henry VII of England also had it, as did Henry VIII and Queen Anne. And in the seventeenth century, the list grew longer and included many famous people who were not born of royal blood: Oliver Cromwell, Samuel Johnson, and John Milton were among the better known gout sufferers in England.

In the field of medicine, Thomas Sydenham, whose works were read by Franklin, was also tortured by gout at this time. In 1683, after more than three decades of living a more restricted life because of his condition, he wrote his famous *Treatise on the Gout*.[9] "The [gout] victim goes to bed and sleeps in good health," Sydenham stated. But "about two o'clock in the morning he is awakened by severe pain in the great toe; more rarely in the heel, ankle, or instep. This pain is like that of a dislocation. . . . Now it is a violent stretching and tearing of the ligaments—now it is a gnawing pain, and now a pressure and tightening. So exquisite and lively meanwhile is the feeling of the part affected, that it cannot bear the weight of the bedclothes nor the jar of a person walking in the room. . . . He wakes freer from pain, and finds the part recently swollen."[10]

Sydenham considered gout a distinct entity, one different from other forms of arthritis. He concurred with Galen and the other physicians of antiquity that it is a disorder of those who indulge in rich food, abundant wine, and other excesses. "But what is consolation to me, and may be so to other gouty persons of small fortunes and slender abilities," he wrote, "is that kings, great princes, generals, admirals, philosophers and several other great men have thus lived and died. . . . It destroys more rich than poor persons, and more wise men than fools."[11]

Sydenham had little faith in divine healing or in the concoctions that had been prescribed by physicians of the previous century, some of which might have seemed like witches' brews to him. Andrew Boorde, for example, called for stockings of dog skin and daily applications of baked fermentations of ox dung wrapped in a cabbage leaf.[12] Lorenz Fries, Boorde's predecessor, had a more unthinkable recommendation. "Roast a fat goose and stuff with chopped kittens, lard, incense, wax and flour of rye," he wrote. "This must all be eaten, and the drippings applied to the painful joints."[13]

To Sydenham, it seemed wrong to subject gouty patients to any remedies that would contort and torture their bodies, making them even more miserable than they already were. Hence, he recommended avoiding harsh purges, such as colchicum, and excessive bleeding and other heroic therapies. Instead, he advised his fellow gout sufferers to eat and drink moderately, and to let Nature restore them back to health.

## FRANKLIN'S RISK FACTORS FOR GOUT

"The eighteenth century, known as the Age of Reason, might also be termed the Golden Age of Gout," wrote William Copeman in *A Short History of Gout*. "Its ravages are well documented in both the medical and lay literature and art throughout Europe, and its influence on world history at several important periods can be clearly seen. Everyone who was anybody had it, and those lesser mortals who did not suffer would often simulate what was termed 'the honor of the gout.'"[14] Among the most noteworthy gout sufferers from this era, we find William Pitt, John Wesley, Edward Gibbon, and Benjamin Franklin.

Ironically, Franklin was introduced to gout years before he was afflicted with the disorder. In 1732, his printing press published a book called *The Honour of the Gout*.[15] Its cumbersome subtitle, which left little more to add on the pages that followed, was *A Rational Discourse Demonstrating that the Gout is One of the Greatest Blessings that can Befal Mortal Man; That all Gentlemen that are Weary of it are their own Enemies; That those Practitioners that Offer at the Cure are the Vainest and most Mischievous Cheats in Nature*. "Philander Misaurus," an obvious pseudonym, had originally published the tract in 1699. He claimed, as had others before him, that gouty persons are protected from dangerous fevers and life-threatening disorders, and therefore should endure the pain and not try to be cured.

Franklin had also written about the gout well before he had it. In the first edition of his *Almanack*, Poor Richard warned his readers: "Cheese and salt meat, should be sparingly eat."[16] And in 1734, he opined, "Be temperate in wine, in eating, girls, and sloth; Or the Gout will seize you and plague you both."[17] Poor Richard was not conveying any new thoughts when he wrote these words and, like so many others at the time, he might not have felt that gout could even be cured. As he went on to state in a later edition of the *Almanack*, "*Pride* and the *Gout*, are seldom cur'd throughout."[18]

In a number of ways, Poor Richard's creator was a good candidate for gout, and he understood some of what people today would refer to as risk factors for gout, even if he had little inkling of their underlying mechanisms. For instance, his knew from Sydenham and numerous others that his meaty diet and love of wine made him vulnerable. But it would not be until late in the twentieth century that researchers would learn that purines are released from the DNA in the nuclei of the cells making up the meat and that they are then converted into uric acid. If the uric acid accumulates faster than the kidneys can excrete it, gouty urate deposits may result.

As for drinking wines, the major problem is now known to be that the alcohol triggers the production of lactic acid and beta-hydroxybutarate, which in turn inhibit uric acid excretion by the kidneys. Since the fortified wines, which include port and Madeira, contain about 50 percent more alcohol than ordinary table wines, they would have posed the greatest risk. These were extremely popular in the eighteenth century, and they were the wines Franklin enjoyed most.

The fortified wines also posed a second risk. They could cause chronic lead poisoning, which could ever so slowly seriously damage the kidneys. Surprisingly, Franklin did not shy away from fortified wines, even though George Baker had warned that the thickened wines from Southern Europe were among the most likely to contain dangerous lead. Baker believed that lead frequently leeched into these wines from the equipment used in distilling the thickened spirits, and from their storage in lead-glazed vessels, although he also thought that some casks might have had lead deliberately added to sweeten the taste of the wines.[19]

In this context, a study of previously unopened bottles of fortified wines imported into England in the late-eighteenth and early-nineteenth centuries is noteworthy.[20] Although the sample was small, the lead values ranged from 320 (Malaga) to 1,900 (Old Canary Wine) micrograms per liter. To put these numbers in perspective, drinking water with a lead concentration exceeding 15 micrograms per liter is considered unhealthy in the United States today.

It was not unusual for Franklin to down one or two bottles of Madeira each day while he was in England and during much of his stay in France, although the bottles were about half the size they are now. The effects of ingesting lead on the kidney are now well known, and they include damaging the proximal convoluted tubules, which will impair the elimination of uric acid and raise serum uric acid levels.[21]

Franklin's age also put him at risk, because the kidneys become less efficient with age. Glomerular filtration rate, a key measure of kidney function, drops about 1 percent a year after age forty-five, and the drop proceeds with greater rapidity after age sixty-five.[22] Thus, normal aging leads to a diminished ability of the kidneys to process uric acid, raising the risk of clinical manifestations. In this context it is worth noting that Franklin first complained of his gout when he was middle aged, and that his attacks became more painful and protracted as he grew older.

Finally, Franklin had a risk factor for gout that he could not have been aware of at all. It was his flaky skin condition—the disorder he called the "Scurf" (or scurff). Researchers have now established that disorders associated with rapid cell turnover, such as breakouts of psoriasis, can increase serum uric acid levels.[23] The underlying mechanism has a lot in common with digesting meat. Specifically, when cells die, purines may be released for conversion into uric acid. If the cells die at an exceptionally fast rate, as is the case with pink skin quickly turning white, flaking off, and being replaced, serum uric acid levels can become significantly elevated.

Thus, Benjamin Franklin had his diet, love of wine, age, and a psoriasis-like condition working against him. Each of these conditions had the potential to elevate his uric acid levels. But just how important each of these factors might have been in causing or adding to the agonies of his gout is impossible to say. For all we know, some of the risk factors mentioned might have been insignificant, while others, such as his genetic background, could have been of greater importance. Still, there can be no doubt that, given the number of risk factors that Franklin had, he was a likely candidate to be frequented by the gout. And the gout repeatedly visited him.

## FRANKLIN'S GOUT ATTACKS

It is difficult to determine precisely when Franklin had his first encounter with gout, but he tells us he did have attacks when he was in his mid-fifties. They were fairly mild at first, lasting only a few days. On November 11, 1762, for example, he wrote a letter from London to his sister Jane Mecom in which he said that he was well except for "a little Touch of the gout."[24] And in 1767 he told Philadelphia physician Cadwalader Evans: "I thank you for your Remarks on the Gout. They may be useful to me who have already had some Touches of that Distemper."[25]

In his letter to Evans, he also wrote about what gout had done to William Pitt: "As to Lord Chatham [Pitt], it is said that his Constitution is totally destroy'd and gone, partly thro' the violence of the Disease, and partly by his own continual Quacking with it."[26] Indeed, Pitt, who would strongly oppose the way his government would go on to treat the colonists, became so incapacitated by his gout that he would have to miss some crucial legislative sessions, including those when the Stamp Act and the tea tax were passed. It has been suggested that, had it not been for Pitt's gout, England might not have lost the North American colonies when it did.[27]

In 1770, between the Stamp Act and the Boston Tea Party, Franklin complained to Debby about the return of his gout, "from which I had been free Five Years." "My Foot swelled greatly, and I was confined about three weeks," he told her.[28] Sympathetic to what he might have been feeling, she responded: "I only wish I was near aneuef to rub it with a lite hand."[29]

Franklin's gout was growing worse, and he suffered additional painful attacks before he headed home from England. Once back in Philadelphia, he was plagued by it while he and John Adams were trying to help Thomas Jefferson draft the Declaration of Independence. In a letter to George Washington dated June 21, 1776, Franklin explained: "I am just recovering from a severe Fit of the Gout which has kept me from Congress and Company almost ever since you left us, so that I know little of what has pass'd there, except that a Declaration of Independence is preparing."[30]

Franklin's gout appeared to be in remission when he sailed off to France on October 27, 1776, at age seventy. Unfortunately, it returned with a vengeance in 1777. A postscript at the end of a long personal letter from February 1777 reads: "A Fit of the Gout which has confin'd me 5 Days, and made me refuse to see any Company, has given me a little time to trifle."[31] But by April, we find his nephew Jonathan Williams, Jr., beginning a letter to him with the statement "I . . . am happy to find that you are recovered from the Gout."[32]

The gout struck again in 1779, the very year in which John Adams and Arthur Lee were recalled and Franklin became sole minister plenipotentiary to France. Franklin repeatedly had to excuse himself from going to Versailles because of the "G."[33] The most significant cancellation came when he was expected to present his ministerial documents to Louis XVI. He explained to Gabriel de Sartine, the French naval minister: "I was then so ill with the Gout and a Fever, that I could neither write nor think of anything. This necessarily prevented my Attending at Court."[34]

Falling behind in his correspondence, he would continue to make comparable statements, one being "I have been long ill, and unfit to write or think of writing."[35] On March 14th, he sent yet another apologetic note to the Comte de Vergennes, who was hoping Franklin would now be able to present his credentials as minister plenipotentiary. "The Gout having again attacked me, and confined me to my Chair, I find I shall not be able to present myself at Versailles on Tuesday. Your Excellency will have the goodness to excuse me."[36] Three days later, he lamented: "I don't complain much even of the Gout, [but] there seems however some Incongruity in a *Pleni-potentiary* who can neither stand nor go."[37]

It was not until March 23 that Franklin was finally able to travel to Versailles to present his credentials to the king. In a letter written to John Adams, he described the ordeal: "My Gout continued to disable me from walking longer than formerly; but on Tuesday the 23rd past, I thought myself able to go through the Ceremony and accordingly went to Court, had my Audience with the King in the new Character, presented my Letter of Credence, and was received very graciously. After which I went the Rounds with the other Foreign Ministers, in visiting all the Royal Family. The Fatigue however was a little too much for my Feet, and disabled me for near another Week."[38]

During the fall of 1780, Franklin's gout flared up again. Temple now took dictation from his grandfather, beginning the letters with words such as, "My Grandfather is laid up with the Gout & cannot write," and "My Grandfather who is still obliged to keep his Bed and unable to write."[39] Even when Franklin was able to do a little writing, it was from his bed. As he explained to John Adams: "I have other Letters from your Excellency to answer, which I must at present postpone, as I continue ill with the Gout, and write this in my Bed with Difficulty."[40]

Finally, during the last week of 1780, he was able to return to Versailles. Nevertheless, he was in pain and found it agonizing to go up and down the palace stairs. His feet remained so tender over the next few weeks that, when he was obligated to return to the palace, he conducted his business in minimal time, did not partake in "other" events, avoided the stairs as one would an instrument of the Spanish Inquisition, and remained seated whenever possible.

## DIALOGUES WITH "M. GOUT"

Franklin, as we have seen, fully understood the causal relationships between rich foods and abundant wines and the gout. The problem he faced was that his lifestyle changed as he rose to prominence. He was able to heed Poor

Richard's advice early on, but by the time he was deeply involved with politics, club life in England, and the salons of France, Poor Richard, with his wisdom of the ages, was largely forgotten or ignored by "Dr. Fatsides," his now pudgy creator.

"The Roman gourmands found their equals in the gluttonous and bibulous English gentry of the eighteenth and nineteenth centuries," wrote one gout historian. "They had no idea of temperance. . . . The diet of upper-class Englishman consisted largely of meat and port."[41] In France, with its social morays, rich foods, and wine drinking, following Poor Richard's dictates was virtually impossible. This is not to imply that Franklin strove to match the English and French aristocrats when it came to fancy dining. Typically, he did not. But he was also mindful of the company he kept and understood the local customs, and what he consumed would still be staggering by today's standards.

Franklin's wine cellar contained 1,040 bottles in 1779 and 1,203 bottles by 1782. As for his dinner table, it often overflowed with mutton, veal, beef, hors d'oeuvres, cheeses, butter, pastries, bonbons, and other sweets. For the most part, the best he could do was cut back when his gout flared up. Still, Franklin never lost his sense of humor, especially when discussing his infirmity with Madame Brillon, his witty and playful female confidant, with whom he tried to dine once or twice a week.

It was while he was unable to leave his rooms in Passy that he wrote one of his most self-effacing and funniest pieces. Originally composed in French, he sent his bagatelle with his compliments to his charming neighbor. Madame Brillon, in turn, found it amusing, but gave it back to him with some grammatical corrections. The bagatelle's original title was *Dialogue Entre La Goutte et M. F.*, and the stimulus for it was some related poetry that Madame Brillon had, in fact, just sent to Franklin.[42] In her *Le Sage et la Goutte*, which was penned while she was confined with her own *maladie des nerfs* (nervous disorder), Madame Brillon took aim at her famous neighbor's indolence, lifestyle, and amorous disposition. More than just poking fun at the sage next door, her intent might have been to motivate Franklin to take better care of himself without sounding like a parent scolding a misbehaving child.

Historically, Madame Brillon's piece fits into a fairly long line of poetry and cartoons that have poked gentle fun at gout sufferers and their rather "comic disease."[43] Her verses, however, are more amusing than most, because she could not have found a more vulnerable target than Franklin, who loved humor and was not above laughing at his shortcomings and problems, even when they hurt.

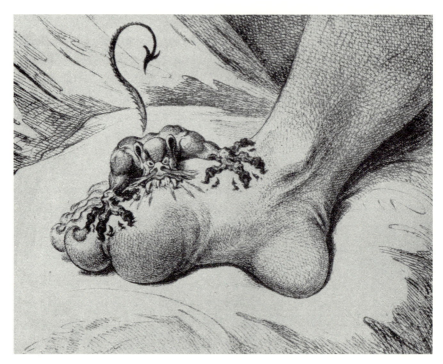

*"Personal Reminiscence," a late eighteenth-century cartoon by James Gilray.*


Translated into English as *The Philosopher and the Gout*, Madame Brillon's verses read:

> The Gout, a fearful plague without a cure,
> Took lodging in a sage and felt quite sure
> Of making him dispair. He *did* complain,
> (Wisdom can't help too much when you're in pain.
> You just don't listen)—but in the end
> Wisdom won out. My philosophic friend
> Started to reason suavely with his Gout.
> Each tried to win a philosophic bout.
> "Dear Doctor," said the Gout. "You must agree
> Prudence is not your strongest point. I see
> You eat too much, you pass the time with dames,
> You hate to take a walk; your long chess games,
> Your drinking and flirtations take up time

And dissipate your powers—it's a crime.
In stopping this I'm doing you a favor.
You should say, 'Thanks friend. You're a life-saver!'"


The sage asserted: "Love can do no wrong
And, softening stern Reason, keeps us young.
I love, I've always loved, I'll always be in love.
And someone still loves me. Heavens above!
Am I to pass my days in dull privation?
No, no. Wisdom must always rest
In relishing the gifts wherein we're blessed.
A glass of punch, a pretty mistress, maybe two
Or three or four—my wife forgave me, why don't you?
Any fair lady I can still delight
Shall not escape me while I stand upright.
Success in chess makes the game amusing,
But I lose interest quickly when I'm losing.
The food renounces pleasures undiminished,
The wise man gives the game up when it's finished."[44]

Franklin did not question the roles of overeating or drinking too much in triggering his attacks of gout, but he questioned whether sexual activity also contributed to the malady, as had once been contended by Galen. In a return letter to Madame Brillon he made the exact opposite case, albeit in jest. He wrote: "One of the characters of your Fable, Madame La Goutte, seems to me to reason pretty well, except when she supposes that Mistresses have had a share in producing this painful Malady. I, for one, believe the exact opposite; and here is my argument. When I was a young man and enjoyed more of the favors of the sex than I do at present, I had no gout. *Hence,* if the ladies of Passy had shown more of that Christian charity that I have so often recommended to you in vain, I should not be suffering from the Gout right now."[45]

Franklin soon began to compose his own *Dialogue Entre La Goutte et M.F.*[46] Setting the stage for the Gothic horror books that would follow, M.F., or Monsieur Franklin, dated his piece "Midnight, the twenty-second of October, 1780." Could the dreaded Gout make its grand appearance at any time other than midnight?

From the Gout's perspective, because of Franklin's miserable lifestyle, with its rich foods, abundant wine, and paucity of exercise—but certainly not from too much sex—the American minister to France was deserving of the worst possible torture. That he was approaching eighty did not matter to the Gout, who was unable to sympathize with a cranky old philosopher whose words and promises rang hollow. The mini-masterpiece opens with Franklin groaning "Eh! Oh! Eh! What have I done to deserve these cruel sufferings?" The Gout's response: "Many things; you have ate and drank too freely, and too much indulged those legs of yours in their indolence."

"Who is it that accuses me?" asks Franklin. And the voice replies, "It is I . . . the Gout." The issue quickly turns to whether the foreboding voice is that of a friend or a foe. Franklin insists the Gout has to be regarded as his enemy, "for you would not only torment my body to death, . . . you reproach me as a glutton and a tippler." The Gout, of course, could not see things more differently. "What may be fine for a man who takes a reasonable amount of exercise would be too much food and wine for another who scarcely moves," Franklin was told. Groaning, the decrepit philosopher insists his desk job limits what he can do, but his adversary will hear none of it. "If your situation in life is a sedentary one, your amusements, your recreations, at least, should be active," insists the Gout. "But let us examine your course of life."

In this context, the Gout admits that the American diplomat was, in fact, tied to his desk part of the day. But, Franklin is reminded, he masterfully avoided exercising even when he had the opportunity to break away. Instead, "you amuse yourself, with books, pamphlets, or newspapers, which for the most part are not worth the reading. Yet you eat an inordinate breakfast, four dishes of tea, with cream, and one or two buttered toasts, with slices of hung beef; which I fancy are not things the most easily digested." After a large dinner, instead of walking, his unsympathetic antagonist continues, "you play hours of chess and wrapt in the speculations of this wretched game, you destroy your constitution." Hence, "What can be expected from such a course of living, but a body replete with stagnant humours, ready to fall prey to all kinds of dangerous maladies, if I, the Gout, did not occasionally bring you relief by agitating those humours, and so purifying or dissipating them?"

Twitching and groaning in pain, Franklin still wants to differ. "It is not fair to say I take no exercise, when I do very often, going out to dine and returning in my carriage." Amused at such a pathetic retort, the Gout fires back with logic reminiscent of what Franklin had once written to his son William on the subject of exercising (see Chapter 2):

That, of all imaginable exercises, is the most slight and insignificant. . . . By observing the degree of heat obtained by different kinds of motion, we may form an estimate of the quantity of exercise given by each. Thus, for example, if you turn out to walk in winter with cold feet, in an hour's time you will be in a glow all over; ride on horseback, the same effect will scarcely be perceived by four hours' round trotting; but if you loll in a carriage, such as you have mentioned, you may travel all day, and gladly enter the last inn to warm your feet at a fire. Flatter yourself then no longer, that half an hour's airing in your carriage deserves the name exercise. Providence has appointed few to roll in carriages, while he has given all a pair of legs . . . be grateful, then, and make proper use of yours.

The Gout continues, now sounding more like a well-trained physician, with the words: "Would you like to know how they forward the circulation of your fluids, in the very action of transporting you from place to place; observe when you walk, that all your weight is alternately thrown from one leg to the other; this occasions a great pressure on the vessels of the foot, and repels their contents; when relieved, by the weight being thrown on the other foot, the vessels of the first are allowed to replenish, and, by a return of this weight, this repulsion again succeeds; thus accelerating the circulation of the blood. The heat produced in any given time, depends on the degree of this acceleration; the fluids are shaken, the humors attenuated, the secretions facilitated, and all goes well; the cheeks are ruddy, and health is established."

After presenting Franklin with a litany of his sins and listening to his feeble replies, the Gout returns to the theme of being his worthy physician. While Franklin reels in pain, the Gout asks: "Is it not I who, in the character of your physician, have saved you from the palsy, dropsy, and apoplexy? one or another of which would have gone for you long ago, but for me."

Franklin submits, admitting that the Gout might serve as his protector from far worse fates. But he humbly begs for no additional help from such a truly wonderful friend. He even argues that he has been a protector of his adversary, never turning to any physician or quack to fight against the Gout's presence. The Gout, not lost for words, fires back: "As to quacks, I despise them, they may kill you indeed, but cannot injure me. And, as to regular physicians, they are at least convinced that the gout, in such a subject as you are, is no disease, but a remedy."

The bewildered, beaten philosopher, now writhing in pain, can only beg for mercy. "Oh! Oh!—for Heaven's sake leave me! and I promise faithfully never more to play at chess, but to take exercise daily, and live temperately." But the Gout knows this victim all too well and replies: "You promise fair;

but, after a few months of good health, you will return to your old habits; your promises will be forgotten like the forms of last year's clouds." The dialogue ends with the Gout gloating triumphantly and getting in the last word: "I leave you with the assurance of visiting you again at a proper time and place; for my object is your good, and you are sensible now that I am your *real friend*."[47]

## FRANKLIN'S GOUT TREATMENTS

Madame Brillon's fable and Franklin's bagatelle again bring up the question of whether the gout should be regarded as a friend or a foe—is it a disorder to be dreaded or a protector from a far worse fate? Franklin had, in fact, asked his physicians the same question about his "Scurf" (see Chapter 16). In a letter written to his sister Jane the year before he composed his bagatelle, Franklin wrote of the gout: "I think it is not settled among Physicians whether that is a Disease or a Remedy."[48]

Perhaps more than any other disorder, many highly respected men of medicine in the eighteenth century thought the gout "was a mascot, talisman, or charm, a disorder inoculating against the worst."[49] Thomas Sydenham, who in the previous century had maintained that when conditions favor one disease a deadlier enemy might be put in abeyance, still remained very influential. And this belief had significant repercussions. Some people, fearing a worse disease, tried to contract gout. For those without the money to buy rich foods and abundant wine, there was always bathing in waters frequented by gout sufferers.[50] A second repercussion was that the true believers did not try to cure their gout; they only wanted to tone it down and do what had to be done to be more comfortable with it as a companion.

Franklin pondered the protection theory, which his personal physicians either endorsed or were unwilling to dismiss. At times, it seemed supported by his own experience. During the summer of 1770, for example, a bothersome swelling and inflammation in his throat disappeared when his gout flared up. And in 1788, he would tell Jan Ingenhousz that, "as these swellings increased and extended, the other malady [scurf] diminished, and at length disappeared entirely."[51] So perhaps "the Gout is one of the Greatest Blessings that can Befal Mortal Man," as stated in the subtitle of the book Franklin published when he was just twenty-six. With the possibility that the gout might be a "real friend," he was not willing to treat his condition aggressively, although he did submit to limited bloodletting and some purging to try to bring it under control on several occasions.

The advice that physician William Cadogan spelled out in his *Dissertation on the Gout* from 1771 appeared to make some sense to Franklin.[52] Cadogan attributed gout to learned habits, not heredity, and he recommended three Galenic non-naturals for it: a plain and sensible diet, a reasonable amount of exercise, and peace of mind. Like Sydenham, Cadogan saw no need to call for painful, dangerous, and usually ineffective medicines—and neither did Franklin.

Although he joked about it in his bagatelle, Franklin did try to moderate his eating and drinking when he had attacks. Additionally, he turned to exercise when his gout allowed him to do so. In the fall of 1780, for example, he began his rehabilitative exercise program by walking with a pair of newly purchased crutches. Once he was able to discard his crutches, he walked rapidly for an hour a day.[53]

He also tried to find gentle ways to reduce his pain, while letting Nature run her course and accepting the protection package offered by the gout. He described one of his experiments from the summer of 1780 in a letter to Alexander Small.

Finding one night that my foot gave me more pain after it was covered warm in bed, I put it out of bed naked; and perceiving it easier, I let it remain longer than I at first designed, and at length fell asleep leaving it there till morning. The pain did not return, and I grew well. Next winter having a second attack, I repeated the experiment; not with such immediate success in dismissing the gout, but constantly with the effect of rendering it less painful, so that it permitted me to sleep every night.

I should mention that it was my son who gave me the first intimation of this practice. He being in the old opinion that the gout was to be drawn out by transportation. And having heard me say that perspiration was carried on more copiously when the body was naked than when clothed, he put his foot out of bed to increase that discharge, and found ease by it, which he thought a confirmation of the doctrine. But this method requires to be confirmed by more experiments, before one can conscientiously recommend it.[54]

Even in his mid-seventies, Franklin was still the medical experimentalist, and still very much aware that single case studies, even on his own body, could be no more than suggestive.

Franklin did not go on to comment on hydrotherapy, a growing fad in the late eighteenth century. In England, taking the mineral waters at Bath was popular among well-to-do gout sufferers, and there were numerous places to go for the water cure on the European continent, such as Spa in Belgium, where Mesmer first resided after leaving France. But taking the water cure was time consuming, and William Heberden, the highly regarded English physician with whom Franklin had worked on smallpox inoculations, did not believe that bathing in spa water did any good in arthritic and gouty cases. "The most perfect cures, of which I have been a witness," stressed Heberden, "have been effected by a total abstinence from spirits and wine, and flesh."[55]

Nothing Franklin did was intended to completely protect him from future attacks. He even presented his recurrent attacks of gout as a principal reason for him to be replaced minister plenipotentiary:

I must now beg leave to say something relating to myself; a Subject with which I have not often troubled the Congress. I have pass'd my 75th Year, and I find that the long & severe Fit of the Gout which I had last Winter, has shaken me exceedingly, and I am yet far from having recovered the bodily Strength I before enjoy'd. I do not know that my mental Faculties are impair'd; perhaps I shall be the last to discover that; but I am sensible of a great Diminution in my Activity; a Quality I think particularly necessary in your Minister for this Court. I am afraid therefore that your Affairs may some time or other suffer by my Deficiency. . . . I have been engag'd in publick Affairs, and enjoy'd public Confidence in some Shape or other, during the long Term of fifty Years, an Honour sufficient to satisfy any reasonable Ambition, and I have no other left, but that of Repose, which I hope the Congress will grant me, by sending some Person to supply my Place.[56]

Congress refused Franklin's request, and he spent several more years serving his country in France, despite the ups and increasing downs of his gout.

## DR. FRANKLIN AND COLCHICUM

One of the questions that some medical historians have asked is whether Franklin tried colchicum in France or anywhere else for his gout. Colchicum, as noted earlier, has been used since ancient times to treat gout and arthritic diseases, and it still considered an effective drug for treating gout. Several writers have suggested that Franklin observed and tried "the wine of colchicum" in Europe, achieving beneficial effects. Moreover, the claim has been made in print that he was the first person to introduce and recommend colchicum to his gouty friends in America.[57]

Nevertheless, not everybody agrees with these assertions, and critics point out that colchicum would have been hard to find on a British apothecary's shelf when Franklin was there.[58] This was largely due to Thomas Sydenham's negative opinion of it, because it was so harsh on the stomach. Further, William Cullen, the most popular teacher in Edinburgh, did not even mention colchicum in his books, including his *Practice of Physic,* which contained a thirty-five-page chapter on gout.

Colchicum did, however, begin a revival in Franklin's lifetime. In 1763, it was "rediscovered" by Baron Anton von Störck, the personal physician of Empress Maria Theresa and head of the Medical Clinic in Vienna. But the influential Störck recommended *Colchicum autumnale* as a diuretic useful for dropsy, not as an agent for gout or arthritis. In 1770, Nicholas Husson patented his *eau d'Husson* as a cure for many diseases, specifically pointing to its excellent effects with arthritic problems.[59] But Husson did not tell anyone that colchicum was the critical ingredient in his formula, and this remained a well-kept secret until well after Franklin's death.[60]

Still, the best evidence of all that Franklin did not use and help popularize colchicum comes from his letters. There is no mention of him knowingly or unknowingly trying it. Further, he told fellow gout sufferer Benjamin Vaughan, in just so many words, that he never had been inclined to try medications, much less patented medicines, for his gout. "I let it take its Course," he informed Vaughan, who had just told him about a new medication.[61]

In summary, Franklin's writings indicate that the way in which he dealt with his gout was fairly consistent with the popular belief, which he never seemed to reject, that the painful disorder could have a beneficial side to it. For this reason, and perhaps because he was so skeptical about new medications and some of the older treatments, he did not turn to the apothecaries to cure his gout. Instead, he tried to manage or control his gout via the Galenic non-naturals: moderating his diet, reducing his wine intake, and doing some basic exercises. In other words, Franklin's main objective was only to convince his so-called "friend" that there was really nothing to be gained by causing him quite so much agony. At the least, the gout should have the consideration to take into account that he also had to contend with a painful bladder stone during the final years of his life.

# CHAPTER 18

# A Debilitating Stone

Being now disabled by the Stone, which in the Easiest Carriage
gives me Pain, wounds my bladder, and occasions me to make
bloody Urine, I find I can no longer pay my Devoirs personally at
Versailles.

—Benjamin Franklin, 1783

In 1785, when Franklin finally received the permission he had long sought to
return home, his movements were severely restricted, not just by his gout but
because of a large kidney stone. He was no longer able to walk even moderate distances, he could not ride a horse, and he could not even handle the
bumping of a carriage ride to Paris without being subjected to intense pain.
So how was he going to make his way from Passy to the coast, where the
ocean-going ships were docked?

Franklin first thought that he might be able to float down the Seine River
on a barge. But the dry summer weather lowered the river's water level and
precluded what would have been the most comfortable of realistic options.
His backup idea was to ride in a litter slung between two large pack animals,
which is what he eventually made up his mind to do. "I found that the motion
of the litter, lent me by the Duke of Coigny, did not much incommode me,"
he would later write. "It was one of the Queen's, carried by two large mules,
the muleteer riding another."[1] And so it was that Franklin made his way to
the French coast, where he boarded a ship to England and then, after a short
stay on land, sailed west to Philadelphia.

In this chapter, we shall look in some detail at Franklin's experience with
stones, and more particularly at the large stone that increasingly immobilized
him. Like gout, stones have a long history. And, as was true for the gout,
Franklin knew a lot about this disorder and possible treatments for it before
he experienced his own problems.

## AN ANCIENT DISORDER

Human remains show that people suffered from urinary stones in antiquity.[2] Early writings further reveal that the ancients had some very specific ideas about what caused them. Greeks at the time of Hippocrates, for example, believed that they were created by the buildup of solid matter in the bladder stemming from impure, muddy waters.

One of the remedies handed down by the Greeks is lithotomy, which literally means "stone removal." Physicians taking the Hippocratic oath would swear, "I will not use the knife, not even on sufferers from the stone, but will withdraw in favor of such men as are engaged in this work."[3] The Hippocratic physicians were not alone. Throughout most of western history, bladder stone removal was considered beneath the dignity of erudite physicians, and hence was left for lithotomists, a lower class of craftsmen that specialized in the art. During the period immediately following Alexander the Great's conquests, lithotomies were performed in Alexandria, Egypt. Ammonius of Alexandria, who practiced approximately 230 B.C., was nicknamed "Lithotomus," or stone cutter. He used a knife and a hook, and, when necessary, first broke the bothersome stones with a blunt-ended instrument, in order to remove them with less difficulty.

Nevertheless, it was not until the first century A.D. that there is a good written description of how to remove a bladder stone with a hook or a finger through an incision. In his authoritative *De re medicina*, Celsus described what to do, but recommended the bladder operation only for patients between nine and fourteen years of age. Like others before him, he advised strongly against trying to operate for kidney stones.

The ancient technique used by Celsus and others for removing bladder stones did not undergo major refinement until the sixteenth century.[4] But high surgical mortality due to infection remained a significant drawback, even after better procedures and improved instruments were developed. This may be one reason why Ambroise Paré, the most innovative barber-surgeon of the Renaissance, probably did not perform the operation himself. Paré did, however, write a chapter on lithotomy in 1564, and he included illustrations showing the surgical technique and the instruments to be used.[5]

Physicians became more skilled in diagnosing urinary stones, determining their locations, and in treating them during Franklin's era. One need only consult the writings of William Heberden, who Franklin had worked with to produce a pamphlet on smallpox inoculations in 1759 (see Chapter 3).[6] Along with other physicians, Heberden knew that the ideal remedy was to have his

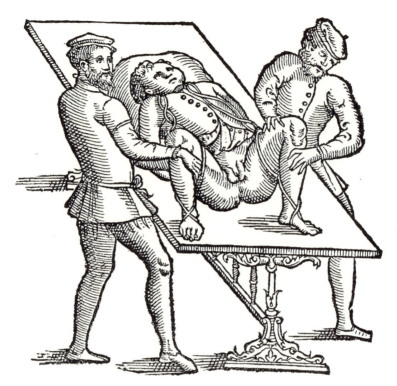

*A man ready to be cut for the stone, as depicted by the French surgeon Paré in 1564. (From Eric W. Riches, "Some Landmarks in the Surgery of Stone,"* Journal of British Urological Surgeons 7 *[1938]: 140–147.)*

patients to pass their stones with their urine. Hence, he first suggested dietary changes and gentle oral medications. If this approach did not work, he tried to dissolve the stone with washes. But here Heberden was more cautious, and he questioned the effectiveness of injecting lime water (calcium hydroxide) and soap into the urinary system. Surgery was the last resort for Heberden, because of the risk of infection and other complications. Franklin, as we shall now see, was in full agreement.

### THE FLEXIBLE CATHETER

It is hard to know for sure whether a propensity for stones was common in Franklin's family, but at least one family member suffered from them. On September 6, 1744, Benjamin Franklin sent a letter to his father and mother in Boston. "I apprehend I am too busy in prescribing, and meddling in the Dr's

Sphere, when any of you complain of Ails in your Letters," he began. "But as I always employ a Physician my self when any Disorder arises in my Family and submit implicitly to his Orders in every Thing, so I hope you will consider my Advice, when I give any, only as a Mark of my good Will, and put no more of it in Practice than happens to agree with what your Dr. directs."[7]

The issue behind these sobering words was how a family member should be treated for stones. The Boston Franklins had already been given some advice, which they passed on to Benjamin in Philadelphia. One suggestion, and a method of choice at the time, was to try lye or soapy solutions to dissolve the deposits. In this domain, Joanna Stephens's once secret and highly touted recipe for the stone had to be considered.[8] It contained eggshells, snails, and soap. Knowing about it, Benjamin Franklin's letter home continued:

Your Notion of the Use of Strong Lee [lye] I suppose may have a good deal in it. The Salt of Tartar, or Salt of Wormwood, frequently prescrib'd as for cutting, opening and cleansing is nothing more than the Salt of Lee procur'd by Evaporation. Mrs. Stephen's Medicine for the Stone and Gravel, the Secret of which was lately purchas'd at a great Price by the Parliament, has for its principle Ingredient, Soap, which Boerhave [sic] calls the most universal Remedy. The same Salt intimately mix'd with Oil of Turpentine, which you also mention, makes the *Sapa Philosophorum*, wonderfully extoll'd by some Chymists, for like Purposes. 'Tis highly probable (as your Dr. says) that Medicines are much alter'd in passing between the Stomach and Bladder; but such Salts seem well fitted in their Nature to pass with the least Alteration of almost any thing we know. And if they will not dissolve Gravel and Stone, yet I am half persuaded that a moderate Use of them may go a great Way towards preventing those Disorders.[9]

Franklin also suggested some remedies that could be found in the kitchen and tasted good, namely honey and molasses. He hypothesized that syrups, often used as stool softeners, might prevent the aggregation of urinary deposits. "As to Honey and Melasses," he wrote, "I did not mention them merely as Openers and Looseners, but also from a Conjecture that as they are heavier in themselves than our common Drink, they might when dissolved in our Bodies, encrease the specific Gravity of our Fluids, the Urine in particular, and by that means keep separate and suspended therein those Particles which when united form gravel, &c."[10]

Last, he raised the possibility of using ginseng root, which was popular in Chinese medicine and was known to his botanist friend John Bartram. "I will enquire after the Herb you mention: We have a botanist here, an intimate Friend of mine, who knows all the plants in the Country. He . . . has twice thro' my Hands sent Specimens of the famous Chinese Ginseng, found here, to Persons who desired it in Boston."[11]

The afflicted family member appeared to be his brother John, the first son from Josiah's marriage to Abiah Folger. Franklin asked his parents to share this information with "Br. John" near the end of his 1744 letter. John was fifty-four years old at the time and living in nearby Rhode Island. Eight years later, John received a letter from his brother in Philadelphia telling him that he would do everything in his power to help him deal with his stones.[12] Part of this letter dealt again with the use of lime water. "I have read Whytt on Lime Water," Benjamin told him, referring to Edinburgh physician Robert Whytt's 1743 essay on the subject, which had just been updated.[13] "You desire my thoughts on what he says. But what can I say? He relates Facts and Experiments; and they must be allow'd good, if not contradicted by other Facts and Experiments."[14]

Franklin's statements are notable because they show his breadth of medical knowledge well before leaving Philadelphia for Europe, and because they reflect his empirical approach to medicine. The most remarkable part of his letter, however, had nothing to do with lime water or Whytt. Rather, it had to do with the construction of a flexible catheter. "Reflecting yesterday on your Desire to have a flexible Catheter, a Thought stuck into my Mind as to how one might possibly be made," he wrote. And he informed John that he "went immediately to the Silversmith's and gave Directions for making one (sitting by 'till it was finish'd), that it might be ready for this Post." Nevertheless, Franklin was a bit uneasy about the device he was sending, so he offered John some brotherly advice.

But now it is done I have some Apprehensions that it may be too large to be easy: if so, a Silversmith can easily make it less by turning it on a smaller Wire, and putting a smaller Pipe to the End, if the Pipe be really necessary. This Machine may either be cover'd with a small fine Gut . . . or perhaps it may be used without the Gut, having only a little Tallow rubb'd over it, to smooth it and fill the Joints.

I think it is as flexible as could be expected in a thing of the kind. . . . The tube is of such a Nature, that when you have Occasion to withdraw [it] its Diameter will lessen, whereby it will move more easily. It is also a kind of Scrue, and may be both withdrawn and introduc'd by turning. Experience is necessary for the right using of all new Tools or Instruments, and that will perhaps suggest some Improvements to this Instrument as well as better direct the Manner of Using it.[15]

Urinary catheters were by no means new in 1752. Bronze catheters were mentioned by Celsus and have been found in the rubble of Pompeii.[16] The early metal catheters, however, were stiff, difficult to insert, and extremely uncomfortable. Consequently, physicians had long been trying to come forth with better instruments. The first flexible catheters might have been made of animal skins treated with agents to make them firm enough for insertion after lubrication. Avicenna, who lived in the eleventh century, mentioned a device of this nature. Fabricius ab Acquapendente, who resided in Italy early in the seventeenth century, tried using horn that would soften when left in place, as well as a tube of cloth impregnated with wax. But these innovations still left a lot to be desired.

During the late 1600s, a Dutch surgeon named Van Solingen made a flexible catheter of wound silver wire that was covered with soft animal skin and treated with wax. Francesco Roncalli-Parolino, early in Franklin's own century, took the next step when he covered a thin spiral tube with fine skin and later silk. Unfortunately, we do not encounter any mention of the new European devices or the names of their inventors or promoters in any of Franklin's writings. Nor are there pictures. Hence, it is almost impossible to know just how much the device he made for John resembled the instruments previously designed by others, or the sources he relied on for its basic construction. Whether Franklin was the person who introduced the flexible catheter in the colonies also remains an open question. The case in favor of Franklin rests on the absence of solid contradictory evidence. But he never claimed that the instrument he had made was the first flexible catheter to be used in America, or even the first one to be constructed in the colonies.

The medical part of the letter to his brother ends with Franklin candidly stating, "I know not what to advise, either as to the Injection or the Operation." By "the Injection," Franklin was alluding to attempts to treat the stone by injecting liquids containing lye into the urethra, with the hope that they could dissolve the stone. But what about the possibility of operating? Historians tell us that an apothecary-surgeon by the name of Sylvester Gardiner, who had been trained by William Cheselden in London, demonstrated how to remove bladder stones to Boston practitioners in 1741.[17] Thus surgery was a viable option for John in 1752. But two factors precluded operating. One was that the operation was still considered dangerous, and the other was that John was now in his sixties.

A letter from Benjamin to his brother, written in January 1753, suggests that John did show some near-term improvement without recourse to surgery. Written in response to a note John sent him in December, Benjamin wrote back that he was happy to be informed "that you are better and have reason to think the Stone either lessen'd or made smoother."[18] John Franklin passed away four years after his younger brother mailed him the flexible metal catheter, about which we know very little.

### BENJAMIN FRANKLIN'S STONES

It may seem ironic that Benjamin Franklin, who was so knowledgeable and tried to be so helpful when it came to helping John deal with his stones, would be tormented by a large stone of his own. But that is exactly what transpired. Thirty years after working on a flexible catheter for John, he found himself reeling from a stone that had lodged in his bladder.

In the interval between his work on the flexible catheter and his first comments about his own bladder stone in 1782, Poor Richard had printed some thoughts about stones. One, dated 1756, related stones to heartburn, indigestion, and unhealthy foods. Poor Richard's "Receipt against the HEART-BURN" reads: "The Heart-burn is an uneasy Sensation of Heat in the Stomach, occasioned by Indigestion, which is the Mother of Gout, Rheumatism, Gravel and Stone. *To prevent it,* Eat no Fat, especially what is burnt or oily; and neither eat or drink any thing sour or acid. *To cure it,* Dissolve a Thimble-full of Salt of Wormwood in a Glass of Water, and drink it."[19]

In numerous ways, Poor Richard's creator was a prime candidate for stones, because most stones are predominantly uric acid in composition. Hence, the risk factors mentioned in the previous chapter for gout also made Franklin vulnerable to stones. Prominent among his risk factors were his rich, meaty diet and love of wines, especially the fortified wines that had 18–20 percent alcohol and might have contained some kidney-damaging lead. Two additional factors mentioned in the context of his gout were his advancing age and his flaky skin condition, which is associated with rapid cell death that in turn can cause uric acid levels to rise. In addition to these factors, stones can run in some families and, as we have seen, at least one of his brothers had stones. Hence, Franklin might also have had a genetic propensity for the disorder, which could have made the other factors just mentioned even more significant in his case.

Additionally, as Franklin well knew, gout sufferers are much more likely to develop stones than people who have never had gout. Historians tell us this important association had been noted by Rufus of Ephesus early in the second century A.D., and by Paul of Aegina in the seventh century.[20] In the seventeenth century, physician Thomas Sydenham first had gout and began to reel from renal calculi a decade later. And Sydenham was by no means alone with gout being followed by stones.

Early in the eighteenth century, physician George Cheyne, who was born and trained in Scotland but practiced in London, wrote that chalk taken from the joints of gouty individuals seemed identical to the gravel stones found in the bladders of these patients. "They both have the same colour, taste and smell, and produce the same internal texture of parts, as far as can be known, and even the same outward shape."[21] Newer studies have, in fact, shown that uric acid-containing stones are some eleven times more likely to be found among gout suffers than among people who have never had gout.[22]

Hence, Franklin was a very good candidate for stones, especially late in his life. Prior to 1782, when his stones first really started to bother him, he seemed to have experienced some small urinary stones or "gravel," but nothing very serious. But in that year, one of his bladder stones began to torment him, and from his perspective its timing could not have been worse. To his horror, it would grow from the size of a small pea to about the size of a pigeon's egg eight years later.[23] This troublesome stone first put him in pain while he was conducting delicate peace negotiations with the British. Lord Sherburne, who represented the Crown, was told by Franklin's friend Benjamin Vaughan, then acting as an envoy, that he had found the American negotiator "very much indisposed this week with gravelly complaints, but today is somewhat better. In the warm bath he has for some days voided small stones."[24]

By mid-August, Franklin was no longer able to travel to Versailles from his home in Passy. The bumps in the roads he traveled by carriage were too much for him to bear. Rather than going to the French court himself, as was his custom on Tuesdays, he was confined to his house and had to ask his grandson Temple to represent him. On December 6, 1783, Franklin wrote apologetically to the Comte de Vergennes. "Being now disabled by the Stone, which in the Easiest Carriage gives me Pain, wounds my bladder, and occasions me to make bloody Urine, I find I can no longer pay my Devoirs personally at Versailles, which I hope will be excused."[25]

Exactly one month later, he philosophized about his medical condition to John Jay, who had served on the peace commission with him. "It is true, as you have heard, that I have the stone, but not that I had thoughts of being cut for it. It is as yet very tolerable. It gives me no pain but when in a Carriage or on the Pavement, or when I make some sudden quick movement. If I can prevent it growing larger, which I hope to do by abstemious living and gentle exercise, I can go on pretty comfortably with it to the end of my Journey, which can now be at no great distance."[26] Franklin also told Jay that he was not taking any special medicines for his stone: "I am cheerful, enjoy the company of my Friends, sleep well, have sufficient appetite, and my stomach performs well its Functions. The latter is very material to the preservation of Health. I therefore take no Drugs lest I should disorder it. You may judge that my Disease is not very grievous, since I am more afraid of the Medicines than of the Malady."[27]

Nevertheless, Franklin was human and, as his condition worsened, he slowly and reluctantly turned to drugs to help him deal with his stone and the pain it was causing. We know this from a letter sent to Jan Ingenhousz on April 29, 1785, in response to several inquiries that had gone unanswered. In his first paragraph, Franklin complained of the uneasiness caused by the stone: "I have been these 20 Months past afflicted with the Stone, which is always giving me more or less Uneasiness, unless when I am laid in Bed; and, when I would write, it interrupts my Train of Thinking, so that I lay down my Pen, and seek some light Amusement." He then explained that he was unable to travel by carriage to Vienna to visit with him, specifically because of his stone, calling it "an insuperable Obstruction to such a journey."

Franklin continued: "I have taken heretofore, and am now again taking the Remedy you mention, which is called *Blackrie's Solvent*. It is the Soap Lie, with Lime Water, and I believe it may have some Effect in diminishing the Symptoms, and preventing the Growth of the Stone, which is all I expect from it. It does not hurt my Appetite; I sleep well, and enjoy my Friends in chearful conversation as usual. But, as I cannot use much Exercise, I eat more sparingly than formerly, and I drink no wine."[28] In another letter we learn that he urged his nephew Jonathan Williams to go to Wilkie's in St. Paul's Churchyard to get him a copy of Alexander Blackrie's *A Disquisition upon Medicines that Dissolve the Stone*.[29]

Blackrie's formula has an interesting story behind it, one that starts with a physician from Bath by the name of Chittick. Early in the 1760s, Chittick devised a formula for treating deposits in the urinary tract, which he, like Joanna Stephens, preferred kept secret so as to control the market. His patients had to come to him with veal broth, and he personally mixed his secret ingredients into the broth. Blackrie, a chemist from Kent, was determined to discover Chittick's secret ingredient. His tests showed that Chittick's solution contained "alkaline fixed salts combined with quicklime, or soap lye." Blackrie was more altruistic than Chittick, and he published his findings in a 1763 issue of *Scots Magazine*.

Three years later, Blackrie published *A Disquisition upon Medicines that*

*Dissolve the Stone*.[30] An expanded version of his *Disquisition* appeared in 1771. Blackrie's instructions were to mix eight ounces of potash and four ounces of fresh quicklime in boiling soft spring water. The mixture had to be stirred occasionally and filtrated. He recommended oyster shell quicklime and noted that tartar salt may be even better than potash. Mixed in veal broth, between thirty drops twice daily and two teaspoons three times a day should be more than sufficient, he informed stone sufferers.

Medical physiology was in its infancy at this time and little was known about the complex nature of the urinary deposits or how to change the content of the urine. In particular, it was not recognized that, even if Franklin's stone had a core of uric acid, which it very likely had, it was also likely to have a coating of calcium and phosphate, which would not be materially affected by these oral alkaline medications.

Nevertheless, three physicians Franklin respected were among those who approved of Blackrie's solvent. They were John Pringle, John Fothergill, and William Hunter. William Heberden, who also bought Blackrie's book, would write: "Lime water has in many cases appeared to communicate a solvent power to the urine. Soap leys perhaps communicate a stronger solvent power to the urine; but it must be owned, that neither of them do so much as is wanted; their effect at best is very slow, and upon some stones they seem to have none at all; for immersed in the strongest undiluted soap leys they hardly seem to waste. But still if they hinder the growth of many stones, and loosen the texture of those already formed, and dissolve, as is probable, their sharp points, which are the chief causes of pain, they must be considered as valuable medicines."[31]

Unfortunately, Franklin was no better off as the winter passed and the sun again began to warm the gentle hills and valleys of Passy. On May 23, 1785, he complained to George Whatley, "I . . . now find at fourscore that three contraries have befallen me, being subject to the gout and the stone and not yet being master of all my passions. Like the proud girl in my country who wished and resolved not to marry a parson nor a Presbyterian nor an Irishman, and at length found herself married to an Irish Presbyterian parson."[32]

## THE NOTES AND THE RESPONSE

Franklin mailed Benjamin Vaughan a complete history of his case two months after sending his note about what happened to the proud girl to George Whatley. "The patient is now in his 79th year," he began.

In the Autumn of 1782, he had a severe Attack accompanied with what was thought to be a Gouty Pain in the Hyp. . . . He daily voided Gravel Stones the Size of small Pease, took now and then some Decoctions of Herbs & Roots that were prescribed him by Friends or Physicians, but persisted constantly in nothing except the Use of Honey at Breakfast instead of or sometimes with Butter on his Bread, he remembering to have heard in the Conversation of Physicians, Honey mentioned as of great Service in Gravelly Cases.

At length, the painful Part of the Disorder left him, and no more large Gravel offer'd; but observing Sand constantly in his Urine, he continued the use of the Honey to the Amount of perhaps a Pound per Week; notwithstanding which the Malady return'd in the Autumn of 1783, when he first perceived after going in his Carriage on the Pavement, that he felt Pain & made bloody Water. At times when he was making Water in full Stream, something came and stopt the Passage; this he suspected to be a small Stone, and he suffered pain by the Stoppage. He found however by Experience that he could by laying down on his Side cause the Obstruction to remove and continue the Operation. He now thinks the Stone is grown bigger & heavier as he is sensible of its falling from Side to Side, as he turns in his Bed.

He had made it a Rule for some Months to walk an hour in his Chamber every Night. This Exercise is of service to him in other Respects; but he has observed that if he has emptied his Bladder just before he begins his Walk, the Stone is apt to hurt him, and he makes bloody Water.

. . . He feels no Pain, nor is at all sensible of the Existence of the Stone, except when it obstructs his Making Water, or when he is in his Carriage on a Pavement, or on some sudden Motion or Turn of the Body; and he enjoys the Conversation of his Friends or his Books as usual.

Thus, if it does not grow worse, it is a *tolerable* Malady, and may be supported for the short time he has a Chance of living. And he would chuse to bear with it rather than have Recourse to dangerous or nauseous Remedies.

If therefore no safe and sure Dissolvent of the Stone is yet known, he wishes to be informed whether there is a Regimen proper to be observ'd for preventing its Increase, as he can without Difficulty conform to any Manner of Living that shall be prescrib's to him.

In the last attack no large Gravel has offer'd, and much less Sand appear'd in the Urine, whence he suspects that it attaches itself to the Stone. His Urine has however been unusually turbid till lately, when a Fit of the Gout came on, & swell'd both Feet, since which the Urine has been very clear.[33]

Franklin sent this formal description of his own case to Vaughan not just because Vaughan had studied medicine in Edinburgh, but because he was

friendly with some of London's most respected physicians. More than anything else, Franklin wanted him to share this information with them, anxious
to know what they might recommend.

As he hoped, Vaughan sprung into action. He showed what Franklin had
written to John Hunter, the leading London surgeon of the day, who had
known Franklin personally and as a fellow member of the Royal Society, and
to a second John Hunter, who practiced in London after receiving his M.D.
from Edinburgh in 1775. He also shared the information with Franklin's
physician friends William Heberden and William Watson, and with Adair
Crawford, then professor and physician to St. Thomas' Hospital.

Watson and the two Hunters met and wrote a single opinion. They began
by stating "From the History of the Case, and the distinct account of the
patient's feelings, we have no doubt that there is a Stone in the Bladder. Taking into consideration the Time of Life of the Patient, and that the Symptoms
are not so urgent as to render Life uncomfortable, we approve of his resolution not to risk an operation, or any course of Medicine that might endanger
his Health."

They went on to state that, "as the patient has already taken Blackrie's Lixivium with some advantage; we would advise him to continue it. . . . It has
some power as a Solvent, and if that should prove sufficient to prevent the farther increase of the Stone without at all diminishing it, it may procure great
relief; For, the painful effects of a stone on the Bladder, do not depend so
much upon size, as the roughness of its Surface, which arises from the constant accretion of new matter."

The three physicians agreed that there were certain other remedies that
might be tried if Blackrie's Lixivium did not help. One was "fixed air," or
carbon dioxide, in water, which originated from the work of Franklin's protégé Joseph Priestley. Another was *Uva Ursi*, or bear berries, a diuretic and
astringent that made the urine even more acid. Still other recommendations
were for laxatives and anodyne clysters to reduce the pressure on his bladder.

In terms of his daily routine, the trio of doctors told Franklin to continue
walking in his room, but to avoid all sudden and rough motions. They also
made it clear that he should watch his diet and daily intake of spirits. "In his
Diet we would advise the patient to avoid salt meats, spirits of all Kinds, pepper, and every thing that is in the smallest degree heating, as they increase the
pain in the bladder, and render it more sensible of any irritation of the Stone.
With regard to Wine, we would advise him never to exceed that quantity,
that habit may have rendered necessary, for the purposes of digestion. . . .
Broths of all kinds are well suited to the Patient's complaint, particularly

white Broths, made with Almonds, which are good for Diet and physick, being of an opening Nature."[34]

Heberden wrote that he concurred with his colleagues—that it would be foolish "to think of an operation at such an advanced age, but to trust wholly to the Levixium, if he can bear it." He also agreed that Franklin should "confine himself to his house and garden, and avoid all riding in Carriages."[35] Crawford's opinion was along the same lines: do not even think of surgery, try gentle remedies such as carbonated water and mild diuretics, use lime water if it can be handled, and employ gentle laxatives to keep the bowels open.

## BACK IN AMERICA

Despite the best efforts of the greatest medical minds of the day and Franklin's own insights, his large bladder stone failed to resolve. There were, however, periods of time in which it did not seem to grow more painful, even after he returned to Philadelphia. For example, during the summer of 1786, he informed Jan Ingenhousz: "My Malady, the Stone, indeed continues, but does not grow worse."[36] Similarly, in a letter to the Abbé de la Roche, he wrote: "My Health continues much in the same State as when I left France, my old malady not growing worse, so that I am able to go through a good deal of Business, and enjoy the Conversation of my Friends as usual."[37]

His letter to the Abbé included a light-hearted philosophical thought about why even good people get sick. "It grieves me to learn that you have been afflicted with Sickness. It is, as you say, the Condition of living, but it seems a hard Condition. I sometimes wonder that all good Men and Women are not by Providence kept free from Pain and Disease. In the best of all possible Worlds, I should suppose it must be so; and I am piously inclin'd to believe that this World's not being better made was owing merely to the Badness of the Materials."[38]

During the spring of 1787, he penned a note to his friend Le Veillard, who acquired a medical degree in 1764 and owned Les Nouvelles Eaux de Passy, a French mineral water business.[39] "As to my malady, concerning which you so kindly inquire, I have never had the least doubt of its being the stone," he told him. "I am sensible that it is grown heavier; but on the whole it does not give me more pain than when at Passy, and except in standing, walking, or making water, I am very little incommoded by it. Sitting or lying in bed I am generally quite easy, God be thanked; and as I live temperately, drink no wine, and use daily the exercise of the dumb-bell, I flatter myself that the stone is kept from augmenting so much as it might otherwise do, and that I may continue to find it tolerable."

Franklin ended his letter to Le Veillard with the words: "People who live long, who will drink of the cup of life to the very bottom, must expect to meet with the usual dregs, and when I reflect on the number of terrible maladies human nature is subject to, I think myself favoured in having to my share only the stone and the gout."[40]

With great respect for his acumen in the field of medicine, many people wanted to know what Dr. Franklin would recommend for their stones. One such person was the Comte de Buffon, who asked his advice in 1787. Franklin wrote back that he could only tell him what might prevent a stone from increasing, not how to dissolve a stone. "I have try'd all the noted Prescriptions for *diminishing* the Stone without perceiving any good Effect. But observing Temperance in Eating, avoiding Wine and Cyder, and using daily the Dumb Bell, which exercises the upper Part of the Body without much moving the Parts in contact with the Stone, I think have prevented its Increase."[41]

Franklin also told his correspondent about his jelly, molasses, and honey remedies, which he had recommended to his brother John more than four decades earlier. "As the Roughness of the Stone lacerates a little the Neck of the Bladder, I find, that when the Urine happens to be sharp, I have much pain in making Water and frequent Urgencies. For Relief under the circumstances, I take, going to Bed, the Bigness of a Pigeon's Egg of Jelly and Blackberries. The Receipt for making it is enclosed. While I continue to do this every Night, I am generally easy the day following, making Water pretty frequently, and with long intervals. I wish most sincerely that this simple Remedy may have the same happy Effect with you. Perhaps Current Jelly, or the Jelly of Apples or Raspberries, may be equally serviceable."[42]

It has been estimated that Franklin's stone might have occupied much of his bladder and weighed as much as five hundred grams, or more than a pound, in 1789.[43] In a letter to Alexander Small, who had passed a stone "as big as a kidney bean," Franklin mentioned that his stone was now enormous. He knew this "by the weight it falls with when I turn in bed." And with it being so large, he told Small, "I have no hope of it being dissoluble by any medicine; and am afraid of tampering."[44]

## FRANKLIN'S USE OF OPIUM

Franklin's inability to bear the increasing pain of his stone led him to try opium very late in his life. Opium was one of the drugs recommended by William Heberden for people with large, inoperable stones, although it came with a price. Franklin was aware of opium's side effects, which included dullness in high doses and emaciation with prolonged use. But the pain had become too hard to endure. On September 5, 1789, at the age of eighty-three, he explained to Le Veillard: "I have a long time been afflicted with almost constant and grievous Pain, to combat which I have been obliged to have recourse to Opium, which indeed has afforded me some Ease from time to time, but then it has taken away my Appetite and so impeded my digestion that I am become totally emaciated, and little remains of me but a Skeleton covered with Skin."[45]

Similar information was conveyed a few months later to Benjamin Vaughan, who thought hemlock might be worth a try. "I thank you much for your intimations of the virtues of hemlock," wrote Franklin, "but I have tried many things with so little effect, that I am quite discouraged, and have no longer any faith in remedies for the stone. The palliating system is what I am now fixed in. Opium gives me ease when I am attacked by pain, and by the use of it I still make life at least tolerable."[46]

Although opium can produce lethargy, especially with prolonged use, Franklin did not allow himself to lose touch with reality or to fall into a stupor. In fact, he took himself off opium when he finally had an opportunity to do so. We know this from a letter written to Jane Mecom on March 24, 1790. "I have been quite free from pain for near three weeks past," he told his sister, "and therefore, not being obliged to take any laudanum, my appetite has returned, and I have recovered some part of my strength. Thus I continue to live on, while all the friends of my youth have left me." Franklin ended his letter to the sibling he loved the most with the thought that he had been lucky to live so long and so well. "I do not repine at my malady, though a severe one," he told her, "when I consider how well I am provided with every convenience to palliate it, and to make me comfortable under it; and how many more horrible evils the human body is subject to; and what a long life of health I have been blessed with, free from them all."[47]

CHAPTER 19

# The Limits of Medicine

Wish not so much to live long as to live well.
—*Poor Richard's Almanack*, 1738

One of the most notable observations about Franklin in his senior years is just how sharp his intellect remained, as exemplified by the prosthetic devices and aids that he developed and his letters, including the highly informative epistle he sent to Benjamin Vaughan in 1786 on lead poisoning (see Chapter 11). His remarkable mental agility can also be gleaned from the numerous activities he turned to with the curiosity and enthusiasm of a much younger man. Even during his final transatlantic crossing, which he doubted he would ever be able to make, he immersed himself in natural philosophy. On some days, he measured water and air temperatures, and examined the grasses floating in the ocean—his early fascination with the Gulf Stream, which was like a warm river running over the colder ocean, having never left him. The same can be said about his interests in better ship designs and more efficient sails.

But health and medicine were never far from his mind, and while he was sailing steadily west he composed his long-awaited treatise on improving poorly designed stoves and fireplaces. Among the reasons Franklin gave for working on stoves, fireplaces, and ventilation systems was that many existing ones caused coughing, irritated eyes, and other health problems (see Chapter 10). In other words, the problem was not just fuel efficiency and economics; it was also a medical one with ties to better hygiene and fresh air. Thus, Franklin wrote about nine basic causes of smoky chimneys, and for each one he prescribed a number of specific solutions. He also committed to paper the basic principles upon which each remedy was based.

Philadelphia was more than ready for Franklin when his ship reached port on September 14, 1785. A faster ship had already brought the news that his vessel was off the coast, dispelling rumors that he had been captured by Barbary pirates and was now a slave in Morocco. In the diary of his voyage, Franklin wrote, "With the flood in the morning came a light breeze, which brought us above Gloucester Point, in full view of dear Philadelphia! ... My son-in-law came with a boat for us; we landed at Market Street wharf, where we were received by a crowd of people with huzzas, and accompanied with acclamations quite to my door. Found my family well."[1]

Honors, banquets, and ceremonies followed for a full week. But it took Franklin considerably less time than this to realize that he would not be able to spend his final years just reading, writing, and conversing about such things as smoky chimneys, Mesmerism, or how medical electricity was now viewed in Europe. Instead, he found himself asked to head a committee to draft a new state constitution almost immediately after arriving. He was then nominated to Pennsylvania's Executive Council, after which he was elected to the first of three one-year terms as President of the State of Pennsylvania. And, if this were not enough, he was elected to represent his state at the Constitutional Convention.

The Constitutional Convention lasted from May 28 to September 17, 1787, at the State House (later called Independence Hall), just a few city blocks from Franklin's home. Yet because of his bladder stone, even walking short distances on the streets produced more pain than he could bear. Hence, the senior delegate from Pennsylvania had to be transported to and from the State House in a sedan chair that he shipped over from Europe. It had flexible supporting rods that made for a fairly smooth ride. Four select prisoners from the Walnut Street Jail provided the power.

While inside the State House, Franklin spent almost all of his time in his seat, while the other delegates moved about to discuss issues with one another. He was about twice the age of the average delegate and was fifteen years older than the next oldest person at the convention. But he confirmed that Poor Richard had it right when his alter ego opined, "The Doors of Wisdom are never shut."[2] In addition to nominating George Washington to chair the convention, Franklin came forth with the compromise that kept the delegates with their various agendas from splitting apart. It called for two legislative bodies: a House of Representatives based on population, and a Senate that would represent all states equally.

In addition to meeting with delegates at the State House, Franklin invited members of the Constitutional Convention, other visitors, and friends to meet with him at his house or, during the warmer months, in his garden. Recognizing his difficulties moving about, a steady stream of visitors did just that. George Washington sat and conversed with him under his shady mulberry tree when he first arrived in Philadelphia in May 1787. Only after

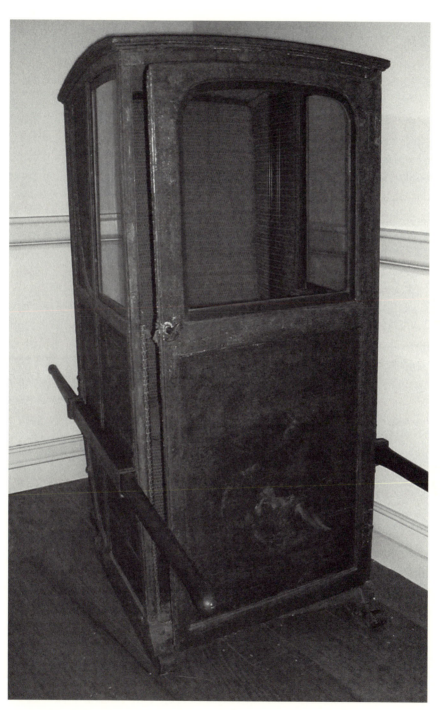

*Franklin's sedan chair*

paying his respects to America's ailing sage did Washington make his way to the nearby State House.

## INVOLVEMENT IN MEDICINE

When he was not engaged in politics, Franklin met with members of the American Philosophical Society and did his best to attend meetings of the organization he had helped to launch in 1743. For decades, he had collected books and papers from Europe for the society's growing library, including the latest works of John Pringle from England and Franz Anton Mesmer from France. While abroad, he had also nominated and supported many of his talented European medical friends for membership. And he had been president of the society since 1769, even though he had been an ocean away the great majority of the time.

The members of the American Philosophical Society were happy to see Franklin return to Philadelphia, and on September 27, 1785, they convened a special meeting to welcome him back in style. In short order, Franklin found himself making some new nominations for membership: French natural philosopher Le Roy, balloonist Jacques-Alexandre-César Charles, "physician of Auteuil" Georges Cabanis, English physician Thomas Percival, and his very close friend, physician to the Emperor of Austria, and fellow experimental natural philosopher, Jan Ingenhousz.

At the time of Franklin's return, many members of the American Philosophical Society wanted to reinvigorate the organization and construct a suitable Philosophical Hall. Not having its own building, the society had been meeting at the college, at Carpenters' Hall, and elsewhere. Franklin thought highly of the idea, presented the motion, and then made a generous contribution and a loan to start construction on a plot of land in State House Yard. He also presented his just completed *On the Causes and Cure of Smoky Chimneys* to the society, which subsequently published it in its *Transactions*.[3]

Benjamin Rush was among the physicians anxious to greet Franklin on his return. Franklin had helped Rush get the best possible medical training in Scotland and England in the 1760s, and they exchanged informative letters over the ensuing years on subjects such as the common cold. Franklin had also helped him secure an appointment at the Pennsylvania Hospital. Among the topics that the two men now discussed was the use of tobacco, and specifically whether smoking and inhaling snuff were dangerous practices. As a Quaker, Rush was not one to use tobacco, but he also favored its restriction for medical reasons. In his diary entry dated August 1786, he wrote:

I waited on the Doctor [Franklin] with a Dr. Minto. He [Franklin] said he believed that Tobacco would in a few years go out of use. That, about thirty years ago, when he went to England, Smoaking was universal in taverns, coffee-houses, and private families, but that it was now generally laid aside, [and] that the use of Snuff, from being universal in France was become unfashionable. . . .

He added that Sir John Pringle and he had observed that tremors of the hands were more frequent in France than elsewhere, and probably from the excessive use of snuff. They once saw in a company of 16 but two persons who had not these tremors at a table in France. He said Sir John was cured of a tremor by leaving off snuff. He concluded that there was no great advantage in using tobacco in any way, for that he had kept company with persons who used it all his life, and no one had ever advised him to use it. The Doctor in the 81st year of his age declared that he had never snuffed, chewed, or smoked.[4]

Rush sent a note to Welsh nonconformist minister Richard Price, who was then in England, informing him that "Our venerable friend Dr. Franklin continues to enjoy as much health and spirits as are compatible with his time in life. I dined with him a few days ago in a most agreeable circle, where he appeared as cheerful and gay as a young man of five-and-twenty. But his conversation was full of the wisdom and experience of mellow old age."[5]

Among the more colorful medical visitors to Franklin's home in 1787 was Dr. Manasseh Cutler of Massachusetts. Cutler was a preacher but had studied medicine and was skilled in the healing arts. In Cutler's biography we find: "He comprehended almost at a glance the leading principles of the science, and in a very short period won for himself among the medical profession the reputation of a safe and skillful practitioner. . . . He read medicine assiduously, studied anatomy, prepared medicines and attended the sick, in addition to his usual pastoral duties."[6] Cutler had long been wishing to meet Franklin, writing, "There was no curiosity in Philadelphia which I felt so anxious to see as this great man, who had been the wonder of Europe as well as the glory of America."[7]

Franklin greeted Cutler in his garden, where a few members of the Constitutional Convention had been sitting and conversing with him. His daughter Sally attended to the guests and served tea, while her children played and made their ever-watchful grandfather smile. After giving Cutler a warm welcome, Franklin showed him a two-headed snake preserved in a large vial. He had previously associated it with the fable of each side not knowing how to compromise at a choice point, and eventually starving to death.

After it turned dark, they went inside to see something just as interesting—

Franklin's personal library, which took up the whole second floor of his home. It contained 4,276 volumes and some unusual pieces of medical equipment. "I presume this is the largest, and by far the best, private library in America," wrote Cutler.

He showed us a glass machine for exhibiting the circulation of the blood in the arteries and veins of the human body. The circulation is exhibited by the passing of a red fluid from a reservoir into numerous capillary tubes of glass, ramified in every direction, and then returning in similar tubes to the reservoir.

He also showed us his long artificial arm and hand, for taking down and putting books up on high shelves which are out of reach; and his great armed chair, with rockers, and a large fan placed over it, with which he fans himself, keeps off flies, etc., while he sits reading, with only a small motion of his foot, and many other curiosities and inventions, all his own, but of lesser note.[8]

Franklin and Cutler enjoyed their time together before Cutler said good-bye and Franklin retired for the night. Franklin understood the importance of getting proper bed rest, especially at his age. Being able to sleep well and balancing sleep with wakefulness had always been an important part of his health regimen. The Roman physician Galen had classified sleep as one of his six "non-naturals," along with eating and drinking moderately, exercising, getting fresh air, and controlling one's passions. These were things that a citizen of Rome should be able to control within reasonable limits to remain in good health (see Chapter 9).

Franklin, who had for decades been talking and writing about the other five non-naturals, had, in fact, just addressed the subject of sleep in an essay.[9] *The Art of Procuring Pleasant Dreams* was one of Franklin's most charming medical pieces, and it was dedicated to Georgiana Shipley, the daughter of his English friend Jonathan Shipley. Franklin had maintained a correspondence with Georgiana since visiting the Shipleys and starting to write his *Autobiography* in their Twyford home in 1771, and Georgiana was among the people who greeted him at Southampton on his voyage home. It was there that she probably asked him to compose the piece, which was written "at her request."

This treatise was not, however, the only notable piece that Franklin had sent to Georgiana. As a young girl, she had become heartbroken when the pet squirrel he had sent her from America escaped and was killed by a dog. To help soothe her, he had another squirrel sent and also wrote a tribute for the poor departed Skugg. The last seven words of the short epitaph he composed in 1772 for her beloved squirrel are still remembered today: "Here Skugg/ Lies snug/ As a bug/ In a Rug!"[10]

Franklin's new essay on sleep opens with a discussion of the importance of adequate sleep for "preserving health." He then turns to how some of the other non-naturals can affect sleep. Here he brings up some old themes he never tired of discussing. He suggests exercising before, not after, eating, and not having a large meal before going to sleep. "The exercise should precede meals, not immediately follow them," he advised; "full feeding" before going to sleep "occasions nightmares and horrors inexpressible." Additionally, "mankind, since the improvement of cookery, eats about twice as much as nature requires. Suppers are not bad, if we have not dined; but restless nights naturally follow hearty suppers after full dinners."

Clearly thinking about another non-natural, Franklin wrote, "Another means of preserving health is the having a constant supply of fresh air in your bed chamber. It has been a great mistake, the sleeping in rooms exactly closed, and in beds surrounded by curtains. No outward air that may come in to you is so unwholesome as the unchanged air, often breathed, of a close chamber." Further, if you are awakened "and you cannot easily sleep again, get out of bed, beat up and turn your pillow, shake the bed-clothes well, with at least twenty shakes, then throw the bed open and leave it to cool; in the meanwhile, continuing undrest, walk about your chamber till your skin has had time to discharge it load. . . . When you begin to feel the cold air unpleasant, then return to your bed, and you will soon fall asleep, and your sleep will be sweet and pleasant."

Franklin concluded his essay by stating, "These are the rules of the art. But, though they will generally prove effectual in producing the end intended, there is a case in which the most punctual observance of them will be totally fruitless . . . . The case is, when a person who desires to have pleasant dreams has not taken care to preserve, what is necessary above all things, A GOOD CONSCIENCE."[11]

Georgiana, who was skilled in the classics, languages, letters, and the fine arts (she studied with Joshua Reynolds), was flattered that Franklin had dedicated this little gem to her. But being well read and inquisitive, she did not hesitate to check on and challenge one of Franklin's facts. She explained to the now elderly American who reminded her of Socrates that she had searched the Bible up and down, but could find no evidence that Methuselem always slept in the open air. Franklin, who still possessed a wonderful sense of humor, must have laughed upon receiving her correction.

THE SLIPPERY SLOPE

Franklin's physical difficulties continued to plague him after he returned to America. Notably, he had more problems with his gout, including one attack in 1787 that resulted in "five Months' painful Confinement."[12] Writing to Le Veillard on October 24, 1788, he complained that he had gotten better only to be sidelined again by the gout during the next summer.[13] Even more significantly, his already huge bladder stone continued to grow larger.

Nevertheless, his mind remained exceptional. To quote Cutler, who saw him in 1787: "I was highly delighted with the extensive knowledge he appeared to have of every subject, the brightness of his memory, and clearness and vivacity of all his mental faculties. Not withstanding his age (eighty-four), his manners are perfectly easy, and everything about him seems to diffuse an unrestrained freedom and happiness. He has an incessant vein of humor, accompanied with an uncommon vivacity, which seems as natural and involuntary as his breathing."[14]

Franklin's remarkable mental status seemed no different to Cutler than it had to John Jay six years earlier. Jay, who had worked with Franklin in France and also served in Spain, sent a public and a private letter to Congress when Franklin first asked to be recalled home because of his health. "I find he has requested Permission to retire, on Account of his Age, Infirmities, &c.," wrote Jay. "How far his Health may be impaired, I know not—The Letters I have received from him bear no Marks of Age, and there is an acuteness and sententious Brevity in them which do not indicate an understanding injured by Years."[15]

Franklin continued composing letters that showed a very acute mind in 1789. One went to Alexander Small, who had a hearing problem. "The deafness you complain of gives me concern," he wrote, "as if great, it must diminish considerably your pleasure in conversation. If moderate, you may remedy it easily and readily by putting your thumb and fingers behind your ear, pressing it outwards, and enlarging it, as it were, with the hollow of your hand. By an exact experiment I found that I could hear the tick of a watch at forty-five feet distance by this means, which was barely audible at twenty feet without it. The experiment was made at midnight when the house was still."[16]

The use of a ticking watch to measure the sensitivity of a person's hearing was common at this time. Pocket watches differed in quality and audibility, but they provided a simple, inexpensive way for physicians to get a reasonable measure of how well a patient could hear. In Small's case, it is not that Franklin offered a new idea, for he did not. Rather, the letter shows just how much Franklin was still in control of his memory and intellect, while his body was clearly faltering.

Benjamin Franklin was a realist and he had long accepted the fact that his body could not last forever. This thought was the subject of a letter he sent to Jonathan Shipley early in 1786. He informed the English cleric that his stone did not seem to be growing worse. Then, turning to the ravages of time, he told the Bishop of St. Asaph: "But the Course of Nature must soon put a period to my present Mode of Existence. This I shall submit to with less Regret, as, having seen during a long Life a good deal of this World, I feel a growing Curiosity to be acquainted with some other; and can cheerfully, with filial Confidence, resign my Spirit to the conduct of that great and good Parent of Mankind, who created it, and who has so graciously protected and prospered me from my Birth to the present Hour."[17]

A year later, Franklin admitted to Jan Ingenhousz that his stone was now growing worse and that he had taken a fall. For weeks, he wrote, he had been "very ill with a severe Fit of the Stone, which follow'd a Fall I had on the Stone Steps that lead into my Garden, whereby I was much bruised, and my Wrist sprained, so as not to be capable of Writing for several Weeks."[18]

Franklin commented on his advancing age and how close he felt to the end of his earthly existence in another letter that was sent just three months later. He explained to George Whatley: "You are now seventy-eight, and I am eighty-two; you tread fast on my heels; but, though you have more strength and spirit, you cannot come up with me till I stop, which must now be soon; for I am grown so old as to have buried most of the friends of my youth, and I now often hear persons whom I knew when children, called old Mr. Such-a-one, to distinguish them from their sons now men grown and in business; so that, by living twelve years beyond David's period, I seem to have intruded myself into the company of posterity, when I ought to have been abed and asleep. Yet," he continued, "had I gone at seventy, it would have cut off twelve of the most active years of my life, employed too in matters of greatest importance."[19]

During the same year, 1787, Franklin was forced to watch the Independence Day parade from his window, with the route altered so he would be able to view the festivities. And he was unable to attend the occasion at Franklin College (later renamed Franklin and Marshall College), when the cornerstone of the school that bears his name was laid.

Sadly, 1788 proved to be even more difficult. In a letter to Miss Flainville he wrote: "I have been harassed with Illness this last Summer, am grown old, near 83, and find myself very infirm, so that I expect soon to be call'd for; and you may, my dear Child, consider this Line as taking Leave."[20] Similarly, in a letter to Elizabeth Partridge, who had asked how he was doing, he responded: "You kindly enquire after my Health. I have not, of late, much reason to boast of it. . . . However, when I consider how many more terrible Maladies the Human Body is liable to, I think myself well off that I have only three incurable ones: the Gout, the Stone, and Old Age."[21]

In March 1789, he would philosophize to Catherine Greene: "I have as much health and cheerfulness, as can be expected at my age, now eighty-three. Hitherto this long life has been tolerably happy; so that, if I were allowed to live it over again, I should make no objection, only wishing for leave to do, what authors do in a second editions of their works, correct some of my errata."[22]

Franklin remained a printer at heart, but he was less than original in what he had just written to Catherine Greene. One of the epitaphs for John Cotton, grandfather of Cotton Mather, also made reference to "a new edition . . . without erratas"—and one more in accord with the "leaves and covers of eternity."[23] In fact, Franklin had previously composed an epitaph for himself along the same lines in 1728.[24]

By this time, Franklin was likely thinking about a letter he had written to Barbeu-Dubourg about death and the possibility of a triumphant return from the Great Beyond. His somewhat humorous piece was probably written in 1773, not long after he received a note from Barbeu-Dubourg that opened a discussion about the possibility of reviving people killed by lightning. Franklin's letter began with some observations, not about humans, but about toads.

A toad buried in sand will live, it is said, till the sand becomes petrified; and then, being enclosed in the stone, it may still live for we know not how many ages. The facts which are cited in support of this opinion are too numerous, and too circumstantial, not to deserve a certain degree of credit. As we are accustomed to see all the animals with which we are acquainted eat and drink, it appears to us difficult to conceive how a toad can be supported in such a dungeon. . . .

A plant, with its flowers, fades and dies immediately, if exposed to the air without having its roots immersed in a humid soil, from which it may draw a sufficient quantity of moisture to supply that which exhales from its substance and is carried off continually by the air. Perhaps, however, if it were buried in quicksilver, it might preserve for a considerable space of time its vegetable life, its smell, and colour.

I have seen an instance of common flies preserved in a manner somewhat similar. They had been drowned in Madeira wine, apparently about the same time when it was bottled in Virginia, to be sent hither [to London]. At the opening of one of the bottles, at the house of a friend where I then was, three drowned flies fell into the first glass that was filled.

Having heard it remarked that drowned flies were capable of being revived by the rays of the sun, I proposed making an experiment upon these; they were therefore exposed to the sun upon a sieve, which had been employed to strain them out of the wine. In less than three hours, two of them began by degrees to recover life. They commenced by some convulsive motions of the thighs, and at length they raised themselves upon their legs, wiped their eyes with their fore feet, beat and brushed their wings with their hind feet, and soon after began to fly, finding themselves in Old England, without knowing how they came thither. The third continued lifeless till sunset, when, losing all hopes of him, he was thrown away.

I wish it were possible, from this instance, to invent a method of embalming drowned persons, in such a manner that they may be recalled to life at any period, however distant; for having a very ardent desire to see and observe the state of America a hundred years hence, I should prefer to any ordinary death, the being immersed in a cask of Madeira wine, with a few friends, till that time, to be then recalled to life by the solar warmth of my dear country![25]

Franklin was not having a delusion or spinning a tall tale when he wrote about the two flies that rose like Lazarus from the dead. Flies, unlike most other insects, seem capable of surviving for considerable lengths of time in bottles of wine. The reason for this is probably that the hairs that densely cover their bodies keep them from sinking into the wine, which would dehydrate their cells and kill them.

Franklin had additional thoughts about the possibility of a glorious resurrection twenty-one years after he joked about being immersed in a cask of Madeira until he could be properly resuscitated. In a playful letter written to George Whatley, he argued tongue-in-cheek that God would never be wasteful. Hence, God would not consider the "annihilation of souls" with the loss of millions of minds, only to turn around and create new ones. Instead, the supreme deity would find it more economical and considerably less troublesome to follow another path, namely to recycle existing souls. The aged but always pragmatic philosopher continued: "Thus finding myself to exist in the World, I believe I shall, in some Shape or other, always exist."[26] Given his religious beliefs, natural philosophy, and a few economic reasons to believe in a meaningful life after death, Franklin found comfort as the sun now set on his long, productive life.

## THE DOCTOR'S DEATH

In a letter to George Washington written during the fall of 1789, Franklin congratulated the first President of the United States on his good recovery from a nagging health problem and on the strength and wisdom of his administration. He then confessed to Washington that it was now difficult for him to even sit up. "For my own personal Ease, I should have died two Years ago; but tho' those Years have been spent in excruciating Pain, I am pleas'd that I have liv'd them, since they have brought me to see our present Situation. I am now finishing my 84th, and probably with it my Career in this Life."[27]

Franklin was actually completing his eighty-third year when he wrote this letter, and Washington was more saddened to hear that he was experiencing pain than he was to learn that Franklin's "Career in this Life" was coming to an end. Like Franklin, he knew that people could not live forever, and he too believed in an afterlife. He replied to his senior countryman that it was his hope, and the hope and prayer of all Americans, that "your existence might close with as much ease to yourself, as its continuance has been beneficial to our country and useful to mankind."[28]

During this obviously difficult time, Franklin's grandson Benny Bache took dictation and penned his letters; his daughter Sally did her best to make him comfortable; and her husband Richard Bache managed his business affairs. Polly Hewson, the widow of English physician William Hewson, had moved to Philadelphia with her children to be near him, and she attempted to keep his spirits up by reading poetry at his bedside. Some of the Founding Fathers of the new republic also stopped by to offer comfort, and they kept him up to date on national and international politics.

One such person was Thomas Jefferson, who had filled Franklin's vacated post when he left France in 1785 and served there until 1789. Jefferson had always had great respect for Franklin. Soon after arriving in France, he was asked: "Il est, Monsieur, qui remplacez le Docteur Franklin?" ("Is it you, Sir, who replaces Doctor Franklin?"). Jefferson's often quoted answer was, "No one can replace him, Sir; I am only his successor."

Jefferson told Franklin that the Ancien Régime of Louis XVI and Marie Antoinette was coming to a more terrifying end than anyone had expected. And he provided one of the last good accounts of Franklin. He had visited him just a few weeks before he composed a note to Le Veillard, their mutual friend who, unfortunately, would not escape the Reign of Terror. Dated April 1790, it read: "I wish I could add to your happiness by giving you a favourable account of the good old Doctor. I found him in bed where he remains almost constantly. He has been clear of pain for some days and was cheerful and in good spirits. He listened with a glow of interest to the details of your revolution and of his friends, which I gave him. He is much emaciated. I pressed him to continue the narration of his life and perhaps he will."[29]

Benjamin Rush wrote about Franklin's final days in 1790. "The evening of his life was marked by the same activity of his moral and intellectual powers which distinguished its meridian," observed America's most influential physician of the era. "Three days before he died he dictated a letter upon very important business relative to the boundaries of the United States to Mr. Jefferson, and three weeks before his death he wrote and published a very agreeable and ingenious parody upon a speech of a member of Congress in favor of the slavery of the Africans."

Rush continued: "His conversation with his family upon the subject of his dissolution was free and cheerful. A few days before he died, he rose from his bed and begged that it be made up for him so that he might 'die in a decent manner.' His daughter told him that she hoped he would recover and live many years longer. He calmly replied: 'He hoped not.' Upon being advised to change his position in bed, that he might breathe *easy*, he said, 'A dying man can do nothing *easy*.'"[30]

Franklin did not die directly from his massive bladder stone, which in turn might be attributed to his diet, wine, and a number of other factors—possibly even lead poisoning. But his stone clearly weakened him considerably and confined him to his bed. In this respect, it predisposed his body for a final illness. According to Dr. John Jones, who was then attending physician at Pennsylvania Hospital, the disease that ultimately killed him was a pulmonary infection.

Franklin had serious lung infections in the past. The most notable occurred at age twenty-one, when he returned from his failed printing equipment buying trip to England to work in Denham's dry goods store. At that time, he came down with an attack of pleurisy that nearly killed him. During 1735, he came down with a second serious lung infection with an abscess on his left lung that suddenly ruptured and almost suffocated him. Now, at age eighty-four, he found himself battling yet another pulmonary infection.

Jones described Franklin's final illness in a black-bordered issue of the *Pennsylvania Gazette*. He wrote that he began to run a "feverish indisposition" about sixteen days before he died. Three or four days later, he started to experience pains in his left breast. The pain grew in intensity and made his breathing more and more laborious. Then, about five days before he died his pain subsided, raising hopes for a recovery. But an abscess that had formed in his lung then burst, producing a great amount of purulent matter. Although he was able to cough up some of the fluid, much remained and, as his strength continued to give out, his breathing became more and more strained. Franklin lost his ability to speak and he quietly passed away at eleven o'clock at night on April 17, 1790.

The funeral took place four days later. As the bells of his adopted city tolled, his casket was lowered into the ground of Christ Church cemetery where it was positioned next to Deborah's. The grave was marked with a marble slab bearing a very simple inscription that Franklin had written shortly before he died: "Benjamin and Deborah Franklin 1790."

Franklin chose not to use the witty printer's epitaph that he had written for himself in 1728, although it was perfectly suited for a man whose professional life began as a printer. It read:

The Body of
B. Franklin, Printer;
(Like the Cover of an old Book,
Its Contents torn out,
And stript of its Lettering and Gilding)
Lies here, Food for Worms.
but the Work shall not be wholly lost:
For it will, (as he believed) appear once more,
In a new & more elegant Edition,
Revised and corrected,
By the Author.[31]

Franklin does not tell us why he chose the simpler epitaph. But one possibility is that, as he approached his own death, he wanted to be remembered as more than just a printer or a writer. He had also been a skilled diplomat, a moralist, an inventor, a naturalist, an experimental natural philosopher, and a man who contributed significantly to health and medicine, and nowhere more so than in enlightened Philadelphia.

It is estimated that Franklin's funeral was attended by approximately half of the population of Philadelphia. The procession had been headed by all denominations of clergy, which seems proper since Franklin had spent his life looking for common grounds that would unite rather than separate people. Next came the local, state, and national politicians. Members of the three organizations associated with medicine followed them: the American Philosophical Society, the College of Philadelphia, and the College of Physicians. The printers of the city had also been present. But more than all these groups and the people he considered his friends and close acquaintances, there were thousands of people who had never met and spoken with him in person.

A number of the mourners knew just how much Franklin's medical contributions had affected their lives; some worked or were treated at Pennsylvania Hospital, others were affiliated with Philadelphia's medical school, and still others had undergone smallpox inoculation at his urging. Numerous others who grieved knew less about the medical side of Franklin, but ate and drank more sensibly, took better care of their bodies, and perhaps treated themselves more effectively, because of the self-help books he published and the sayings of his loveable creation, Poor Richard. And then there were the men, women, and children who might have known nothing about Franklin's medical contributions. Yet, in one way or another, they too benefited by what he did from his youth to the time of his death. Whether these mourners knew it or not, Doctor Franklin's medicine had changed the Western medical landscape for them and for others in many significant ways.

# Franklin's Medical Legacy

*An ill Wound, but not an ill Name, may be healed.*
—*Poor Richard's Almanack,* 1753

In 1706, the year of Franklin's birth, the seeds for the medical Enlightenment that had been planted by Francis Bacon and nurtured by Thomas Sydenham were just starting to break through the ground in Western Europe and were just about to germinate in the British North American colonies. Physicians were beginning to track the weather more carefully in an attempt to understand how changes in the climate may relate to epidemic diseases; remedies calling for stockings of dog skin or goose stuffed with chopped kittens were much less likely to appear in medical texts (see Chapter 17); and astrological medical predictions were no longer taken as seriously as they once had been. But at the same time, medicine, especially academic medicine, was deeply mired in speculation and tied to unsubstantiated theories about bodily humors, the chemical milieu, and internal mechanics.

There were still wild speculations at the time of Franklin's death in 1790, but medicine had changed considerably. There were new tools, such as medical electricity, movements to build hospitals to care for the sick poor, and a growing demand for conclusions and actions to be backed not just by conjecture or casual observations, but by statistics and planned experiments. In almost every way, Franklin was deeply involved with giving preventive medicine, bedside medicine, hospital care, and even hygiene a new look. And what he did and how he did it had a significant impact on his medical contemporaries and helped set the stage for what would follow.

Although he had little formal schooling and never served a medical apprenticeship, Franklin entered medicine with an inquiring mind and an unusual intellect. Because he loved to read and selected printing to be his profession, he became knowledgeable about medical needs, practices, and potential breakthroughs. Early on, he encountered new ideas that begged for more careful study, such as smallpox inoculations, as well as quack remedies and older notions based on loose theorizing, as exemplified by wearing bright red clothes to fight off chilling diseases. His driving force from the start was to be a doer of good—to alleviate human suffering and to be of service to others. With a pragmatic orientation and an optimistic outlook, he approached medicine with a variety of tools, from his printing presses to his electrical machines, but always with mindset of an experimental natural philosopher determined to use science to uncover the truth. And following in the footsteps of the Hippocratic physicians, his first rule was to do no harm.

What Franklin accomplished in medicine did not take place in a vacuum. He was clearly influenced by the writings and personal contacts he had with practitioners, and his ability to make friends with people trained in medicine or in closely related areas provided him with a large, formidable network for developing and exchanging new thoughts. This network included the leading physicians, botanists, and chemists of his day. Peter Collinson, John Fothergill, John Pringle, William Heberden, George Baker, William and John Hunter, Georges Cabanis, Jan Ingenhousz, Joseph Priestley, Antoine-Laurent Lavoisier, Thomas Bond, and Benjamin Rush were among the better-known people he worked with in Europe and America. Franklin also used his medical associates in another important way. Rather than write thick books of his own, he sent many of these people, and others as well, detailed letters filled with new information. He asked them for feedback and to help him disseminate his findings and carefully reasoned conclusions.

Franklin's forays into medicine often started with something another person wrote or said, such as how his adopted city might benefit from a new hospital or how electricity was starting to be used medically in Europe. To his credit, he had an exceptional ability to evaluate new ideas and to single out the good ones from those with little potential. Although he was a skilled "institutionalizer" of good and useful ideas, he also showed exceptional creativity on numerous occasions, and he made many original contributions, even in his final years when his own body was failing him.

Many of Franklin's writings dealt with improving regimens for living, or what we might think of hygiene, habits, and behaviors that an individual should be able to control. Early on, he used Poor Richard to tell people how to eat and drink moderately, as well as how to avoid things that might be dangerous to their health, such as rum punch, which might cause the "West India Dry-Gripes." Similarly, he actively promoted exercising as a means of both staying fit and warding off diseases, even calling for exercise programs in schools. The benefits of fresh air were also never far from his mind. And after returning to America for the last time, he wrote an essay enumerating various ways to get a good night's sleep, so as to function better the next day.

Franklin also devoted himself throughout his life to preventing specific diseases and disorders. In part to reduce eye and lung irritations, he improved stoves and furnaces and invented better ventilation systems. He also helped to give people fresh insights about occupational lead poisoning and other perils of lead. In addition, he did his best to educate people on how to avoid catching colds, shifting attention from cold and wet weather to minute infectious matter that could be transmitted from one person to another by sneezing, coughing, and even just breathing in closed, cramped quarters.

Particularly significant in the prevention domain was Franklin's support of variolation. Drawing on what he witnessed as a printer's apprentice in Boston, stimulated by the loss of his own son, and with the help of his pen and printing press in Philadelphia, he became a leading supporter of inoculation as the best way to prevent naturally occurring smallpox. His efforts to reduce the death toll from the most feared illness of his day were firmly grounded in the statistics he collected. As a good citizen, he was particularly concerned about educating and inoculating the poor, recognizing that this segment of the population was least likely to understand the procedure and to be able to pay for professional services, whether in America, England, or elsewhere.

Franklin also applied his intellect and skills to curing diseases. Some of his work in this area involved "clinical trials" that he personally conducted on patients. He was, in fact, one of the first electrotherapists. Although the "common paralytic disorder" cases that he dealt with in the colonies convinced him that electricity was not a panacea, he successfully treated a woman with hysteria. Moreover, he and his friend Jan Ingenhousz broke new ground when they suggested applying strong electrical shocks to the heads of people with depressive disorders, or what was then called melancholia. Further, Franklin was probably the first person to describe the retrograde amnesia that can accompany such shocks.

Franklin dealt with treating diseases in other ways too. A notable example would be the clever means he used to evaluate Mesmerism, arguably one of the greatest fads in the history of clinical medicine. Franz Anton Mesmer had been claiming that he could cure patients of a wide variety of ills with an invisible force that he called animal magnetism. Franklin first tried to detect the force with instruments and, when this failed, he carefully designed a series of "trick" experiments to find out why some people seemed to get better as a result of their treatments. Employing blind protocols that would be adopted by subsequent investigators of the human mind, he and his fellow commissioners showed Mesmerism for what it really was: a cure based on the manipulation of a gullible person's imagination.

It is worth noting that Franklin had used suggestion to cure sick minds well before he was called upon in 1784 to evaluate Mesmer's cure. In one instance, he had skillfully combined suggestion with relaxing music therapy to help a distraught Polish princess. To Franklin, suggestion and placebo effects had legitimate places in medicine. With his understanding of the human mind, which was derived in part from John Locke's writings, Franklin can even be thought of as a pioneer in psychotherapy.

Franklin obviously knew that not all of mankind's ills could be cured, which is why he also worked on several inventions to make life easier for the aged and afflicted. His bifocals are the best known, and they made it easier for some visually impaired people, beginning with himself, to see both near and far objects clearly without having to change eyeglasses. He also invented the "long arm," which is extremely useful to people who are unsteady on their feet and unable to climb ladders to grasp out-of-reach objects, and he envisioned how hot-air balloons could be used to move the disabled.

Additionally, based upon his ability to see a need, his people skills, and his ability to turn good ideas into reality, Franklin assisted in founding two important medical institutions. One is Pennsylvania Hospital, the first major charity hospital in the colonies, which opened its doors to poor but deserving physically and mentally ill patients on its permanent site in 1756. Franklin secured the needed funding for the hospital, helped design its bylaws, and served as one of its first governors. After going to Europe, he continued to study hospital care and to funnel cash donations to its coffers and medical books to its library.

A second landmark institution that owed much to Franklin is the first medical school in the colonies, which dates from 1765. Initially associated with the College of Philadelphia, it would later become a part of the University of Pennsylvania. Franklin played two important roles in the establishment and success of the first American medical school. On the one hand, he was involved with, and supportive of, such an institution from the time the idea appeared to be informally launched in London, perhaps even by him, in 1759. And on the other, with his contacts in London and Edinburgh, he made sure that the American medical students who would go on to open and staff the new school would get the best practical and theoretical training then available. Notably, he personally urged them to study natural philosophy, in order to gain a better appreciation of how medicine could best be rooted in empirical science.

Several other institutions started by Franklin also had important ties to medical education, although the healing arts was not their sole purpose. The Library Company, for instance, disseminated medical tracts in Philadelphia to the tradesmen and others who subscribed. In contrast, the American Philosophical Society, which grew out of Franklin's Junto, fostered new explorations and the exchange of medical information to a much wider audience. It included not only Pennsylvanians, but members from distant colonies and even foreign associates, and in 1769 it launched its own journal, which was disseminated not just in America but also in Europe.

Franklin's medical legacy also includes its share of intangibles. He viewed what he was doing as something that transcended local and even national boundaries. Hence, he did not hesitate to encourage the exchange of medical information between countries, including those that were, or had recently been, at war. Through his personal efforts, influential people in France, Great Britain, and the new United States became acutely aware of ways to prevent malnutrition, the means by which staggering childhood mortality statistics might be decreased, and ideas that would make hospitals and foundling homes better, safer, and more patient oriented.

Additionally, Franklin set a striking example for others to follow by how he first considered all sides of a complex issue before voicing an opinion. His work served as a model for how conclusions should stem from facts, not theories or conjectures, and he showed that the best strategy was never to be argumentative or dogmatic. In this context, he deliberately used language that has become fundamental to good medical science today, but which was not common in his own day—phrases such as "I conceive" or "I apprehend," or words to the effect that his findings might "indicate" or "suggest." As a rule, Franklin always left the door open for new and better ideas—provided they could be substantiated by careful observations and, ideally, convincing experiments.

It was his abhorrence of dogmatism, empirical orientation, and passion for systematically collecting new facts that gave Franklin's medicine its relatively modern look in comparison to the speculations of many of his contemporaries. What Franklin strove to build was not just another theoretical edifice that would soon be toppled, but a structure constructed with blocks of scientific facts and solidly mortared conclusions—one on which future stories could be erected by ensuing generations.

In closing, it seems fitting to return to Poor Richard's words in the epigraph to the Introduction to this book. Always wise, never lost for words, and fond of rhyming, Poor Richard opined that to be remembered one must "Either write things worth reading, Or do things worth the writing."[1] Poor Richard's creator, with his empiricism, pragmatism, and public-spirited approach to medicine, clearly wrote things worth reading and did things worth the writing. With an assortment of skills and tools, and in a myriad of ways, Benjamin Franklin changed the medical landscape around him, and left an impressive medical legacy on which a healthier future could be built.

# Notes

The major source of material for this book is *The Papers of Benjamin Franklin*, edited successively by Leonard W. Labaree, William Willcox, Barbara B. Oberg, and Ellen R. Cohn (New Haven: Yale University Press, 1959–2004) (*Papers*). Because the volumes after 2004 were not completed at the time this book went to press, the earlier *Writings of Benjamin Franklin* by Alfred Henry Smyth (New Haven: Yale University Press, 1905–1907) has also been used (*Writings*), as was a more complete prepublication computer disk of the *Papers*. The *Autobiography of Benjamin Franklin* was another frequently consulted primary source (Mineola, N.Y.: Dover, 1996) (*Autobiography*).

There are many good biographies of Franklin. The classic in the field is Carl Van Doren's *Benjamin Franklin* (New York: Viking Press, 1938). Among the newer biographies that provide good general background are H. W. Brands's *The First American* (New York: Anchor, 2002), Walter Isaacson's *Benjamin Franklin* (New York: Simon & Schuster, 2003), and Gordon S. Wood's *The Americanization of Benjamin Franklin* (New York: Penguin Press, 2004).

The following abbreviations are used in the notes.

| | |
|---|---|
| AHR | *American Historical Review* |
| AIM | *Annals of Internal Medicine* |
| AMH | *Annals of Medical History* |
| BHM | *Bulletin of the History of Medicine* |
| BJHH | *Bulletin of the Johns Hopkins Hospital* |
| GM | *Gentleman's Magazine* |
| HS | *History of Science* |
| JAMA | *Journal of the American Medical Association* |
| JHBS | *Journal of the History of the Behavioral Sciences* |
| JHM(AS) | *Journal of the History of Medicine (and Allied Sciences)* |
| MOI | *Medical Observations and Inquiries* |
| NEJM(S) | *New England Journal of Medicine (and Surgery)* |
| NEQ | *New England Quarterly* |
| NR | *Notes and Records of the Royal Society of London* |
| PMHB | *Pennsylvania Magazine of History and Biography* |
| PAPS | *Proceedings of the American Philosophical Society* |
| PMHS | *Proceedings of the Massachusetts Historical Society* |
| PT | *Philosophical Transactions of the Royal Society of London* |
| WMQ | *William and Mary Quarterly* |

## Introduction

Note to epigraph: *Papers 2:* 194.

1. Benjamin Franklin et al., *Report of Dr. Benjamin Franklin, and Other Commissioners . . .* (London: Printed for J. Johnston, St. Paul's Churchyard, 1785). Reprinted in *Foundations of Hypnosis,* ed. Maurice M. Tinterow (Springfield, Ill.: Charles C. Thomas, 1970), 107.

2. Franklin, *Report,* 108.

3. There have been two earlier tracts on Franklin and medicine, both small and written almost a century ago: William Pepper, *The Medical Side of Benjamin Franklin* (Philadelphia: Campbell, 1911); Theodore Diller, *Franklin's Contribution to Medicine* (Brooklyn, N.Y.: Huntington, 1912).

4. Whitfield J. Bell, Jr., "A Portrait of the Colonial Physician," in *The Colonial Physician and Other Essays* (New York: Science History Publications, 1977), 5–25; Richard H. Shryock, *Medicine and Society in America, 1660–1860* (New York: New York University Press, 1960).

5. Genevieve Miller, "A Physician in 1776," *JAMA 236* (1976): 26–30.

6. William Douglass, *A Summary, Historical and Political, of the . . . Present State of the British Settlements in North-America,* vol. 2 (London: R. Baldwin, 1755), 351.

7. Richard H. Shryock, "Early Licensing and Subsequent Decadence," in *Medical Licensing in America, 1650–1965* (Baltimore: Johns Hopkins University Press, 1967), 3–42.

8. For more on competition in the medical marketplace, see Paul Starr, "Medicine in a Democratic Culture: 1760–1850," in *The Social Transformation of American Medicine* (New York: Basic Books, 1982), 30–59.

9. William Smith, *History of the Province of New York . . .* (London: Thomas Wilcox, 1757), 212.

10. Albert Deutsch, "The Sick Poor in Colonial Times," *AHR 46* (1941): 560–579; Bryan F. LeBeau, "The 'Angelical Connection' Revisited," *Journal of American Culture 18* (1995): 1–12.

11. Cotton Mather, *Bonifacius: An Essay Upon the Good* (1710; Cambridge: Harvard University Press, 1966), 82.

12. Patricia Ann Watson, *The Angelical Connection* (Knoxville: University of Tennessee Press, 1991).

13. Otho T. Beale, Jr., "Cotton Mather, the First Significant Figure in American Medicine," *BHM 26* (1952): 103–116; Otho T. Beale, Jr., and Richard H. Shryock, *Cotton Mather* (Baltimore: Johns Hopkins University Press, 1954); Kenneth Silverman, *The Life and Times of Cotton Mather* (New York: Columbia University Press, 1985).

14. Lester S. King, *The Medical World of the Eighteenth Century* (Huntington, N.Y.: Krieger, 1971).

15. Keith Thomas, *Religion and the Decline of Magic* (New York: Charles Scribner's Sons, 1971).

16. Herbert Leventhal, *In the Shadow of the Enlightenment* (New York: New York University Press, 1976).

17. Shigehisa Kuriyama, "Interpreting the History of Bloodletting," *JHMAS 50* (1995): 11–46.

18. Allen G. Debus, *The Chemical Philosophy* (New York: Science History Publications, 1977); Lester S. King, *The Road to the Medical Enlightenment* (London: MacDonald, 1970);

Lester S. King, "Iatrochemistry," in *The Philosophy of Medicine* (Cambridge: Harvard University Press, 1978), 64–94.

19. King, "Iatromechanism," 95–124.

20. Douglass, *Present State of the British Settlements*, 252.

21. Guy Williams, *The Age of Agony* (Chicago: Academy Chicago, 1986).

22. Colin G. Calloway, "Healing and Disease," in *New Worlds for All* (Baltimore: Johns Hopkins University Press, 1997), 25–41.

23. Thomas L. Hankins, *Science and the Enlightenment* (Cambridge: Cambridge University Press, 1985), 2.

24. Ernest Cassara, *The Enlightenment in America* (New York: Twayne, 1975); Dorinda Outram, *The Enlightenment* (Cambridge: Cambridge University Press, 1995); Roy Porter, *The Enlightenment* (Atlantic Highlands, N.J.: Humanities Press International, 1990).

25. Francis Bacon, *The New Organon*, Lisa Jardine and Michael Silverthorne, eds. (1620; Cambridge: Cambridge University Press, 2000); Loren Eiseley, *The Man who Saw Through Time* (New York: Charles Scribner's Sons, 1973); Antonio Pérez-Ramos, *Francis Bacon's Idea of Science and the Maker's Knowledge Tradition* (Oxford: Clarendon Press, 1988).

26. *Papers 3:* 339.

27. Thomas Sydenham, *The Works of Thomas Sydenham*, 2 vols. (London: Sydenham Society, 1848, 1850); Kenneth Dewhurst, "Thomas Sydenham, Reformer of Clinical Medicine," *MH 6* (1962): 101–118; Kenneth Dewhurst, *Dr. Thomas Sydenham* (Berkeley: University of California Press, 1966); King, *Medical Enlightenment*, 113–138.

28. F. N. L. Poynter, "Sydenham's Influence Abroad," *MH 17* (1973): 223–234; Richard B. Sher and Jeffrey R. Smitten, *Scotland and America in the Age of the Enlightenment* (Princeton: Princeton University Press, 1990); R. R. Trail, "Sydenham's Impact on English Medicine," *MH 9* (1965): 356–364.

29. *Autobiography*, 62.

30. *Papers 2:* 171.

31. *Papers 3:* 105.

32. *Papers 3:* 257.

33. Mather, *Bonifacius*.

34. *Writings 9:* 208.

35. *Autobiography*, 68.

36. *Writings 1:* 117.

*Chapter 1. Poor Richard's Medicine*

Note to epigraph: *Papers 1:* 352.

1. *Papers 4:* 243–247.

2. *Autobiography*, 5.

3. *Autobiography*, 10–11.

4. *Autobiography*, 13.

5. *Autobiography*, 13.

6. *Autobiography*, 17.

7. Carl Bridenbaugh and Jessica Bridenbaugh, *Rebels and Gentlemen* (New York: Oxford University Press, 1962).

8. *Autobiography*, 33.

9. *Papers 1:* 72–100.

10. *Papers 1:* 195.

11. *Autobiography*, 76.

12. *Autobiography*, 28.

13. *Autobiography*, 39.

14. Jennifer R. Fry, "Extraordinary Freedom and Great Humility: A Reinterpretation of Deborah Franklin," *PMHB 127* (2003): 167–196.

15. Helmut Lehmann-Haupt, *The Book in America* (New York: Bowker, 1952); Lawrence C. Wroth, *The Colonial Printer* (Charlottesville: University Press of Virginia, 1964).

16. *Papers 1:* 219.

17. Oscar Reiss, *Medicine and the American Revolution* (Jefferson, N.C.: McFarland, 1998), 193–204.

18. M. A. Montesu and F. G. C. Cottoni, "Bonomo and D. Cestoni: Discoverers of the Parasitic Origin of Scabies," *American Journal of Dermatopathology 13* (1991): 425–427; Ruben Friedman, "The 250th Anniversary of His [Bonomo's] Discovery of the Parasitic Nature of Scabies," *Medical Life 44* (1937): 3–26; Giovan Cosimo Bonomo, "Letter of Giovan Cosimo Bonomo to Francisco Redi Concerning the Discovery of the Parasitic Origin of Scabies," *Medical Life 44* (1937): 1–17.

19. Richard Mead, "An Abstract of Part of a Letter from Dr. Bonomo to Signior Redi," *PT 23* (1703): 1298.

20. Mead, "An Abstract," 1296–1299.

21. For the early history of self-help medical books in America, see Robert B. Austin, *Early American Medical Imprints* (Bethesda, Md.: National Library of Medicine, 1961); John B. Blake, "The Compleat Housewife," *BHM 49* (1975): 30–42; John B. Blake, "Early American Medical Literature," *Clio Medica 11* (1976): 147–160; Francesco Guerra, "Medical Almanacs of the American Colonial Period," *JHMAS 16* (1961): 234–255; Charles E. Rosenberg, "Health in the Home," in *Right Living*, ed. Charles E. Rosenberg (Baltimore: Johns Hopkins University Press, 2003), 1–20.

22. *Every Man His Own Doctor* (Philadelphia: B. Franklin, 1734).

23. Whitfield J. Bell, Jr., "John Tennent (1710–1748)," in *Patriot Improvers* (Philadelphia: American Philosophical Society, 1997), 159.

24. *Papers 2:* 188.

25. Thomas Short, *Medicina Britannia*, 3rd ed. (Philadelphia: B. Franklin and D. Hall, 1751).

26. Milton Drake, *Almanacs of the United States* (New York: Scarecrow Press, 1962); Thomas A. Horrocks, "Rules, Remedies, and Regimens," in *Right Living*, ed. Charles E. Rosenberg (Baltimore: Johns Hopkins University Press, 2003), 112–146; Thomas A. Horrocks, "Rules, Remedies, and Regimens" (Ph.D. diss., University of Pennsylvania, 2003); Robb Sagendorph, *America and Her Almanacs* (Boston: Little, Brown, 1970); Marion Barber Stowell, *Early American Almanacs* (New York: Burt Franklin, 1977).

27. *Papers 3:* 100.

28. *Autobiography*, 75.

29. *Papers 1:* 311.

30. *Papers 1:* 280–283.

31. *Papers 3:* 100–101.

32. *Papers 2:* 218.

33. H. W. Brands, *The First American* (New York: Anchor, 2002), 130.

34. *Papers 2:* 137, 138, 168, 169; *4:* 252; *3:* 449; *2:* 140, 140; *4:* 405.

35. *Papers 4:* 251.

36. Herbert Leventhal, "Astrology," in *In the Shadow of the Enlightenment* (New York: New York University Press, 1976), 13–65; Keith Thomas, *Religion and the Decline of Magic* (New York: Charles Scribner's Sons, 1971).

37. Thomas, *Religion*, 333.

38. Jon Butler, "Magic, Astrology, and the Early American Religious Heritage, 1600–1760," *AHR 84* (1979): 317–346; Patrick Curry, "Astrology in Early Modern England," in *Science, Culture, and Popular Belief in Renaissance Europe*, ed. Stephen Pumfrey, Paolo L. Rossi, and Maurice Slawinski (Manchester: Manchester University Press, 1991), 274–291; Anna Marie Roos, "Luminaries in Medicine," *BHM 74* (2000): 433–457; William D. Stahlman, "Astrology in Colonial America," *WMQ 1* (1956): 551–563; Thomas, *Religion;* Michael P. Winship, "Cotton Mather, Astrologer," *NEQ 63* (1990): 308–314.

39. *Papers 1:* 311.

40. *Papers 1:* 350–351.

41. Horrocks, "Rules," 124.

42. *Papers 2:* 9.

43. Ludwig Edelstein, "The Dietetics of Antiquity," in *Ancient Medicine*, ed. Oswei Temkin and C. Lilian Temkin (Baltimore: Johns Hopkins University Press, 1967), 303–316; Steven Shapin, "How to Eat like a Gentleman," in *Right Living*, ed. Charles E. Rosenberg (Baltimore: Johns Hopkins University Press, 2003), 21–58; Oswei Temkin, "Nutrition from Classical Antiquity to the Baroque," in *On Second Thought* (Baltimore: Johns Hopkins University Press, 2002), 180–194.

44. Temkin, "Nutrition," 182.

45. *Papers 3:* 448, 251; *2:* 337; *1:* 314; *7:* 354; *1:* 314.

46. *Papers 1:* 352; Henry Peacham, *The Complete Gentleman*, ed. Virgil B. Heltzel (1622, 1634; Ithaca: Cornell University Press, 1962), 152.

47. *Papers 2:* 339–341.

48. *Papers 3:* 337.

49. *Papers 3:* 104.

50. *Papers 3:* 249.

51. *Papers 2:* 338.

52. *Papers 2:* 142, 139.

53. *Papers 1:* 312, 314.

54. *Papers 2:* 169; *4:* 252.

55. *Papers 1:* 316.

56. *Papers 2:* 245, 254–256; for more on Tennent, see Bell, "John Tennent."

57. *Papers 2:* 245.

58. *Papers 3:* 449.

59. *Papers 6:* 339.

*Chapter 2. In Praise of Exercise*

Note to epigraph: *Autobiography,* 37.

1. Laurence Brockliss and Colin Jones, *The Medical World of Early Modern France* (Oxford: Clarendon Press, 1997), 464.

2. *Writings 5:* 545.

3. *Papers 20:* 131–133; translated in *Writings 5:* 542–545.

4. *Writings 5:* 543.

5. *Autobiography,* 37.

6. Melchisédec Thévenot, *The Art of Swimming* (London: Brown, Midurnter, Leigh, and Knaplock, 1699).

7. *Autobiography:* 38.

8. *Papers 1:* 82.

9. *Papers 1:* 90.

10. *Writings 5:* 543.

11. *Writings 5:* 543.

12. *Papers 20:* 544.

13. *Writings 5:* 544.

14. *Papers 15:* 295–296.

15. Benjamin Franklin. *Experiments and Observations on Electricity,* 4th ed. (London: F. Newberry, 1769).

16. Benjamin Franklin, "Useful Hints for Learning to Swim," *GM 47* (1777): 474–476. C. Lennart Carlson, *The First Magazine: A History of* Gentleman's Magazine (Providence: Brown, 1938); Roy Porter, "Lay Medical Knowledge in the Eighteenth Century," *MH 29* (1985): 138–168.

17. *Papers 1:* 260.

18. *Papers 3:* 402.

19. *Papers 3:* 402–403.

20. Kenneth Dewhurst, *John Locke* (London: Wellcome Historical Medical Library, 1963), 160–162.

21. *Papers 3:* 403.

22. Erasmus Darwin, *A Plan for the Conduct of Female Education in Boarding Schools* (Dublin: J. Chambers, 1798); Desmond King-Hele, *Erasmus Darwin* (London: Giles de la Mare, 1999), 283.

23. *Papers 13:* 383.

24. *Papers 18:* 118.

25. *Papers 18:* 207; also see 213.

26. *Papers 34:* 351.

27. *Papers 19:* 256–257.

28. *Papers 6:* 331.

29. *Papers 19:* 256.

30. *Papers 19:* 256–257.

31. *Papers 34:* 13–20; *Writings 8:* 154–162.

32. Thomas Sydenham, *Opera Ommia* (1742; London: Sydenham Society, 1844).

33. Guenter B. Risse, "Hysteria at the Edinburgh Infirmary," *MH 32* (1988): 19–21.

34. Thomas Cadwalader, *An Essay on the West-India Dry-Gripes* (Philadelphia: Franklin, 1745), 15–17.

35. *Papers 33:* 45.

36. John Adams, *The Works of John Adams,* vol. 3 (Boston: Little, Brown, 1851), 326.

37. *Papers 44:* 602.

38. *Papers 45:* 278.

39. The story can be found in Claude-Anne Lopez's "The Only Founding Father in a Sports Hall of Fame," in *My Life with Benjamin Franklin* (New Haven: Yale University Press, 2000), 17–23.

## Chapter 3. The Smallpox Wars

Note to epigraph: *Papers 8:* 285–286.

1. *Papers 19:* 28.

2. *Papers 2:* 154.

3. *Autobiography,* 79.

4. Donald R. Hopkins, *Princes and Peasants* (Chicago: University of Chicago Press, 1983); Charles Kahn, "History of Smallpox and Its Prevention," *American Journal of Diseases of Children 106* (1963): 597–609.

5. Nicolau Barquet and Pere Domingo, "Smallpox," *AIM 127* (1997): 635–642; Cyril W. Dixon, *Smallpox* (London: J. & A. Churchill, 1962).

6. Ann G. Carmichael and Arthur M. Silverstein, "Smallpox in Europe Before the Seventeenth Century," *JHMAS 42* (1987): 147–168.

7. John Duffy, "Smallpox and the Indians in the American Colonies," *BHM 25* (1951): 324–341; E. W. Stearn and A. E. Stearn, *The Effect of Smallpox on the Destiny of the Amerindian* (Boston: Humphries, 1945).

8. Oscar Reiss, *Medicine and the American Revolution* (Jefferson: McFarland, 1998), 118.

9. Anna Marie Roos, "Luminaries in Medicine," *BHM 74* (2000): 449.

10. Dixon, *Smallpox;* Kahn, "History of Smallpox"; Arnold C. Klebs, "The Historic Evolution of Variolation," *BJHH 24* (1913): 69–83; Genevieve Miller, *The Adoption of Inoculation for Smallpox in England and France* (Philadelphia: University of Pennsylvania Press, 1957); Raymond P. Stearns, "Remarks upon the Introduction of Inoculation for Smallpox in England," *BHM 24* (1950): 103–122.

11. Emanuele Timoni, "An Account, or History, of the Procuring of the Smallpox by Incision, or Inoculation," *PT 29* (1714): 72–82; Jacobus Pylarinus, "Nova et tuta variolas excitandi per transplantationem methodus, nuper inventa et in usum tracta," *PT 29* (1716): 393–399.

12. Robert Halsband, *The Life of Lady Mary Wortley Montague* (Oxford: Clarendon Press, 1956); Miller, *Adoption of Inoculation;* Genevieve Miller, "Putting Lady Mary in Her Place," *BHM 55* (1981): 2–16; Stearns, "Remarks."

13. Mary Wortley Montagu, *Letters of the Right Honourable Lady M—y W—y M—e,* vol. 1, letter 36. (Aix: Anthony Hencricy, 1796), 167–169.

14. Edward was not the first English child to undergo the procedure in Constantinople. The sons of the secretary of the previous ambassador had been engrafted a few years earlier, although little was made of it.

15. Charles Maitland, *Mr. Maitland's Account of Inoculating the Small Pox* (London: Downing, 1722); Stearns, "Remarks."

16. John T. Barrett, "The Inoculation Controversy in Puritan New England," *BHM 12* (1942): 169–190.

17. Cotton Mather, *Several Reasons Proving that Inoculation or Transplanting Small-Pox is a Lawful Practice* (Boston, 1721). Also see: Barrett, "Inoculation Controversy"; Solon S. Bernstein, "Smallpox and Variolization," *Journal of the Mount Sinai Hospital 18* (1951): 228–244; George L. Kittredge, "Some Lost Works of Cotton Mather," *PMHS 45* (1911–12): 418–479.

18. Reginald H. Fitz, "Zabdiel Boylston, Inoculator, and the Epidemic of Smallpox in Boston in 1721," *BJHH 22* (1911): 315–327.

19. For more on what transpired in Boston, see Otho T. Beale, Jr., and Richard H. Shryock, *Cotton Mather* (Baltimore: Johns Hopkins University Press, 1954); John B. Blake, "The Inoculation Controversy in Boston, 1721–1722," *NEQ 25* (1952): 489–506; Ola Winslow, *A Destroying Angel* (Boston: Houghton-Mifflin, 1974).

20. For a very different portrait of Mather, see Kenneth Silverman, *The Life and Times of Cotton Mather* (New York: Columbia University Press, 1985).

21. Christine Lee Heyrman, *Commerce and Culture* (New York: Norton, 1984).

22. Cotton Mather, *An Account of the Method and Success of Inoculating the Small-Pox* (London, 1722); Zabdiel Boylston, *An Historical Account of the Small-Pox Inoculated in New England* (London: S. Chandler, 1726).

23. Andrea Rusnock, "'The Merchant's Logick," in *The Road to Medical Statistics*, ed. Eileen Magnello and Anne Hardy (Amsterdam: Rodopi, 2002), 37–54.

24. Thomas Nettleton, "A Letter from Dr. Nettleton," *PT 32* (1722): 51; Thomas Nettleton, "Part of a Letter from Dr. Nettleton," *PT 32* (1722): 209–212; Andrea Rusnock, *The Correspondence of James Jurin (1784–1750)* (Amsterdam: Rodopi, 1996).

25. Andrea Rusnock, "The Weight of Evidence and the Burden of Authority," in *Medicine in the Enlightenment*, ed. Roy Porter (Amsterdam: Rodopi, 1995), 289–315; Andrea Rusnock, *Vital Accounts* (Cambridge: Cambridge University Press, 2002); Rusnock, "Merchant's Logick."

26. *Papers 10:* 46.

27. *Papers 1:* 186–187.

28. *Papers 1:* 200.

29. *Papers 3:* 78.

30. *Papers 3:* 78.

31. *Papers 3:* 78.

32. *Papers 3:* 79.

33. *Papers 4:* 41–42, 63–64, 71–72.

34. Henry L. Smith, "Dr. Adam Thompson, the Originator of the American Method of Inoculation for Small-pox," *BJHH 20* (1909): 49–52.

35. *Papers 4:* 80–82.

36. Adam Thompson, *A Discourse on the Preparation of the Body for the Small-pox* (Philadelphia: Franklin and Hall, 1750).

37. *Papers 4:* 337, 340, 358.

38. *Papers 2:* 166.

39. *Papers 3:* 445.

40. *Papers 3:* 445.

41. C. Lennart Carlson, *The First Magazine: A History of Gentleman's Magazine* (Providence: Brown, 1938); Roy Porter, "Lay Medical Knowledge in the Eighteenth Century," *MH 29* (1985): 138–168.

42. Edward Cave, Note accompanying "Success of the Bark in a Deplorable Smallpox," *GM 22* (1752): 210.

43. William Heberden, *Some Account of the Success of Inoculation for the Small-Pox in England and America* . . . (London: Strahan, 1759).

44. Miller, *Adoption of Inoculation,* 146–156.

45. *Papers 8:* 285–286.

46. *Papers 8:* 286.

47. *Papers 11:* 356.

48. *Papers 12:* 198; *21:* 205.

49. Elizabeth A. Fenn, *Pox Americana* (New York: Hill and Wang, 2001).

50. *Papers 24:* 15.

51. Benjamin Franklin, *Writings* (New York: Library of America, 1987), 1127; Fenn, *Pox Americana,* 132–133.

52. John C. Long, *Lord Jeffrey Amherst* (New York: Macmillan, 1933).

53. At the time of the Revolutionary War, Amherst was sympathetic to the colonists' plight, and believing that they were fighting for the rights of all Englishmen, he resigned his commission.

54. Edward Jenner, *An Inquiry into the Causes and Effects of the Variolae Vaccinae* (London: Low, 1798); Edward Jenner, *Further Observations on the Variolae Vaccinae* (London: Low, 1799). Also see Hervé Bazin, *The Eradication of Smallpox* (San Diego: Academic Press, 2000); Richard B. Fisher, *Edward Jenner* (London: André Deutsch, 1991); Henry J. Parish, *Victory with Vaccines* (Edinburgh: E. and S. Livingston, 1968).

*Chapter 4. The Citizen and the Hospital*

1. *Autobiography,* 45.

2. *Papers 1:* 260.

3. *Papers 1:* 257.

4. *Papers 1:* 262–263.

5. *Autobiography,* 46.

6. *Autobiography,* 53.

7. *Autobiography,* 60–61.

8. *Autobiography,* 61.

9. *Autobiography,* 53.

10. Whitfield J. Bell, Jr., "John Bartram (1699–1777)," in *Patriot Improvers* (Philadelphia: American Philosophical Society, 1997), 48–62.

11. *Papers 2:* 380–383.

12. For the early history of the APS, see Whitfield J. Bell, Jr., "History of the Society," in *Patriot Improvers* (Philadelphia: American Philosophical Society, 1997), 3–8; Edward C. Carter, II, *One Grand Pursuit* (Philadelphia: American Philosophical Society, 1993); Brooke

Hindle, *The Pursuit of Science in Revolutionary America* (Chapel Hill: University of North Carolina Press, 1956).

13. Whitfield J. Bell, Jr., "Cadwallader Colden (1688–1776)," in *Patriot Improvers* (Philadelphia: American Philosophical Society, 1997), 111–119.

14. *Papers 3:* 36.

15. William H. Williams, *America's First Hospital* (Wayne, Pa.: Haverford House, 1976). Francis R. Packard, "The Pennsylvania Hospital," in *History of Medicine in the United States* (New York: Hoeber, 1931), 181–230.

16. Anthony Deutsch, "The Sick Poor in Colonial Times," *American Historical Review* *46* (1941): 560–579; David J. Rothman, "Charity and Correction in the Eighteenth Century," in *The Discovery of the Asylum* (Boston: Little, Brown, 1971), 30–56.

17. Dieter Jetter, *Geschichte des Hospitals, Band 3* (Wiesbaden: Franz Steiner Verlag, 1972).

18. Simon P. Newman, *Embodied History* (Philadelphia: University of Pennsylvania Press, 2003).

19. The birth of the so-called "modern" hospital is usually thought of as starting in Padua during the mid-sixteenth century. The idea, with its potential for research and education, then spread north from Italy to Leyden and Vienna. Several growing British cities followed, as healthcare for the poor began to be institutionalized under the auspices of charitable foundations. Othmar Keel, "The Politics of Health . . .," in *William Hunter and the Eighteenth-Century Medical World*, ed. William F. Bynum and Roy Porter (Cambridge: Cambridge University Press, 1985), 207–256; Guenter B. Risse, *Mending Bodies, Saving Souls* (New York: Oxford University Press, 1999).

20. Robert Nelson, *Address to Persons of Quality and Estate* (London: James, 1715).

21. John Bellers, *Essay Toward the Improvement of Physick* (London: Sowle, 1714).

22. Guenter B. Risse, ed., *Hospital Life in Enlightenment Scotland* (Cambridge: Cambridge University Press, 1986); Guenter B. Risse, "Enlightenment," in *Mending Bodies, Saving Souls*, 231–273.

23. Andrew Hook, "Scottish Thought and Culture in Early Philadelphia," in *Scotland and America in the Age of the Enlightenment*, ed. Richard B. Sher and Jeffrey R. Smitten (Princeton: Princeton University Press, 1990), 227–241.

24. *Papers 9:* 3.

25. Roy Porter, "Lay Medical Knowledge in the Eighteenth Century," *MH 29* (1985): 154–156.

26. "A View *of the Many* Peculiar *Advantages* of a Public Hospital," *GM 11* (1741): 476–477.

27. Whitfield J. Bell, Jr., "Thomas Bond (1713–1784)," in *Patriot Improvers* (Philadelphia: American Philosophical Society, 1997), 37–47; Elizabeth H. Thompson, "Thomas Bond, 1713–1784," *Journal of Medical Education 33* (1958): 614–624.

28. Whitfield J. Bell, Jr., "Phineas Bond (1717–1773)," in *Patriot Improvers* (Philadelphia: American Philosophical Society, 1997), 79–85.

29. *Autobiography,* 96.

30. *Autobiography,* 96.

31. *Autobiography,* 96.

32. Conevery Bolton Valencius, *The Health of the Country* (New York: Basic Books, 2002).

33. *Papers 5:* 316–317.

34. *Papers 5:* 312.

35. Lyman H. Butterfield, *Letters of Benjamin Rush*, vol. 2 (Princeton: Princeton University Press, 1951), 1063.

36. Andrew Scull, *The Most Solitary of Afflictions* (New Haven: Yale University Press, 1993), 57.

37. For more on the social, political, and economic factors behind British mental institutions, see Jonathan Andrews and Andrew Scull, *Customers and Patrons of the Mad-Trade* (Berkeley: University of California Press, 2003); Andrew Scull, *Undertaker of the Mind* (Berkeley: University of California Press, 2001).

38. *Papers 5:* 283–330.

39. *Papers 5:* 320–321.

40. Francis R. Packard, "Medical Case Histories in a Colonial Hospital," *BHM 12* (1940): 145–168.

## Chapter 5: Electricity and the Palsies

Note to epigraph: *Papers 7:* 299.

1. W. D. Hackmann, *Electricity from Glass* (Alphen aan den Rijn: Sijthoff & Noordhoff, 1978); John Heilbron, *Electricity in the Seventeenth and Eighteenth Centuries* (Berkeley: University of California Press, 1979).

2. Otto von Guericke, *Experimenta nova (ut vocantur) Magdeburgica . . .* (Amsterdam: Jansson-Waesberg, 1672).

3. Francis Hawksbee, *Physico-Mechanical Experiments on Various Subjects* (London: Printed for the author, 1709).

4. Stephen Gray, "A Letter to Cromwell Mortimer," *PT 37* (1731): 18–44.

5. Mary Brazier, *A History of Neurophysiology in the Seventeenth and Eighteenth Centuries* (New York: Raven Press, 1984), 178–180; C. Dorsman and C. A. Grommelin, "The Invention of the Leyden Jar," *Janus 46* (1957): 275–280; Hackmann, *Electricity from Glass*, 90–103.

6. *Autobiography*, 120; I. Bernard Cohen, "Benjamin Franklin and the Mysterious 'Dr. Spence,'" *Journal of the Franklin Institute 235* (1943): 1–25; I. Bernard Cohen, *Benjamin Franklin's Science* (Cambridge: Harvard University Press, 1990), 40–60; N. H. de V. Heathcote, "Franklin's Introduction to Electricity," *Isis 46* (1955): 29–35.

7. *Autobiography*, 120–121.

8. Cohen, "Mysterious 'Dr. Spence,'" 6.

9. Anonymous, "An Historical Account of the Wonderful Discoveries, Made in Germany, &c Concerning Electricity," *GM 15* (1745): 192–197.

10. *Papers 3:* 118–119.

11. *Papers 4:* 9.

12. *Papers 3:* 472–473.

13. *Papers 15:* 166.

14. *Papers 3:* 156–165, 356; *5:* 71; also see Heinz O. Sibum, "The Bookkeeper of Nature,"

in *Reappraising Benjamin Franklin*, ed. J. A. L. Lemay (Newark: University of Delaware, 1993), 221–241.

15. *Papers 5:* 523–524.

16. *Papers 4:* 20.

17. Cohen, *Franklin's Science*, 66–158.

18. *Papers 4:* 366–367; also see Joseph Priestley, *History and Present State of Electricity*, 3rd ed., vol. 1 (London: Bathurst and Lowndes, 1775; reprint,New York: Johnson, 1966), 217.

19. For a history of the pamphlet with original text, see I. Bernard Cohen, *Benjamin Franklin's Experiments* (Cambridge: Harvard University Press, 1941).

20. David Yerkes, "Franklin's Vocabulary," in *Reappraising Benjamin Franklin*, ed. J. A. L. Lemay (Newark: University of Delaware, 1993), 396–411.

21. *Papers 17:* 259.

22. Carl Van Doren, *Benjamin Franklin* (New York: Viking Press, 1938), 171.

23. Peter Kellaway, "The Part Played by Electric Fish in the Early History of Bioelectricity and Electrotherapy," *BHM 20* (1946): 112–137; David C. Schechter, "Origins of Electricity," *New York State Journal of Medicine* (1971): 997–1008.

24. Johann Gottlob Krüger, *Zuschrift an seine Zuhörer* . . . (Halle: Hemmerde, 1744). Translated in Licht, *History of Electricity*, 5. See Paola Bertucci, "The Electrical Body of Knowledge," in *Electric Bodies*, ed. Paola Bertucci and Giuliano Pancaldi (Bologna: University of Bologna, 2001), 43–68; Sidney Licht, "History of Electrotherapy," in *Therapeutic Electricity and Ultraviolet Radiation*, 2nd ed., ed. Sidney Licht (Baltimore: Waverly Press, 1967), 1–70.

25. Christian Gottlob Kratzenstein, *Schreiben von dem Nutzen der Electricität in der Arzneywissenschaft* (Halle: Hemmerde, 1745).

26. Priestley, *History of Electricity*, 472.

27. Jean-Antoine Nollet, *Essai sur l'Electricité des Corps* (Paris: Guerin, 1746); also see Priestley, *History of Electricity*, 472.

28. Jean-Antoine Nollet, "Extract of a Letter from the Abbé Nollet," *PT* 46 (1749–50): 368–397.

29. *Papers 3:* 483.

30. Jean Louis Jallabert, *Expériences sur l'Electricité* (Geneva: Barrillot & Fils, 1748).

31. Priestley, *History of Electricity*, 473.

32. Bertucci, "The Electrical Body."

33. Nollet, *Essai sur l'Electricité;* Jean-Etienne Deshais, *De Hemiplegia per Electricitatem Curanda* (Montpellier: Martel, 1749).

34. "An Historical Account," 197.

35. "An Historical Account," 197.

36. Joannes B. Bohadsch, "An Account of Dr. Bohadsch's Treatise . . .," *PT 47* (1751): 345–351; quotation, 350–351.

37. Frederick B. Tolles, *James Logan and the Culture of Provincial America* (Boston: Little, Brown, 1957).

38. Tolles, *James Logan*, 211.

39. *Papers 3:* 110.

40. *Papers 3:* 111.

41. Tolles, *James Logan*, 211.

42. *Papers 3:* 433.

43. *Papers 3:* 483.

44. Michael C. Batinski, *Jonathan Belcher* (Lexington: University Press of Kentucky, 1966).

45. Clifford K. Shipton, *Sibley's Harvard Graduates* (Cambridge: Harvard University Press, 1933), 448; *Papers 4:* 198.

46. William S. Middleton, "Thomas Cadwalader and His Essay," *AMH 3* (1941): 102.

47. New Jersey Historical Society, "Jonathan Belcher Governor," *Collections of the New Jersey Historical Society 5* (1858): 294.

48. New Jersey Historical Society, "Jonathan Belcher," 274.

49. *Papers 4:* 197–198.

50. *Papers 4:* 198.

51. *Papers 4:* 197–198.

52. *Papers 4:* 205.

53. *Papers 4:* 216.

54. *Papers 4:* 255–256.

55. Sydney Selwyn, "Sir John Pringle," *MH 10* (1982): 266–274.

56. Patrick Brydone, "An Instance of the Electrical Virtue in the Cure of a Palsy," *PT 50* (1757): 392–395.

57. Cheney Hart, "Part of a Letter from Cheney Hart . . .," *PT 49* (1754): 558–563; Cheney Hart, "An Account of a Cure of a Paralytic Arm, by Electricity," *PT 49* (1756): 558–563.

58. Benjamin Franklin, "An Account of the Effects of Electricity in Paralytic Cases," *PT 50* (1758): 481–483; Benjamin Franklin, *Experiments and Observations on Electricity*, 5th ed. (London: Newberry, 1774); *Papers 7:* 298–300.

59. *Papers 16:* 144.

60. *Papers 16:* 153.

61. *Papers 16:* 230.

62. *Papers 16:* 231.

63. *Papers 16:* 230.

64. *Papers 18:* 90.

65. *Papers 20:* 449–450.

66. *Papers 21:* 210.

67. *Papers 21:* 303.

68. *Papers 21:* 402–403.

69. *Writings 9:* 656.

70. William Heberden, *Commentaries on the History and Cure of Diseases* (1782; New York: Hafner, 1962).

71. John Wesley, *The Desideratum* (London: Flexney, 1760), 63.

72. Oliver Hochadel, "My Patient Told Me How to Do It," in *Electric Bodies*, ed. Paola Bertucci and Giuliano Pancaldi (Bologna: University of Bologna, 2001), 69–90.

*Chapter 6. Electricity, Mental Disorders, and a Modest Proposal*

Note to epigraph: Cadwallader Evans, "A Relation of a Cure Performed by Electricity. Communicated October 21, 1754," *MOI 1* (1757): 84–85.

1. Michel Foucault, *Madness and Civilization* (New York: Vintage, 1965); Roy Porter, *Mind-Forg'd Manacles* (Cambridge: Harvard University Press, 1987); E. Trillat, "Conversion Disorder and Hysteria," in *A History of Clinical Psychiatry*, ed. German E. Berrios and Roy Porter (New York: New York University Press, 1995), 433–450; Ilza Veith, *Hysteria* (Chicago: University of Chicago Press, 1970).

2. George Cheyne, *The English Malady* (London: Strahan and Leake, 1733).

3. John Wesley, *Primitive Physic*, 22nd ed. (Philadelphia: Parry Hall, 1791), xii.

4. George Baker, *Medical Tracts* (London: Bulmer, 1818), 338–339.

5. Wesley, *Primitive Physic*, 70.

6. Randolph S. Klein, "Dr. Cadwalader Evans (1716–1773)," *Transactions and Studies of the College of Physicians of Philadelphia 35* (1967): 30–36; James Thacher, "Cadwallader Evans," in *American Medical Biography* (Boston: Richardson et al., 1828), 265.

7. Thacher, "Cadwallader Evans," 265.

8. Evans, "Cure by Electricity," 83–86; "Account of a Cure by Electricity," *GM 37* (1757): 260.

9. Thacher, "Cadwallader Evans," 265.

10. Christian Gottlob Kratzenstein, *Schreiben von dem Nutzen der Electricität in der Arznei-wissenschaft* (Halle: Hemmerde, 1745); Kratzenstein's words are translated in Sidney Licht, "History of Electrotherapy," in *Therapeutic Electricity and Ultraviolet Radiation*, 2nd ed., ed. Sidney Licht (Baltimore: Waverly Press, 1967), 6.

11. For more on the imagination in the history of medicine, see G. S. Rousseau, "Science and the Discovery of the Imagination in Enlightened England," *Eighteenth-Century Studies 3* (1969): 108–135; Beverley C. Southgate, "The Power of Imagination," *HS 30* (1992): 281–294.

12. John Webster, *The Displaying of Supposed Witchcraft. . . .* (London: J.M., 1677), 323–324.

13. *Papers 1:* 356.

14. John Locke, *Essay on Human Understanding* (1690; New York: Dover, 1959).

15. Patrick Brydone, "An Instance of the Electrical Virtue in the Cure of a Palsy," *PT 50* (1757): 392–395.

16. Stanley W. Jackson, "Melancholia and the Waning of Humoral Theory," *JHMAS 33* (1978): 367–376.

17. Robert Burton, *The Anatomy of Melancholy* (1621; New York: Tudor, 1948).

18. Everett Mendelsohn, "John Lining and His Contribution to Early American Science," *Isis 51* (1960): 278–292.

19. *Papers 5:* 525. This letter also appears in the fifth edition of Franklin's *Experiments and Observations on Electricity* (London: Newbery, 1774) as Letter XVII.

20. *Papers 5:* 525. For details of Franklin's first electrical accident, see *Papers 4:* 82–83; 112–113 (letter of December 20, 1750, presumably to John Franklin and one dated February 4, 1751, to Peter Collinson). In the former letter, Franklin wrote: "The company present . . . Say that the flash was very great and the crack as loud as a Pistol; yet my Senses being instantly gone, I neither Saw the one nor heard the other . . . I tho't the Bottles must be discharged but could not conceive how, thill at last I perceived the Chain in my hand, and Recollected what I had been about to do."

21. *Papers 5:* 525.

22. P. Smit, "Jan Ingen-Housz," *Janus 67* (1980): 126–139.

23. Timothy K. Conley and Melissa Brewer-Anderson, "Franklin and Ingenhousz: A Correspondence of Interests," *PAPS 141* (1997): 276–296.

24. *Papers 40:* unit 209.

25. *Papers 40:* unit 209.

26. *Writings 9:* 308–309.

27. *Writings 9:* 309.

28. *Writings 9:* 309.

29. *Papers 40:* 209.

30. John Birch, "A Letter to Mr. George Adams," in *An Essay on Electricity . . . by George Adams,* 4th ed. (London: Hindmarsh, 1792), 519–573.

31. Birch, "Letter," 565–566.

32. Giovanni Aldini, *An Account of the Late Improvements in Galvanism* (London: Wilks and Taylor, 1803).

33. T. Gale, *Electricity, or the Ethereal Fire, Considered* (Troy: Moffitt and Lyon, 1802); for more on Gale see James Delbourgo, "Electrical Humanitarianism in North America," in *Electric Bodies,* ed. Paola Bertucci and Giuliano Pancaldi (Bologna: University of Bologna, 2001), 117–156.

34. Gale, *Electricity,* 129–131.

35. Ugo Cerletti, "Electroshock Therapy," *Journal of Clinical and Experimental Psychopathology 15* (1954): 191–217. Interestingly, Cerletti believed that convulsions were critical for the cure. The reports that came soon after Franklin and Ingenhousz urged such experiments, however, clearly suggested otherwise.

## Chapter 7. Friends and Medical Connections

Note to epigraph: *Autobiography,* 123.

1. *Papers 5:* 334.

2. *Papers 21:* 582.

3. R. Hingston Fox, *Dr. John Fothergill and His Friends* (London: Macmillan, 1919); M. Jefferson, "Dr. John Fothergill, Physician and Humanist," *BMJ* 2 (1966): 637–644; F. Clifford Rose, "John Fothergill (1712–1780)," in *A Short History of Neurology,* ed. F. Clifford Rose (Oxford: Butterworth Heinemann, 1999), 88–92.

4. *Papers 21:* 599.

5. *Writings 9:* 16.

6. Sydney Selwyn, "Sir John Pringle," *MH 10* (1982): 266–274.

7. "Historical Chronicle, March 1, 1766," *GM 36* (1766): 147.

8. *Papers 14:* 96–97.

9. *Papers 14:* 95.

10. John L. Heilbron, "Franklin as an Enlightened Natural Philosopher," in *Reappraising Benjamin Franklin,* ed. J. A. L. Lemay (Newark: University of Delaware, 1993), 196–219; quotation from p. 212.

11. For Franklin's nominees, consult *Papers 9:* 356–360. For more on Hewson, see George Gulliver, *The Collected Works of William Hewson* (London: Sydenham Society,

1846); Ralph H. Major, "William Hewson, the Hunters and Benjamin Franklin," *JHM 8* (1953): 324–328.

12. Claude-Anne Lopez, "The Patriarch of Craven Street," in *The Private Franklin* (New York: Norton, 1975), 149–157.

13. Roy Porter, "William Hunter: A Surgeon and a Gentleman," in *William Hunter and the Eighteenth-Century Medical World*, ed. William F. Bynum and Roy Porter (Cambridge: Cambridge University Press, 1985), 7–34.

14. Paul Knapman, "Benjamin Franklin and the Craven Street Bones," *Transactions of the Medical Society of London 116* (1999): 9–17.

15. John Walsh, "On the Electric Property of the Torpedo," *PT* 63 (1773): 461–477. Quotation p. 462.

16. John Hunter, "Anatomical Observations on the Torpedo," *PT 63* (1773): 481–489. Quotation p. 481. For a scholarly treatise on electric fish in the eighteenth century, see Marco Piccolino, *The Taming of the Ray* (Firenze: Leo S. Olschki, 2003).

17. Hunter, "Anatomical Observations," 486.

18. Walsh, "Electric Property"; "Of Torpedos Found on the Coast of England," *PT* 64 (1774): 464–473; Hunter, "Anatomical Observations"; "An Account of the *Gymnotus electricus*," *PT 65* (1775): 395–407.

19. Hunter, "Anatomical Observations," 486.

20. Tiberius Cavallo, *A Complete Treatise of Electricity . . .*, vol. 2, 4th ed. (London: Dilly, 1795), 309.

21. V. W. Crane, "The Club of Honest Whigs," *WMQ 23* (1966): 210–233.

22. Joseph Priestley, *Autobiography of Joseph Priestley* (1806; Teaneck, N.J.: Fairleigh Dickinson University Press, 1970), 116.

23. Priestley, *Autobiography*, 117.

*Chapter 8. Scotland and the First American Medical School*

Note to epigraph: *Papers 8:* 279.

1. J. Bennett Nolan, *Benjamin Franklin in Scotland and Ireland* (Philadelphia: University of Pennsylvania Press, 1956).

2. *Papers 8:* 279.

3. Nolan, *Franklin in Scotland*, 76–83.

4. *Writings 9:* 21–22.

5. *Papers 39:* 23.

6. Roger L. Emerson, "Medical Men, Politicians, and the Medical Schools at Glasgow and Edinburgh, 1685–1803," in *William Cullen and the Eighteenth Century Medical World*, ed. A. Doig et al. (Edinburgh: Edinburgh University Press, 1993), 186–215; Christopher Lawrence, "Ornate Physicians and Learned Artisans," in *William Hunter and the Eighteenth-Century Medical World*, ed. William F. Bynum and Roy Porter (Cambridge: Cambridge University Press, 1985), 153–176.

7. *Papers 10:* 385–386.

8. A. Johnstone, "William Cullen," *MH 3* (1959): 33–46; Andrew Doig et al., eds., *William Cullen and the Eighteenth-Century Medical World* (Edinburgh: Edinburgh University

Press, 1993); Guenter B. Risse, "Clinical Instruction," in *Hospital Life in Enlightenment Scotland* (Cambridge: Cambridge University Press, 1986), 240–278.

9. Francis R. Packard, *History of Medicine in the United States* (New York: Hoeber, 1931), 143.

10. *Papers 9:* 219–220.

11. *Papers 9:* 373–374.

12. *Papers 9:* 377.

13. *Papers 9:* 221.

14. *Papers 23:* 387–388.

15. *Papers 13:* 471.

16. *Papers 13:* 532.

17. *Papers 13:* 530.

18. *Papers 13:* 530.

19. William F. Bynum and Roy Porter, eds., *William Hunter and the Eighteenth-Century Medical World* (Cambridge: Cambridge University Press, 1985).

20. Whitfield J. Bell, Jr., "Philadelphia Medical Students in Europe, 1750–1800," *PMHB* 67 (1943): 1–29.

21. Betsy C. Corner, *William Shippen, Jr.* (Philadelphia: American Philosophical Society, 1951); William S. Middleton, "William Shippen, Junior," *AMH 4* (1922): 440–452; Oscar Reiss, *Medicine and the American Revolution* (Jefferson, N.C.: McFarland, 1998).

22. Corner, *Shippen*, 7.

23. J. R. Elkinton, "Betty Fothergill and Her 'Uncle Doctor'," *AIM 85* (1976): 637–640; F. H. Fox, *Dr. John Fothergill and His Friends* (London: Macmillan, 1919).

24. George W. Corner, *Two Centuries of Medicine* (Philadelphia: Lippincott, 1965), 19.

25. Corner, *Two Centuries*, 28, 33–34.

26. Packard, *History of Medicine*, 220–224, 319.

27. Whitfield J. Bell, Jr., *John Morgan* (Philadelphia: University of Pennsylvania Press, 1965); William S. Middleton, "John Morgan, Father of Medical Education in North America," *AMH 9* (1927): 13–26.

28. *Papers 10:* 146.

29. Deborah C. Brunton, "The Transfer of Medical Education," in *Scotland and America in the Age of the Enlightenment*, ed. Richard B. Sher and Jeffrey R. Smitten (Princeton: Princeton University Press, 1990), 242–258.

30. *Papers 12:* 203.

31. *Papers 12:* 307.

32. Middleton, "William Shippen," 446.

33. Corner, *Shippen*, 9.

34. P. D. Olch, "The Morgan-Shippen Controversy," *Review of Surgery 22* (1965): 1–8.

35. E. H. Thompson, "Thomas Bond, 1713–1784," *Journal of Medical Education 33* (1958): 614–624.

36. John Duffy, *The Healers* (Urbana: University of Illinois Press, 1979), 65.

37. J. B. Blake, "The Anatomical Lectures of William Shippen, 1776," *Transactions and Studies of the College of Physicians of Philadelphia 42* (1974): 61–66; Brunton, "Medical Education," 247–248.

38. Carl Bridenbaugh and Jessica Bridenbaugh, *Rebels and Gentlemen* (New York: Oxford University Press, 1962), 300.

39. *Papers 19:* 65.

*Chapter 9. Colds, the Weather, and the Invisible World*

Note to epigraph: *Papers 20:* 444–445.

1. *Papers 7:* 272–279.

2. *Papers 3:* 346–347.

3. *Papers 6:* 339; *Papers 7:* 350.

4. *Papers 18:* 161.

5. *Papers 9:* 25.

6. *Papers 9:* 35–36.

7. *Papers 9:* 36.

8. Nicolaas A. Rupke, ed., *Medical Geography in Historical Perspective* (London: Wellcome Trust, 2000); Frederick Sargent, II, *Hippocratic Heritage* (New York: Pergamon Press, 1982).

9. Genevieve Miller, "'Airs, Waters, and Places' in History," *JHMAS 8* (1962): 129–140.

10. Robert M. Green, *Galen's Hygiene* (Springfield, Ill.: Charles C. Thomas, 1951).

11. Saul Jarcho, "Galen's Six Non-naturals," *BHM 44* (1970): 372–377; Peter H. Niebyl, "The Non-naturals," *BHM 45* (1971): 486–492; L. J. Rather, "The Six Things Non-natural," *Clio Medica 3* (1968): 337–347; Oswei Temkin, *Galenism* (Ithaca, N.Y.: Cornell University Press, 1973). The "naturals" included the humors and were intrinsic to the body.

12. Vivian Nutton, "The Seeds of Disease," *MH 27* (1983): 1–34.

13. Nutton, "Seeds,"

14. Thomas Sydenham, *The Works of Thomas Sydenham*, trans. R. G. Latham (London: Sydenham Society, 1848–1850); Kenneth Dewhurst, *Dr. Thomas Sydenham* (Berkeley: University of California Press, 1966).

15. Kenneth D. Keele, "The Sydenham-Boyle Theory of Morbific Particles," *MH 18* (1974): 240–248; Dewhurst, *Sydenham,* 65–67.

16. Keele, "Sydenham-Boyle Theory," 245; Sargent, *Hippocratic Heritage,* 154–156.

17. Kenneth Dewhurst, "Locke's Contribution to Boyle's Researches on the Air and on Human Blood," *NR 17* (1962): 198–206; "John Locke's Medical Notes During His Residence in Holland (1683–1689)," *Janus 50* (1962): 176–192; *John Locke* (London: Wellcome Historical Library, 1963).

18. William E. K. Middleton, *Invention of the Meteorological Instruments* (Baltimore: Johns Hopkins University Press, 1969).

19. For more on the first decades of medical meteorology in America, see James H. Cassedy, "Meteorology and Medicine in Colonial America," *JHMAS 24* (1969): 193–204. For how later American settlers saw themselves in relation to the environment, see James R. Fleming, *Meteorology in America* (Baltimore: Johns Hopkins University Press, 1990); Conevery Bolton Valencius, *The Health of the Country* (New York: Basic Books, 2002).

20. *Papers 1:* 252–254.

21. T. Molyneux, "Historical Account of the Late General Coughs and Colds," *PT 18* (1694): 105–111.

22. Everett Mendelsohn, "John Lining and His Contribution to Early American Science," *Isis 51* (1960): 278–292.

23. John Lining, "Extracts of Two Letters from Dr. John Lining," *PT 42* (1742–43): 491–509; "A Letter from Dr. John Lining," *PT 43* (1744–45): 318–330; "A Letter from Dr. John Lining," *PT 45* (1748): 336–344; "Extract of a Letter from the Ingenious Dr. John Lining," *GM 23* (1753): 431.

24. John Lining, "A Description of the American Yellow Fever," *Essays and Observations, Physical and Literary 1* (1756): 386–389; *2,* 370–395.

25. Sydney Selwyn, "Sir John Pringle," *MH 10* (1982): 266–274.

26. John Pringle, *Observations on the Nature and Cure of Hospital and Jayl-Fevers* (London: Millar and Wilson, 1750); *Observations on the Diseases of the Army in Camp and Garrison* (London: Millar et al., 1752).

27. John Pringle, *Observations on the Diseases of the Army in Camp and Garrison,* 4th ed. (London: Millar et al., 1764).

28. Clifford Dobell, *Anthony Van Leeuwenhoek and His Little Animals* (New York: Dover, 1960).

29. Benjamin Marten, *A New Theory of Consumptions* (London: Knaplock et al., 1720).

30. Richard H. Shryock, *Medicine and Society in America* (New York: New York University Press, 1960), 57.

31. Otho T. Beale, Jr., and Richard H. Shryock, *Cotton Mather* (Baltimore: Johns Hopkins University Press, 1954), 149–154.

32. Beale and Shryock, *Cotton Mather,* 150.

33. *Papers 3:* 257.

34. *Papers 4:* 91–94.

35. *Papers 4:* 90–94.

36. *Papers 18:* 203.

37. *Papers 18:* 206.

38. H. L. Ganter, "William Small, Jefferson's Beloved Teacher," *WMQ 4* (1947): 505–511.

39. *Papers 18:* 198.

40. *Papers 20:* 103.

41. *Papers 20:* 251.

42. *Papers 20:* 193.

43. *Papers 20:* 315–316.

44. *Papers 20:* 405.

45. *Papers 20:* 444–445.

46. *Papers 20:* 538.

47. *Papers 20:* 533–534.

48. John Adams, *The Works of John Adams,* vol. 3 (Boston: Little, Brown, 1851), 75–76.

49. *Writings 9:* 436–437.

*Chapter 10. Fresh Air and Good Health*

Note to epigraph: *Papers 15:* 180.

1. For more on what smells meant throughout history, see Alain Corbin, *The Foul and the Fragrant* (Cambridge: Harvard University Press, 1986).

2. *Papers 7:* 379.

3. *Papers 20:* 444.

4. *Papers 2:* 331.

5. *Papers 2:* 365.

6. *Papers 2:* 419–446.

7. *Autobiography*, 78.

8. *Papers 15:* 50–51.

9. *Papers 40:* 209.

10. *Writings 9:* 425–426.

11. *Writings 9:* 435–436.

12. *Papers 15:* 180.

13. Desmond King-Hele, *Erasmus Darwin* (London: Giles de la Mare, 1999).

14. King-Hele, *Darwin*, 48.

15. Erasmus Darwin, *A Plan for the Conduct of Female Education in Boarding Schools* (Dublin: Chambers, 1798).

16. John Pringle, *Observations on the Diseases of the Army in Camp and Garrison* (London: Millar et al., 1752); Sydney Selwyn, "Sir John Pringle," *MH 10* (1982): 266–274.

17. *Papers 7:* 74–75.

18. *Papers 23:* 486.

19. *Papers 23:* 487.

20. *Papers 23:* 489–490.

21. *Papers 23:* 498.

22. *Papers 46:* 140.

23. *Papers 46:* 216.

24. Henry S. Commager, *The Spirit of Seventy-Six* (Cambridge: Da Capo Press, 1985), 835–836.

25. *Papers 20:* 241–242.

26. Laurence Brockliss and Colin Jones, *The Medical World of Early Modern France* (Oxford: Clarendon Press, 1997), 756–757.

27. Joseph Priestley, *History and Present State of Electricity* (London: Dodsley et al., 1767).

28. F. W. Gibbs, *Joseph Priestley* (New York: Doubleday, 1967); Robert E. Schofield, *The Enlightenment of Joseph Priestley* (University Park: Pennsylvania State University Press, 1997).

29. Joseph Priestley, "Observations on Different Kinds of Air," *PT 62* (1772): 147–264.

30. *Papers 19:* 173.

31. *Papers 19:* 200–201.

32. *Papers 19:* 215.

33. Kenneth Thompson, "Trees as a Theme in Medical Geography and Public Health," *Bulletin of the New York Academy of Medicine 54* (1978): 517–531.

34. Conevery Bolton Valencius, *The Health of the Country* (New York: Basic Books, 2002).

35. John Woodward, "Some Thoughts and Experiments Concerning Vegetation," *PT 21* (1708): 193–277.

36. *Papers 38:* 439.

37. *Papers 19:* 214–215.

38. Priestley, "Observations," 194.

39. Priestley could not have known that Karl Wilhelm Scheele, a Swedish apothecary, had discovered oxygen shortly before he did, since Scheele did not make his findings public until 1777.

40. A. H. Harken, "Oxygen, Politics and the American Revolution," *Annals of Surgery 184* (1976): 645–650; Schofield, *Priestley,* 997.

41. Howard S. Reed, "Jan Ingenhousz," *Chronica Botanica 11* (1947–48): 288–391.

42. A. Donovan, *Antoine Lavoisier* (Cambridge: Cambridge University Press, 1993).

43. Priestley, however, contended that he had already recognized the importance of sunlight. See Jack Lindsay, *Autobiography of Joseph Priestley* (Teaneck, N.J.: Fairleigh Dickinson University Press, 1970), 20–21.

44. Jan Ingenhousz, *Experiments upon Vegetables* (London: Elmsley and Payne, 1779).

45. Donovan, *Lavoisier,* 184.

46. *Papers 21:* 188–189.

47. Joseph Priestley, "On the Noxious Quality of the Effluvia of Putrid Marshes," *PT 64* (1774): 90–95.

48. Richard Price, "Farther Proof of the Insalubrity of Marshy Situations," *PT 64* (1774): 97.

49. *Papers 32:* 396–400.

50. *Papers 40:* 365.

*Chapter 11. The Perils of Lead*

Note to epigraph: *Writings 9:* 531.

1. *Papers 14:* 222.

2. R. M. S. McConaghey, "Sir George Baker and the Devonshire Colic," *MH 11* (1967): 345–360.

3. William Musgrave, *De arthritide symptomatica* (Exoniae: Farlcianis et al., 1703); John Huxham. *Opusculum de Morbo Colico Damnoniorum* (London: John Hinton, 1738).

4. George Baker, *An Essay Concerning the Cause of Endemial Colic of Devonshire* (London: Hughs, 1767).

5. George Baker, *Medical Tracts* (London: Bulmer, 1818), 125–127.

6. Jerome O. Nriagu, *Lead and Lead Poisoning in Antiquity* (New York: John Wiley, 1983).

7. *Papers 1:* 311.

8. S. Colum Gilfillan, "Lead Poisoning and the Fall of Rome," *Journal of Occupational Medicine 7* (1965): 53–60; *Rome's Ruin by Lead Poison* (Long Beach: Wenzel Press, 1990); Nriagu, *Lead Poisoning;* "Saturnine Gout Among Roman Aristocrats," *NEJM 38* (1983): 660–663.

9. J. Scarborough, "The Myth of Lead Poisoning Among the Romans," *JHMAS 39* (1984): 469–475.

10. Eberhard Gockel, *Eine curiose Beschreibung dess An. 1694, 95, und 96* (Ulm, 1697); Josef Eisinger, "Lead and Wine, " *MH 26* (1982): 279–302; Erik Skovenborg, "Lead in Wine Through the Ages," *Journal of Wine Research 6* (1995): 49–64.

11. Baker, *Medical Tracts,* 125–127.

12. For more on lead toxicity, see R. L. Singhal and J. A. Thomas, eds., *Lead Toxicity* (Baltimore: Urban and Schwartzenberg, 1980). Alfred B. Garrod conducted some of the most important early studies relating lead to gout and stones: "On Gout and Rheumatism," *Medico-Chirurgical Transactions 19* (1854): 181–220; *The Nature and Treatment of Gout and Rheumatic Gout* (London: Walton Maberly, 1859); *A Treatise on Gout and Rheumatic Gout,*

3rd ed. (London: Longmans, Green, 1876). For newer studies on lead and the kidneys, see David D. Choie and Goetz W. Richter, "Effects of Lead on the Kidney," in *Lead Toxicity,* ed. R. L. Singhal and J. A. Thomas (Baltimore: Urban and Schwartzenberg, 1980), 187–212; Robert A. Goyer, "Lead and the Kidneys," *Current Topics in Pathology 55* (1971): 147–176; Vecihi Batuman et al., "The Role of Lead in Gout Nephropathy," *NEJM 304* (1981): 520–523.

13. Baker, *Medical Tracts,* 131.

14. Baker, *Medical Tracts,* 187.

15. Gene V. Ball, "Two Epidemics of Gout," *BHM 45* (1971): 401–408.

16. *Writings 10:* 407; Claude-Anne Lopez and Eugenia W. Herbert, *The Private Franklin* (New York: Norton, 1975), 25.

17. *Papers 38:* 2.

18. Otho T. Beale, Jr., and Richard H. Shryock, *Cotton Mather* (Baltimore: Johns Hopkins University Press, 1954), 56–57.

19. *Writings 9:* 530–531.

20. Carey P. McCord, "Lead and Lead Poisoning in Early America," *Internal Medicine and Surgery 22* (1958): 397–399; A. H. Whittaker, "Acts and Laws of His Majesty's Province of the Massachusetts-Bay in New-England," *Industrial Medicine and Surgery 10* (1941): 532–535.

21. Thomas Cadwalader, *An Essay on the West-India Dry-Gripes* (Philadelphia: Franklin, 1745).

22. Cadwalader, *Dry-Gripes,* 1–2.

23. When it came to treating patients with the "West-India Dry-Gripes," Cadwalader recommended lubricating the intestines to make passing feces easier, while strengthening the tone of the digestive tract with various drugs. He also saw merit in exercise (especially horseback riding) and music, both of which were then classified as stimulants.

24. *Papers 1:* 356.

25. *Papers 6:* 339.

26. *Writings 9:* 531–532.

27. *Papers 2:* 419.

28. *Papers 14:* 214.

29. *Papers 14:* 312–313.

30. *Papers 15:* 51–52.

31. Baker, *Medical Tracts,* 161–162, 168–169.

32. Baker, *Medical Tracts,* 209, 396.

33. Baker, *Medical Tracts,* 113–114.

34. Baker, *Medical Tracts,* 385.

35. Baker. *Medical Tracts,* 124–125.

36. Claude-Anne Lopez, "Saltpeter, Tin and Gunpowder," *Annals of Science 16* (1960): 83–92.

37. Baker, *Medical Tracts,* 137–141.

38. *Papers 19:* 71.

39. *Writings 9:* 530–533.

*Chapter 12. French Medicine and Health Imperatives*

Note to epigraph: *Papers 31:* 455.

1. *Papers 32:* 366–367.

2. Carl Van Doren, *Benjamin Franklin* (New York: Viking, 1938), 570–571.

3. I. Bernard Cohen, *Science and the Founding Fathers* (New York: Norton, 1995), 188.

4. A. O. Aldridge, *Franklin and His French Contemporaries* (New York: New York University Press, 1957); Susan M. Alsop, *Yankees at the Court* (Garden City, N.Y.: Doubleday, 1982); David Schoenbrun, *Triumph in Paris* (New York: Harper & Row, 1976).

5. Oscar Reiss, *Medicine and the American Revolution* (Jefferson, N.C.: McFarland, 1998).

6. George W. Corner, *Two Centuries of Medicine* (Philadelphia: Lippincott, 1965), 28.

7. *Papers 26:* 223.

8. *Papers 32:* 547.

9. *Writings 9:* 74.

10. Arthur L. Donovan, *Antoine Lavoisier* (Cambridge: Cambridge University Press, 1993); Denis I. Duveen and Herbert S. Klickstein, "Benjamin Franklin (1706–1790) and Antoine Laurent Lavoisier (1743–1794)," *Annals of Science 11* (1955): 103–128, 271–308; Sidney J. French, *Torch and Crucible: The Life and Death of Antoine Lavoisier* (Princeton: Princeton University Press, 1941).

11. Donovan, *Lavoisier,* 188–210; Claude-Anne Lopez, "Saltpeter, Tin and Gunpowder," *Annals of Science 16* (1960): 83–92.

12. Peter Heering, "John Paul Marat," in *Electric Bodies,* Paola Bertucci and Giuliano Pancaldi, eds. (Bologna: University of Bologna, 2001), 91–116; Sidney L. Phipson, *Jean Paul Marat* (London: Methuen, 1924).

13. Lester King, *The Medical World of the Eighteenth Century* (Huntington: Krieger, 1971), 27.

14. Jean-Paul Marat, *Recherches Physiques sur l'Electricité* (Paris: Clousier, 1782); *Mémoires sur l'Electricité Médicale* (Paris: Méquignon, 1784).

15. P. J. C. Mauduyt de la Verenne, "Premier Mémoire sur l'Electricité," *Histoire et Mémoires* (1776): 461–513; Caroline Hannaway, "The Société Royale de Médecine and Epidemics in the Ancien Régime," *BHM 46* (1972): 257–273.

16. Laurence Brockliss and Colin Jones, *The Medical World of Early Modern France* (Oxford: Clarendon Press, 1997), 754–755.

17. *Papers 35:* 292–294.

18. *Writings 9:* 313.

19. Melvin A. Gravitz, "Mesmerism and Masonry," *American Journal of Clinical Hypnosis 39* (1997): 266–270; Claude-Anne Lopez, "Franklin and the Nine Sisters," in *My Life with Benjamin Franklin* (New Haven: Yale University Press, 2000), 148–157.

20. Genevieve Miller, *The Adoption of Inoculation for Smallpox in England and France* (Philadelphia: University of Pennsylvania Press, 1957).

21. Aldridge, *Franklin,* 11.

22. Claude-Anne Lopez, *Mon Cher Papa* (New Haven: Yale University Press, 1966), 243–302.

23. William Coleman, "Health and Hygiene in the Encyclopédie," *JHM 19* (1974): 399–421; Thomas L. Hankins, *Science and the Enlightenment* (Cambridge: Cambridge University Press, 1985), 163–170.

24. Pierre Jean Georges Cabanis, *On the Relations Between Physical and Moral Aspects of Man* (Baltimore: Johns Hopkins University Press, 1981); Theodore L. Sourkes, "Light and the Enlightenment," *Journal of the History of the Neurosciences 5* (1996): 254–264.

25. Bernard Mackler, *Philippe Pinel* (New York: Watts, 1968); Walther Riese, *The Legacy of Philippe Pinel* (New York: Springer, 1969).

26. Ernest Caulfield, *The Infant Welfare Movement in the Eighteenth Century* (New York: Hoeber, 1931); Fielding H. Garrison, "History of Pediatrics," in *Abt-Garrison History of Pediatrics,* Isaac A. Abt, ed. (Philadelphia: Saunders, 1965), 1–170.

27. Brockliss and Jones, *Medical World,* 467–470.

28. Stephen Hales, "Observations of the Very Ingenious Dr. Hales in His Treatise of Ventilators," *GM 13* (1743): 432–433.

29. William Cadogan, *An Essay upon Nursing and the Management of Children* (London: Roberts. 1747); Caulfield, *Infant Welfare,* 101–124; J. Rendle-Short, "Infant Management in the Eighteenth Century with Special Reference to the Work of William Cadogan," *BHM 34* (1960): 97–122.

30. Jean Jacques Rousseau, *Emile,* B. Foxley, trans. (London: Dent, 1911). (Originally published in 1762.)

31. Mary Jacobus, "Incorruptible Milk," in *Rebel Daughters,* Sara. E. Meltzer and Leslie W. Rabine, eds. (New York: Oxford University Press, 1992), 54–78.

32. Caulfield, *Infant Welfare,* 140.

33. *Writings 9:* 265.

34. *Writings 9:* 334–335.

35. *Writings 9:* 335.

36. *Papers 6:* 321.

37. John Gascoigne, *Joseph Banks and the English Enlightenment* (Cambridge: Cambridge University Press, 1994).

38. *Writings 8:* 592–593.

39. *Writings 9:* 80.

40. *Writings 9:* 81–82.

41. *Writings 9:* 106.

42. *Writings 9:* 115–116.

43. *Writings 9:* 117–118.

44. *Writings 9:* 155.

45. *Writings 9:* 83.

46. *Papers 31:* 455.

47. *Writings 9:* 82–83.

48. *Writings 9:* 83.

49. *Papers 44:* 224.

50. *Writings 9:* 572.

*Chapter 13. The Folly of Mesmerism*

1. Vincent Buranelli, *The Wizard from Vienna* (New York: Coward, 1975); Frank A. Pattie, *Mesmer and Animal Magnetism* (Hamilton: Edmonston, 1994); Donald M. Whalmsley, *Anton Mesmer* (London: Hale, 1967).

2. Frank A. Pattie, "Mesmer's Medical Dissertation," *JHM 11* (1956): 175–287.

3. Richard Mead, *De Imperio Solis ac Lacunae in Corpora Humana, et Morbis Oriundis* (Londoni: Smith, 1704).

4. Richard Mead, *A Treatise Concerning the Influence of the Sun and Moon Upon Human Bodies* (London: Brindley, 1748), 82–83.

5. Nicholas Culpeper, *Pharmacopoeia Londinensis* (London: Printed by a Well-Wisher, 1654), A3-A4.

6. Robert Darnton, *Mesmerism and the End of the Enlightenment in France* (Cambridge: Harvard University Press, 1968), 10–11.

7. Geoffrey Sutton, "Electric Medicine and Mesmerism," *Isis 72* (1981): 375–392.

8. Franz Anton Mesmer, *Mémoire* (Paris: Fuchs, 1779). (Translated as *Memoir of F. A. Mesmer on His Discoveries* [Mt. Vernon: Eden Press, 1957].) Translated in Buranelli, *Wizard*, 62.

9. For more on the imagination at this time, see Beverley C. Southgate, "The Power of Imagination," *HS 30* (1992): 281–294.

10. R. Angermueller, "Paradies, Maria Theresa von," in *The New Grove Dictionary of Music and Musicians*, vol. 14, S. Sadie, ed. (London: Macmillan, 1995), 175.

11. *Papers 27:* 506.

12. Carl Van Doren, *Benjamin Franklin* (New York: Viking, 1938), 713).

13. *Papers 31:* 5–6. The story is also told by Claude-Anne Lopez, "Franklin and Mesmer," *Yale Journal of Biology and Medicine 66* (1993): 325–331; Kevin M. McConkey and Campbell Perry, "Benjamin Franklin and Mesmerism," *International Journal of Clinical and Experimental Hypnosis 33* (1985): 122–130.

14. *Writings 10:* 428–429.

15. *Papers 31:* 186–187 (translated by the author).

16. *Writings 9:* 182–183.

17. Melvin A. Gravitz, "Mesmerism and Masonry," *Americal Journal of Clinical Hypnosis 39* (1997): 266–270.

18. Robert C. Fuller, *Mesmerism and the American Cure of Souls* (Philadelphia: University of Pennsylvania Press, 1982), 16.

19. Edward E. Hale and Edward E. Hale, Jr., *Franklin in France*, vol. 2 (Boston: Roberts Brothers, 1888), 308.

20. Alan Gauld, *A History of Hypnotism* (Cambridge: Cambridge University Press, 1992).

21. Darnton, *Mesmerism*.

22. Stephen J. Gould, "The Chain of Reason vs. the Chain of Thumbs," *Natural History 7* (1989): 14.

23. Benjamin Franklin et al., *Rapport des Commissaires* (Paris: Marchands de Nouveautés, 1784).

24. Benjamin Franklin et al., *Report of Dr. Benjamin Franklin, and Other Commissioners*

(London: Johnston, 1785). (Reprinted in *Foundations of Hypnosis,* Maurice M. Tinterow, ed. [Springfield, Ill.: Charles C. Thomas, 1970], 82–128.)

25. Franklin, *Report,* xv.

26. Franklin, *Report,* 87–88.

27. Franklin, *Report,* 95.

28. Franklin, *Report,* 95.

29. Franklin, *Report,* 102.

30. Franklin, *Report,* 102.

31. Franklin, *Report,* 108.

32. Franklin, *Report,* 114, 117, 123.

33. Franklin, *Report,* 124.

34. Charles D'Eslon, "Observations on the Two Reports," in *The Nature of Hypnosis,* Robert E. Shor and Martin T. Orne, eds. (New York: Holt, Rinehart, & Winston, 1965). (Originally published in 1784.) Steven J. Lynn and Scott Lilienfeld, "A Critique of the Franklin Commission Report," *International Journal of Clinical and Experimental Hypnosis 50* (2002): 369–386.

35. *Writings 9:* 268.

36. *Writings 9:* 320.

37. *Papers 1:* 316.


*Chapter 14. From Music Therapy to the Music of Madness*

Note to epigraph: Translated from Friedrich Rochlitz, *Allgemeine Musikalische Zeitung* (Amsterdam: Israel-Frits, Knuf, 1798).

1. *Papers 10:* 126–130; Giambattista Beccaria, *Dell' Elettricismo Artificiale* (Turin: Campana, 1753).

2. Previous publications by the author on this topic include David A. Gallo and Stanley Finger, "The Power of a Musical Instrument," *History of Psychology 3* (2000): 326–343; Stanley Finger and David Gallo, "The Music of Madness," in *Neurology of the Arts,* F. Clifford Rose, ed. (London: Imperial College Press, 2004), 207–235.

3. For the history of glass music, see A. Hyatt King, "The Musical Glasses and the Glass Harmonica," *Proceedings of the Royal Musical Association,* session 72, London, 1946.

4. Franchino Gafori, *Theoria Musicae* (Milan, 1492).

5. Galileo Galilei, *Two New Sciences* (Toronto: Wall & Thompson, 1989). (Originally published in 1638.)

6. Thomas D. Rossing, "Acoustics of the Glass Harmonica," *Journal of the Acoustical Society of America 95* (1994): 1106.

7. Anne Ford, *Instructions for the Playing of the Musical Glasses* (London, 1761).

8. Oliver Goldsmith, *The Vicar of Wakefield* (Boston: Houghton Mifflin, 1985), 60. (Originally published in 1771.)

9. Ellen R. Cohn, "Benjamin Franklin and Traditional Music," in *Reappraising Benjamin Franklin,* J. A. L. Lemay, ed. (Newark: University of Delaware Press, 1993), 290–318.

10. *Papers 8:* 359–360.

11. Paget Toynbee and Leonard Whibley, eds., *Correspondence of Thomas Gray,* vol. 2 (Oxford: Clarendon Press, 1935), 664.

12. *Papers 10:* 127.

13. *Papers 10:* 130.

14. Esmond Wright, *Benjamin Franklin* (Cambridge: Harvard University Press, 1990), 159.

15. *Papers 10:* 204.

16. Leigh Hunt, *The Autobiography of Leigh Hunt* (New York: Harper, 1850), 28.

17. *Papers 10:* 385.

18. Carl Van Doren, *Benjamin Franklin* (New York: Viking, 1938), 299.

19. Frank A. Pattie, *Mesmer and Animal Magnetism* (New York: Edmonston, 1994), 30.

20. Vincent Buranelli, *The Wizard from Vienna* (New York: Coward, 1975), 56.

21. King, "Musical Glasses," 109.

22. C. F. Pohl and K. M. Pisarowitz, "Kirchgässner, Marianne," in *The New Grove Dictionary of Music and Musicians,* vol. 10, S. Sadie, ed. (London: Macmillan, 1995), 74.

23. Brockhill Newburgh, *Essays Poetical Moral and Critical* (Dublin: M'Culloh, 1759), 241.

24. Richard Browne, *Medicina Musica* (London: Cooke, 1727).

25. Richard Brocklesby, *Reflections on Ancient and Modern Music* (London: Cooper, 1749).

26. *Papers 12:* 64.

27. A. Aleksandrowicz, *Izabela Czartoryska* (Lublin: Wydawnictwo, 1998); G. Pauszer-Klonowska, *Pani na Pulawach* (Warsaw: Czytelnik, 1980).

28. Nancy Sinkoff, "Benjamin Franklin in Jewish Eastern Europe," *Journal of the History of Ideas 61* (2000): 133–152.

29. Z. J. Lipowski, "Benjamin Franklin as a Psychotherapist," *Perspectives in Biology and Medicine 27* (1984): 361–366; "Benjamin Franklin and Princess Czartoryska," *Pennsylvania History 51* (1984): 167–171.

30. Lipowski, "Princess," 362.

31. Thomas Cadwalader, *An Essay on the West-India Dry-Gripes* (Philadelphia: Franklin, 1745), 33–34.

32. Lipowski, "Princess," 170.

33. Winslow C. Watson, *Men and Times of the Revolution* (New York: Dana, 1856), 154–155.

34. *Writings 10:* 429–430.

35. Karl Leopold Röllig, *Über die Harmonika: ein Fragment* (Berlin: Ohne, 1787), translated in King, "Musical Glasses," 114.

36. Pohl and Pisarowitz, "Kirchgässner," 74.

37. *Papers 25:* 543.

38. Johann Christian Müller, *Anleitung zum Selbstunterricht an der Harmonika* (Leipzig, 1788).

39. Rochlitz, *Allgemeine Musikalische.*

40. *Writings 9:* 360–361.

41. O. G. Sonneck, "Benjamin Franklin's Relation to Music," *Music 19* (1900): 1–14.

42. King, "Musical Glasses," 110.

43. Franz Anton Mesmer, *Mémoire* (Paris: Fuchs, 1779). (Translated as *Memoir of F. A. Mesmer on his Discoveries* [Mt. Vernon: Eden Press, 1957].)

44. Laurence Brockliss and Colin Jones, *The Medical World of Early Modern France* (Oxford: Clarendon Press, 1997), 783.

45. Pattie, *Mesmer*, 73.

46. Pattie, *Mesmer*, 103.

47. King, "Musical Glasses," 110.

48. Étienne-Gaspard Robertson, *Mémoires* (Paris: Auteur et à la Librairie de Wurtz, 1831–1833) (reissued by Philippe Blon, Langres: Café Clima, 1985); Terry Castle, "Phantasmagoria and the Metaphorics of Modern Reverie," in *The Female Thermometer* (New York: Oxford University Press, 1995), 140–167.

49. Castle, "Phantasmagoria," 150.

50. Gerhard Finkenbeiner and Vera Meyer, "The Glass Harmonica," *Leonardo 20:* (1987): 139–142. King, "Musical Glasses," 113–115; Vera Meyer and Kathleen J. Allen, "Benjamin Franklin and the Glass Armonica," *Endeavour 12* (1988): 185–188.

*Chapter 15. Bifocals and the Aging Inventor*

Note to epigraph: *Papers 9:* 265.

1. *Papers 32:* 57.

2. *Writings 9:* 209.

3. Richard Corson, *Fashions in Eyeglasses* (Chester Springs, Pa.: Dufour, 1967); H. W. Holtmann, "A Short History of Spectacles," in *Atlas on the History of Spectacles*, W. Poulet, ed. (Bonn: Wayenborgh, 1978), i-xxi; Edward Rosen, "The Invention of Eyeglasses," *JHMAS 11* (1956): 13–46, 183–218; J. William Rosenthal, *Spectacles and Other Vision Aids* (San Francisco: Norman Publishing, 1996).

4. Austen H. Layard, *Discoveries in the Ruins of Nineveh and Babylon* (New York: Putnam, 1853).

5. George Sines and Yannis Sakellarakis, "Lenses in Antiquity," *American Journal of Archeology 91* (1987): 191–196.

6. Corson, *Eyeglasses*, 19.

7. Nicolaus Cusanus, *Opuscula varia Nicolai de Cusa* (Norimbergae, 1741); Vincent Ilardi, "The Role of Florence in the Development and Commerce of Spectacles," *Atti deall Fondazione Giorgio Ronchi 56* (2001): 163–176.

8. *Writings 9:* 248.

9. C. A. Wood, "The First Scientific Work on Spectacles," *AMH 3* (1921): 150–155.

10. *Papers 18:* 185–186.

11. *Papers 18 :*186.

12. *Papers 18 :*186.

13. Whitfield J. Bell, Jr., "John Bartram (1699–1777)," in *Patriot Improvers* (Philadelphia: American Philosophical Society, 1997), 60.

14. *Papers 18:* 180–181.

15. *Papers 19:* 28–29.

16. Johann Zahn, *Oculus Artificialis Teledioptricus sive Telescopium* (Herbipolis: Quirini Heyl, 1685); Christian Gottlieb Hertel, *Vollständige Answeisung zum Glass-Schleiffen* (Halle: Rengerischen Buchhandlung, 1716).

17. A. G. Bennett, "Christian Gottlieb Hertel," *Ophthalmic Optician 8* (1968): 462, 467–469, 818–820.

18. John R. Levine, "Benjamin Franklin, F.R.S., Sir Joshua Reynolds, F.R.S., P.R.A.,

Benjamin West, P.R.A., and the Invention of Bifocals," *Notes and Records of the Royal Society of London 27* (1972): 141–163.

19. *Papers 29:* 378.

20. *Writings 9:* 265–266.

21. *Writings 9:* 337–338.

22. Charles E. Letocha, "The Invention and Early Manufacture of Bifocals," *Survey of Ophthalmology 35* (1990): 226–235. Quote on pp. 231–232.

23. Levine, "Benjamin Franklin."

24. Letocha, "Bifocals," 235.

25. Letocha, "Bifocals," 233.

26. D. Waldstreicher, "The Long Arm of Benjamin Franklin," in *Artificial Parts, Practical Lives*, Katherine Ott et al., eds. (New York: New York University Press, 2002), 300–326.


*Chapter 16. Skin and "Scurf"*

Note to epigraph: *Papers 2:* 497.

1. *Papers 23:* 256.

2. *Papers 25:* 77–80.

3. *Papers 25:* 78.

4. *Papers 25:* 78–79.

5. *Papers 25:* 79.

6. *Papers 25:* 79–80.

7. *Papers 25:* 80.

8. *Papers 25:* 80.

9. *Papers 25:* 80.

10. For more on medical diaries in Franklin's century see Joan Lane, "'The Doctor Scolds Me': The Diaries and Correspondence of Patients in Eighteenth Century England," in *Patients and Practitioners*, Roy Porter, ed. (Cambridge: Cambridge University Press, 1985), 205–248.

11. *Papers 27:* 496–497.

12. *Papers 26:* 68.

13. *Papers 26:* 68.

14. *Papers 27:* 497–498.

15. *Papers 27:* 498.

16. *Papers 27:* 498–499.

17. *Papers 27:* 499.

18. *Writings 9:* 670.

19. Robert James, *A Medicinal Dictionary* (London: Osborne, 1743); George Motherby, *A New Medical Dictionary*, 3rd ed. (London: Johnson, 1791).

20. Robert Hooper, *Dictionary Medicum* (New York: Duyckinck et al., 1824).

21. Motherby, *New Medical Dictionary* , 379.

22. *Papers 25:* 77–78.

*Chapter 17: The Gout as Your Friend?*

Note to epigraph: *Writings 9:* 99.

1. William Copeman, *A Short History of the Gout and the Rheumatic Diseases* (Berkeley: University of California Press, 1964).

2. Gerald P. Rodnan and Thomas G. Benedek, "Ancient Therapeutic Arts in the Gout," *Arthritis and Rheumatism 6* (1963): 317–340; Maurice. A. Schnitker, "A History of the Treatment of Gout," *BHM 4* (1936): 89–120.

3. Edward F. Hartung, "History of the Use of Colchicum and Related Medicaments in Gout," *Annals of Rheumatoid Diseases 13* (1954): 190–220; Stanley L. Wallace, "Colchicum," *Bulletin of the New York Academy of Medicine 49* (1968): 130–135; "Benjamin Franklin and the Introduction of Colchicum into the United States," *BHM 42* (1973): 312–320.

4. Copeman, *Gout,* 2.

5. William Eamon, "The Tale of Monsieur Gout," *BHM 55* (1981): 564–567.

6. Richard Hawes, *The Poore-Mans Plaster-Box* (London: Cotes, 1634).

7. Eamon, "Tale," 566–567.

8. Thierry Appelboom and J. Claude Bennett, "Gout of the Rich and Famous," *Journal of Rheumatology 13* (1986): 618–622.

9. Thomas Sydenham, "Treatise on the Gout," in *Thomas Sydenham, The Works,* vol. 2 (London: Sydenham Society, 1850), 119–162. (Originally published in 1683.)

10. Sydenham, "Treatise," 124–125.

11. Copeman, *Gout,* vii.

12. Andrew Boorde, *The Breviary of Helthe* (London: East, 1575).

13. Lorenz Fries, *Spiegel der Artzny* (Strasbourg: Beck, 1518).

14. Copeman, *Gout,* 80.

15. Philander Misaurus, *The Honour of the Gout* (Philadelphia: Franklin, 1732).

16. *Papers 1:* 316.

17. *Papers 1:* 352.

18. *Papers 3:* 104.

19. George Baker, *Medical Tracts* (London: Bulmer, 1818), 187–189.

20. Gene V. Ball, "Two Epidemics of Gout," *BHM 45* (1971): 401–408. For more on wine, lead, and gout, see Gene V. Ball and L. B. Sorensen, "Pathogenesis of Hyperuricemia in Saturnine Gout," *NEJM 280* (1969): 1199–1202; L. A. Healey, "Port Wine and the Gout," *Arthritis and Rheumatism 18* (1975): 661; Erik Skovenborg, "Lead in Wine Through the Ages," *Journal of Wine Research 6* (1995): 62.

21. For an early anatomical study on lead and the kidney, see Jean-Martin Charcot and P. H. Gombault, "Note Relative à l'Etude Anatomique de la Néphrite Saturnine Expérimentale," *Archives de Physiologie Normale et Pathologique 8* (1881): 126, 154. For more recent anatomy, see David D. Choie and Goetz W. Richter, "Effects of Lead on the Kidney," in *Lead Toxicity,* R. L. Singhal and J. A. Thomas, eds. (Baltimore: Urban and Schwartzenberg, 1980), 187–212; Robert A. Goyer, "Lead and the Kidneys," *Current Topics in Pathology 55* (1971): 147–176; Kim Cramer et al., "Renal Ultrastructure, Renal Function, and Parameters of Lead Toxicity in Workers with Different Periods of Lead Exposure," *British Journal of Industrial Medicine 31* (1974): 113–127; Ruth Lilis et al.,

"Nephropathy in Chronic Lead Poisoning," *British Journal of Industrial Medicine 25* (1968): 196–202. For research on lead and renal physiology see Choie and Richter, "Lead"; Rokho Kim et al., "A Longitudinal Study of Low-level Lead Exposure and Impairment of Renal Function," *JAMA 275* (1996): 1177–1181; Ruth Lilis et al., "Renal Function Impairment in Secondary Lead Smelter Workers," *Journal of Environmental Pathology and Toxicology 2* (1979): 1447–1474; Marinelle Payton et al., "Low-level Lead Exposure and Renal Function in the Normative Aging Study," *American Journal of Epidemiology 140* (1994): 821–829; Jan A. Staessen et al., "Impairment of Renal Function with Increasing Blood Lead Concentrations in the General Population," *NEJM 327* (1992): 151–156; Richard P. Wedeen et al., "Occupational Lead Neuropathy,"

22. J. W. Rowe et al., "The Effect of Age on Creatinine Clearance in Men: A Cross-sectional and Longitudinal Study," *Journal of Gerontology 31* (1976): 155–163.

23. Robert R. Baumann and Otis F. Jillson, "Hyperuricemia and Psoriasis," *Journal of Investigative Dermatology 36* (1961): 105–107; Arthur Z. Eisen and J. E. Seegmiller, "Uric Acid Metabolism in Psoriasis," *Journal of Clinical Investigation 40* (1961): 1486–1493.

24. *Papers 10:* 153.

25. *Papers 14:* 222.

26. *Papers 14:* 222.

27. Appelboom and Bennett, "Gout," 621.

28. *Papers 17:* 168.

29. *Papers 17:* 205.

30. *Papers 22:* 484.

31. *Papers 23:* 205.

32. *Papers 23:* 572.

33. *Papers 28:* 511, 589, 601.

34. *Papers 28:* 607.

35. *Papers 29:* 132.

36. *Papers 29:* 121.

37. *Papers 29:* 143.

38. *Papers 29:* 252.

39. *Papers 33:* 464, 502.

40. *Papers 33:* 518.

41. Skovenborg, "Lead in Wine," 59.

42. *Papers 33:* 530–531.

43. Roy Porter, "Gout: Framing and Fantasizing Disease," *BHM 68* (1994): 1–28.

44. Benjamin Franklin, *The Bagatelles from Passy* (New York: Eakins Press, 1967), 32–33. (Originally published in 1784.)

45. *Papers 34:* 20–22; *Writings 10:* 414–415.

46. *Papers 34:* 13–20.

47. *Writings 8:* 154–162.

48. *Papers 29:* 357.

49. Porter, "Gout," 12.

50. Copeman, *Gout,* 93.

51. *Writings 9:* 670–671.

52. William Cadogan, *A Dissertation on the Gout* (London: Dodsley, 1771).

53. John Adams, *The Works of John Adams*, vol. 3 (Boston: Little, Brown, 1851), 326.

54. *Papers 33:* 97–98.

55. William Heberden, *Commentaries on the History and Cure of Diseases* (New York: Hafner, 1962), 48. (Originally published in 1782.)

56. *Papers 34:* 446.

57. Houston M. Kimbrough, Jr., "Benjamin Franklin," *Investigative Urology 12* (1975): 509–510; Schnitker, "History"; John H. Talbott, *Gout and Gouty Arthritis* (New York: Grune and Stratton, 1953).

58. Wallace, "Colchicum."

59. Hartung, "History"; Nicholas Husson, *Collection de Faits et Recueil d'Expériences sur le Spécifique et les Effets de l'Eau Médicinale* (Bouillon: Brasseur, 1783). Also see Edwin Jones, *An Account of the Remarkable Effects of the Eau Medicinale d'Husson in the Gout* (London: White & Cochrane, 1810).

60. J. Moore, "A Letter to Dr. Jones on the Composition of Eau Medicinale," *NEJMS 1* (1812): 97; James Want, "Composition of Eau Medicinale," *Medical and Physical Journal 32* (1814): 77–78. (Also in *NEJMS 4* [1814]: 88–90).

61. *Papers 29:* 438.

## Chapter 18. A Debilitating Stone

Note to epigraph: *Writings 9:*124.

1. *Papers 32:* 57.

2. Leonard Murphy, *The History of Urology* (Springfield, Ill.: Charles C. Thomas, 1972); Eric W. Riches, "The History of Lithotomy and Lithotrity," *Annals of the Royal College of Surgeons of England 43* (1968): 185–199; Francis Twinem and Benjamin Langdon, "Surgical Management of Bladder Stone," *Journal of Urology 66* (1951): 201–210.

3. Ludwig Edelstein, *Ancient Medicine* (Baltimore: Johns Hopkins Press, 1967), 6.

4. Eric W. Riches, "Some Landmarks in the Surgery of Stone," *Journal of British Urological Surgeons 7* (1938): 140–147.

5. Ambroise Paré, *Ten Books of Surgery* (Athens: University of Georgia Press, 1969). (Originally published in 1564.)

6. William Heberden, *Commentaries on the History and Cure of Diseases* (New York: Hafner, 1962). (Originally published in 1782.)

7. *Papers 2:* 413.

8. Anon, "Mrs. Stephens' Recipe for the Stone," *GM 9* (1739): 298–299; E. Lee Strohl, "Parliament Hoodwinked by Joanna Stephens," *Surgery, Gynecology, and Obstretrics 116* (1963): 509–511.

9. *Papers 2:* 413–414.

10. *Papers 2:* 414.

11. *Papers 2:* 414.

12. *Papers 4:* 385–387.

13. Robert Whytt, *An Essay on the Virtues of Lime Water in the Cure of the Stone* (Edinburgh: Hamilton et al., 1752).

14. *Papers 4:* 526–527.

15. *Papers 4:* 385–386.

16. Murphy, "History."

17. Henry R. Viets, "Some Features of the History of Medicine in Massachusetts During the Colonial Period," *Isis 23* (1935): 389–405.

18. *Papers 4:* 409.

19. *Paper 6:* 320.

20. William S. C. Copeman, *A Short History of the Gout and the Rheumatic Diseases* (Berkeley: University of California Press, 1964); Murphy, *Urology;* Leonard P. Wershub, *Urology* (St. Louis: Green, 1970).

21. George Cheyne, *An Essay of the True Nature and Due Method of Treating the Gout,* 6th ed. (London: Strahan, 1724), 72.

22. W. E. Kittredge and Ralph Downs, "The Role of Gout in the Formation of Urinary Calculi," *Journal of Urology 67* (1952): 841–849.

23. George W. Corner and William E. Goodwin, "Benjamin Franklin's Bladder Stone," *JHMAS 8* (1953): 359–377.

24. Susan M. Alsop, *Yankees at the Court* (Garden City, N.Y.: Doubleday, 1982), 246.

25. *Writings 9:* 124.

26. *Writings 9:* 150–151.

27. *Writings 9:* 151.

28. *Writings 9:* 308- 318.

29. *Writings 9:* 329.

30. Alexander Blackrie, *A Disquisition upon Medicines that Dissolve the Stone* (London: Wilson, 1766).

31. Heberden, *Commentaries,* 89–90.

32. *Writings 9:* 333.

33. Corner and Goodwin, "Bladder Stone," 365–366.

34. Corner and Goodwin, "Bladder Stone," 366–367.

35. Corner and Goodwin, "Bladder Stone," 367–368.

36. *Writings 9:* 520.

37. *Writings 9:* 504.

38. *Writings 9:* 506.

39. Claude-Anne Lopez, *Mon Cher Papa* (New Haven: Yale University Press, 1966), 141–142.

40. *Writings 9:* 560–561.

41. *Writings 9:* 622.

42. *Writings 9:* 622.

43. Corner and Goodwin, "Bladder Stone," 376.

44. *Writings 10:* 1.

45. *Writings 10:* 35.

46. *Writings 10:* 49–50.

47. *Writings 10:* 91–92.

## Chapter 19. The Limits of Medicine

Note to epigraph: *Papers 2:* 195.

1. *Papers 43:* 310.

2. *Papers 5:* 473.

3. *Writings 9:* 413–443.

4. *Writings 1:* 116.

5. Lyman H. Butterfield, *Letters of Benjamin Rush,* vol. 1 (Princeton: Princeton University Press, 1951), 389.

6. William P. Cutler and Julia P. Cutler, *Life, Journals and Correspondence of Rev. Manasseh Cutler,* vol. 1 (Cincinnati: Robert Clarke, 1988), 72–73.

7. Cutler and Cutler, *Life,* 267.

8. Cutler and Cutler, *Life,* 269.

9. Although it was originally thought to have been written in Passy, Franklin scholars now believed that his piece on sleep and dreaming was composed in mid-1786 in Philadelphia.

10. *Papers 19:* 302.

11. *Writings 10:* 132–137.

12. *Writings 9:* 640.

13. *Writings 9:* 673–674.

14. Cutler and Cutler, *Life,* 270.

15. *Papers 35:* 387.

16. *Writings 10:* 2.

17. *Writings 9:* 491.

18. *Papers 45:* 395.

19. *Writings 9:* 588–589.

20. *Writings 9:* 667.

21. *Writings 9:* 682–683.

22. *Writings 10:* 4.

23. Mitchell R. Breitwieser, *Cotton Mather and Benjamin Franklin* (Cambridge: Cambridge University Press, 1984), 270.

24. *Papers 41:* 539.

25. *Papers 20:* 189–190; translated in *Writings 6:* 42–44.

26. *Writings 9:* 334.

27. *Writings 10:* 41.

28. *Writings 10:* 41.

29. *Writings 9:* 488.

30. Butterfield, *Rush,* 564.

31. *Papers 41:* 539.

## *Epilogue. Franklin's Medical Legacy*

Note to epigraph: *Papers 4:* 405.

1. *Papers 2:* 194.

# Index